Using this book may strengthen your immune system, cause permanent weight loss, add years to you life and life to your years, give you energy, prevent disease and illness, make you feel and look great and slow the aging process.

The information in this book is not intended to replace the recommendations of your health-care practitioner. any application of information in this book is at the reader's discretion and sole responsibility.

Editor:	Linda Neese
Production Assistant:	Chris Babbitt
Page Design:	Linda Neese & David Clark
Graphics:	Dover Publications, Inc.
Cover Design:	Vision Pointe Graphics

Library of Congress Cataloging-in-Publication Data

Balch, James F., 1933-
　　Prescription for Cooking & Dietary Wellness

　　Includes index.
　　1. Reducing diets 2. Immunity --- Nutritional aspects
3. Nutrition 4. Health I. Balch, Phyllis, 1930-
II. Title [DNLM: 1. Diet---popular works 2. Immune
System---drug effects---popular works QT 235 B174d]
RM222.2B35 1987　　　　　613.2'5　　　　　87-8397
ISBN 0-942023-00-5 (pbk.)

10 9 8 7 6 5 4 3

Printed in the United States of America

Rx

Prescription for *Cooking* and

Dietary Wellness

P.A.B. Publishing, Inc.

610 West Main Street, Greenfield, Indiana 46140

Contents

Wellness Charts

Powerful Nutrition

Healthy Recipes

Index & Recipe Index

Introduction to Health

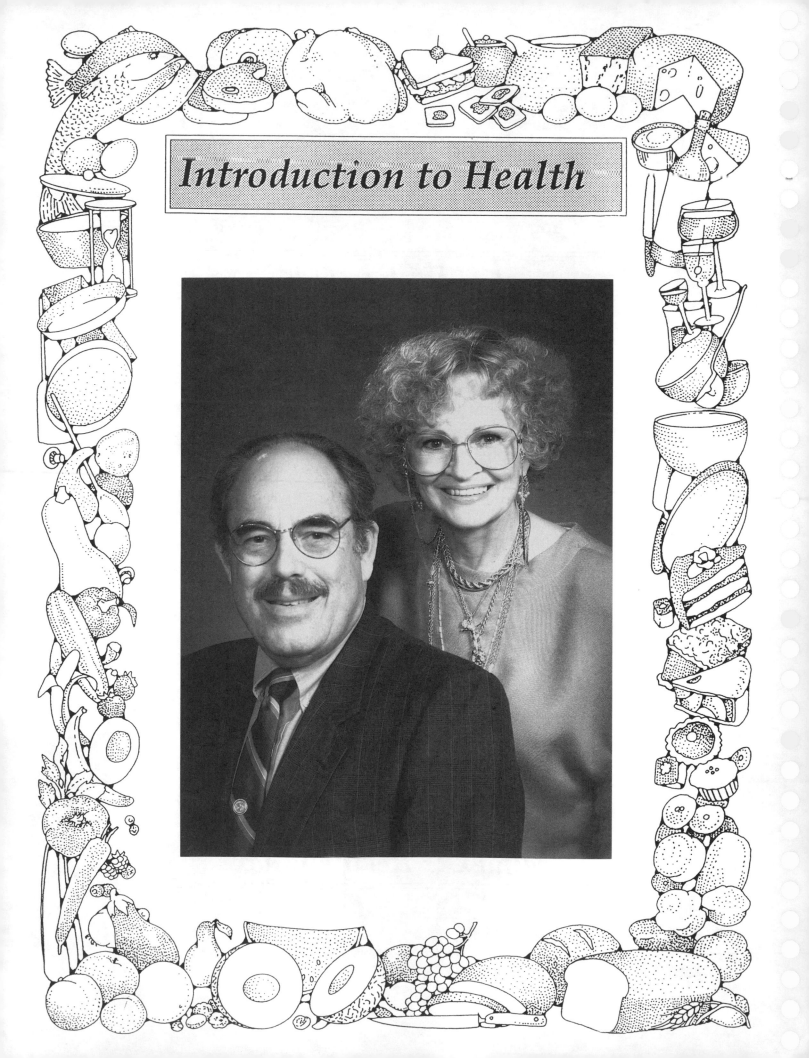

About the Authors and This Book

Thirteen years ago Dr. and Mrs. Balch began their journey in search of more effective ways to provent and cure degenerative diseases. They traveled around the world, visiting clinics and talking with doctors and healers of all kinds. Their book, *Prescription for Nutritional Healing*, has been a best-seller in the field of preventive health since its publication in 1990. It is a companion book to *Prescription for Cooking and Dietary Wellness* and *Powerful Prescription Diets*. Together these books present a complete library on health, including: nutrition research, vitamins, designed diets, herbs, diseases, and a revolutionary cookbook with healing recipes. This library is truly ahead of its time, when it comes to the prevention of disease using natural healing methods.

The Balches extensive experience has been gained through worldwide travel, investigation, and the treatment of thousands of patients. This book presents many findings that they actually witnessed, not just things they read or heard from others.

Dr. Balch, Jr. presently practices genito-urinary surgery in Greenfield, Indiana. He graduated from Indiana University Medical School with honors and spent four years in surgical residency at the Indiana University Medical Center.

He began his private practice in urology in 1966. Presently he is a member of the American Medical Association, is certified by the American Board of Urology, and is a fellow in the American College of Surgeons. He has endeavored to instill in his patients the concept of "maintaining their good health, using their own wisdom in action."

Through radio and TV appearances and his newspaper column, *Exploring Life,* he has educated the public about the basics of maintaining good health as a triune being--body, soul, and spirit. His insight into health problems in these stressful times has been well received.

Phyllis Balch is a certified nutritional consultant. She received her certification from the American Association of Nutritional Consultants, has counseled clients for over a decade, served as nutritional consultant in her husband's practice, and also contributes to his health column. Her interest in natural foods led to the establishment of her nutritional center, and a natural foods restaurant that flourished for over a decade.

Dr. Balch tells us, "As a physician and surgeon, I am involved with sick people every day. A significant percentage of these people have preventable disorders. Many of these disorders are caused by routine violations of good health and nutritional habits."

> **"It is unfortunate but true that the average doctor today is not trained to diagnose most diseases in their early stages. Even with the U.S.'s sophisticated investigative tools, most diseases are not readily recognized until they have advanced beyond the point of cure."**

An ill person's insufficient or inaccurate knowledge, the inability to obtain nutritious foodstuffs and supplements, and/or indifferent attitudes toward self care are the most common underlying reasons behind poor eating habits and resulting sickness.

All substances on the earth which are consumed in excess are toxic to the body! Even water, if consumed in excess, can destroy life, as demonstrated by the Chinese, who committed suicide by drinking too much water.

It is no wonder that even in this day, man has so many allergies. Consuming the same foods day-after-day, saturates the body and intoxicates (poisons) it. Rather than nourishing, these foods repeatedly cause the body to react negatively.

In our travels, we discovered that many diseases span the world's cultures, thriving on vastly different but always nutritionally deficient diets. **Six out of**

ten deaths in our country are directly related to diet. Many people believe that diet is only important as it relates to weight loss and body building. The media has "programmed" us to pay scant attention to the fact that diet is also an important factor in overall health and well being. Unfortunately, there is a great division in the health care marketplace. The orthodox medical physician proclaims that he has all the answers, while the nutritionally- oriented physician claims that he has all the answers. At the same time results in confusion and ultimately, we lose sight of our common goal: the improved health of mankind.

> *We urge you to let your Healing Power Within work to its fullest potential through a diet designed just for You!*
>
> *"What truly matters most when our lives touch others, is not only what things we give, but what we give of ourselves. There can be no warmer feeling than that of sharing information about man's most valuable asset--health."*
>
> *Phyllis Balch, C.N.C*

Maybe you don't have any health problems now, and you want to avoid future problems. Or you have wanted to learn how to make nutritious healthy foods that taste as good as junk foods (nutritionally deficient, high calorie foods). Maybe you want to change your diet, but don't understand how to use all the items in health food stores. If you want to know how to prepare nutritious meals without spending all day in the kitchen and how to put a meal together quickly in the middle of a busy schedule, then this book is for you! It is designed not only to help you increase your energy, but also as a resource, that through use will add many quality years to your life because you have maintained a healthy body.

A typical American diet consists of 90% cooked, processed, packaged, adulterated, and even irradiated and possibly genetically-engineered foods. It is filled with chemicals and preservatives, grown in nutrient-depleted soil, and stored on shelves for long periods of time, resulting in massive nutritional loss. All of this adds up to a "dead-food diet." The body cannot build strong new cells and maintain a healthy immune system to prevent disease, when it's receiving lifeless food. Continuing these misguided eating habits will prevent the body from functioning normally as The Creator intended-- dead foods do not produce life.

Malnutrition is already manifesting itself in our children, obesity and high blood cholesterol are examples. The young may turn to drugs because of depression resulting from their poor diets, looking for a way to feel good. Many children never eat raw fruits or vegetables, but subsist on a diet high in fat, sugar and salt. We even see children with colas in their hands at breakfast time!

The right foods do have the power to heal; just as the wrong foods can cause sickness, rapid aging, and in time, premature death.

Prescription for Cooking and Dietary Wellness is designed to lead you, precept-by-precept, to a power-filled healthy state, by helping you to better understand what nutritional resources to provide your Healing Power Within.

Discover power foods for longevity, energy, the immune system, healing-specific disorders and brain food.

Prescription for Cooking and Dietary Wellness is designed to assist anyone and everyone to lead a more healthful life.

Here's to your health! Dr. James & Phyllis Balch

In the future, food will be used as preventive medicine. Growing evidence points in the direction that certain foods fight disease --the way of the future is prevention.

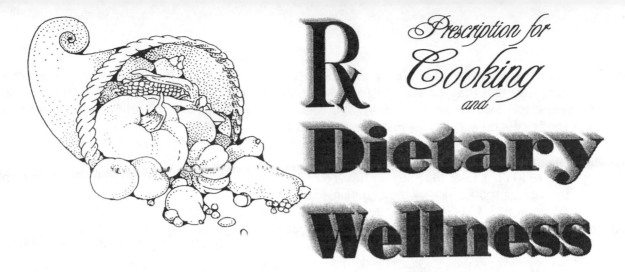

R℞ Prescription for Cooking and Dietary Wellness

Nearly every ancient culture has used plants for the prevention and cure of disease. Even in the United States these remedies were widely used until the late 1800's when American medicine became exclusively committed to allopathic medical therapy. Allopathy attempts to remedy illness by producing a condition in the body that does not allow the disease to live or thrive; chemotherapy is a good example of this approach to treating diseases. Since the 1900's, alternatives like using foods to heal the body, have been discredited by orthodox medical practitioners, and drug therapy remains supreme for most of them.

Herb and plant food therapy has been successful through the ages, but man has not known why. Now with our advanced technology, science has selected and isolated key components from plants, and has some of the answers to why plants have helped heal for centuries. But is it wise to isolate these compounds that heal? Did the Creator create them whole for a reason? "I have given every green herb for food, . . .and God saw that everything He made was very good," *Bible*, Gen 1:30-31. Undoubtedly, all the plant parts are present to work together, as buffers and regulators, minimizing side effects and aiding assimilation.

The drug industry isolates or synthesizes a part of the whole plant, and during use, this may produce undesirable side effects. The most powerful drug used in cancer chemotherapy was isolated from the plant Madagascar periwinkle. It is an effective agent against breast and lymph cancers, but it's side effects may be debilitating and dangerous. Another extreme example is *TPA, Genetech's* blood clot dissolver, so potent in its action that it can only be used in dire emergencies, such as heart attacks. Unfortunately, *TPA* also disrupts normal clotting mechanisms, with internal hemorrhage as a major complication.

In critical cases, drugs do save lives. In fact, it may be necessary to give exceptionally high amounts of one particular substance, in order to save a life.

Massive, organism specific antibiotic IVs, for a bloodstream infection, are a good example. But drugs can be dangerous, especially when over used and/or incorrectly prescribed or dispensed.

Since we know herbs and plant foods are God's powerful pharmacopoeia, we need to know which ones have therapeutic applications for various disorders. The powerful prescription foods discussed in this book, are basically fresh vegetables, fruits, sea vegetables, whole grains, nuts, seeds, beans, legumes, soybean products and herbs. You never need to worry about counting calories or watching your fat intake with these foods. You can eat all that you like, whether raw, fresh,

> "Leave your drugs in the chemist's pot if you can heal the patient with food." **Hippocrates Father of medicine**

steamed, boiled, baked, poached,or sauteed. This diet detoxifies and eliminates cancer-causing chemicals from your body and prevents degenerative disease. These foods are full of vitamins and minerals, enzymes, fiber, protein and all the nutrients needed for a healthy body. Many of these power foods contain specific immune-boosting potential.

The **Magnificent 12 Cruciferous Vegetables** contain *indoles* and *isothiocyanates,* triggering enzymes that prevent the activation of many carcinogens including those we breath in, for example tobacco smoke and city pollution. They also contain *lutein, lycopene,* and *carotene.* Scientists at the *National Cancer Institute* are doing a five-year study to identify the cancer-fighting components in vegetables and fruits. They are attempting to substantiate research done on the *indoles,* found in the **Magnificent 12 Vegetables,** that produce such powerful protection. Researchers at the *American*

Health Foundation have produced a highly active form of *isothiocyanate* that may be used to fortify foods. *Lee Wattenberg, of the University of Minnesota*, believes most foods contain substances that prevent cancer in laboratory animals, but the **Magnificent 12**, especially the broccoli variety stand out. He states, "All you have to do is taste the pungent flavor of broccoli or brussels sprouts to know they contain potent chemical factors." Cruciferous vegetables are loaded with *indole-3 carbonals*, substances which block carcinogens before they can harm the body. The *indoles* also trigger enzymes that dismantle the female hormone estrogen and protect against breast cancer. *H. Leon Bradlow, Institute for Hormone Research in New York* says, "We know that in areas of rural China where cabbage is a staple, breast cancer is exceedingly rare." In addition, he states, "It has been shown that capsules of purified indoles (equivalent to 1/2 head of cabbage) speed the breakdown of estrogen in humans."

Science is now investigating the chemical constituents of the leafy greens, orange and yellow vegetables, fruits and grains and not just focusing on vitamins, proteins, fibers, and fats. The phytochemicals in many of the foods tested, showed potent anti-carcinogenic activity. More than 1,000 chemicals have been identified with the ability to prevent cancer by themselves or in combinations--*polyacetylenes, flavonoids, ellagic acid, T. Geraniol, phenolic acids, limonoids, coumarins,* and *glucarates* are just a few of these chemicals. The characteristic odors and tastes of foods are because of the unique combinations of the phytochemical terpenoids. Scientists are now looking closely at carrots, parsley, broccoli, garlic, licorice root, flaxseed, celery, and citrus fruits.

Animals showed a shrinkage of mammary tumors when fed high amounts of *limonene* at the *University of Wisconsin, Clinical Cancer Center*. *Limonene* is an oil in the citrus fruit rind of lemons, oranges, and grapefruit. *Phenolic acid,* found in citrus fruits, neutralizes carcinogens (cancer causing substances) like nitrosamines and additionally stimulates the synthesis of *glutathione*, a natural detoxifier.

Flavonoids in citrus fruits also have been found to enhance the body's detoxification activity. Antioxidants in the *flavonoids* protect the cell membranes by helping to regulate enzymes--these go unchecked when a cell turns malignant. *Saponins* and *triterpenoids* may work like the drug, Tomoxifen, which is prescribed to many women with breast cancer and works by blocking estrogen, usually absorbed by the breast cells. *Saponins and triterpenoids* inhibit cancer in rodents. This is possible because of the *saponins* ability to block cell receptors for estrogen. Estrogen encourages certain breast tumors to grow. Studies have shown 3 mg. of *boron* daily could double blood levels of estrogen, this is not good if one has estrogen receptors. It is good for those suffering from *osteoporosis*, as estrogen aids in the assimilation of calcium. Polyunsaturated fats and animal fats increase the production of cellular hormones, thus accelerating the rate of cell production, leading to possible tumor growth which *esculetin* prevents within the body's blood and cells. *Esculetin* is found in grapefruits, blueberries, carrots, basil, and many fruits and vegetables.

The *carotenoid* family of nutrients is found in many of the same foods as those rich in beta-carotene. But they are not found in beta-carotene supplements. Research suggests that *carotenoids* are even more important to good health than beta-carotene. *Beta-carotene* is found in high amounts in carrots, sweet potatoes, yellow winter squash, and most vegetables. Many studies have shown beta-carotene protects against lung, prostate and pancreatic cancer. An increased risk of cancer has been linked to below normal levels of beta-carotene in the blood. Beta-carotene retards the growth of tumors in animals. Presently the *National Cancer Institute* is funding 10 studies to determine whether beta-carotene can prevent cancer, primarily skin and lung cancers. Many types of cancers cannot only be prevented but kept under control by the vegetable kingdom.

Flaxseed contains a high content of *alpha-linolenic acid*, fatty acids similar to those in fish oil. It also contains *lignans*, a type of fiber, that has anti-estrogenic activity. The urine of vegetarian women contains a high content of *lignans,* and their risk of developing breast cancer is low, *Herbert Pierson, Ph.D, National Cancer Institute*. Countries where a high amount of flaxseed is consumed, have a lower risk of breast and colon cancer, *University of Toronto*. Stabilized flaxseed contains more *lignans* than any other food. Buckwheat and wheat are next, with vegetables containing smaller amounts.

High amounts of *geraniol* are found in ginger and rosemary, and lower amounts are found in peas and corn. A study by *Dr. Charles Ellson of the University of Wisconsin, Nutrition Science Department,* found that only 0.1 percent of *geraniol* increased the survival rate of rats with malignant tumors. *Triterpenoids and phenolics* found in licorice root (not candy), inhibit the key enzymes that are over productive in cells undergoing conversion to cancer.

4

These protease inhibitors are found in kidney beans, chick-peas, and tofu in high amounts. These foods, containing protease inhibitors, can block natural carcinogens from forming tumors, *Dr. Ken Carol, University of Ontario*. Another substance that hinders the growth of cancer in animals is vitamin E, this has been proven in two independent studies. Other research suggests that it protects against cancer in humans as well as in animals.

Isoflavones in soybeans, inhibit the activity of *tyrosine kinase enzymes* that tend to overproduce and transform normal cells into cancer cells. The Netherlands reported certain breast cells become increasingly malignant when the activity of *tyrosine kinase enzymes* increases.

Science has found the bark and needles of the Pacific yew tree to aid healing. Research shows it to be effective in reducing ovarian cancer tumors, *Dr. Ken Swenerton*. Bristol-Myers Squibb, a drug company, signed an agreement with 75 federal agencies to obtain supplies of this rare tree bark to produce Taxol for chemical trials. Taxol is most promising as a new anti-cancer drug for ovarian and breast cancer, *The Choice*, Fall/ Winter 1991.

Just last year approximately 45,000 women died of breast cancer. Still, if they could have found it before it had spread and sought out alternative treatments like those available from American Biologics Hospital near San Diego in Mexico, many of these women could have lived useful and longer lives.

Drugs can turn environmental pollutants, food contaminants, and some substances manufactured by the body into carcinogens. Many of the phytochemicals mentioned stimulate the body to detoxify and excrete drugs before they become carcinogens. Steroids, prostaglandins, and many other drugs have been linked to cancer. Prostaglandin-E2 was potentially very harmful and linked to tumor production in every study. Foods that inhibit E2 are garlic, licorice root extract, citrus fruits, flaxseed and many umbelliferous vegetables like parsley, celery, and carrots.

Undoubtedly future designer foods, like *Star Trek*-type super capsules, will contain these potent disease-fighting phytochemical isolates. However, we must also remember the whole is superior to the isolated parts, and the **Magnificent 12** are the proof. They contain great sources of beta-carotene and vitamin C, protecting us against cancer and many other diseases. Vitamins A and C are powerful anti-oxidants, as is the trace mineral *selenium*.

Because of ill-advised farming techniques, *selenium* is lacking in most of our soils, and our foods are depleted of this important nutrient. A deficiency of this mineral is linked to cancer and heart disease, the foremost killer diseases in our country. Garlic contains the important trace mineral selenium.

Garlic is one of the many **Power Foods** and possibly is the most potent healing herb we have on our planet. In fact, more studies on garlic have been done and are presently being done, than on any other food or herb. Two examples reveal the therapeutic and preventative potential of garlic. In 1983, *Sidney Belman of New York University Medical Center*, placed garlic oil on skin tumors of animals, the tumor growth was slowed considerably, and many disappeared. In another experiment, *diallyl sulfide*, a chemical abundant in garlic was given to mice. The mice were then exposed to chemicals that caused colon cancer. A dramatic 75% fewer tumors were found in those mice exposed to the chemicals than those fed a diet only of grains, *Michael Wargovich, Biologist , M.D. Anderson Cancer Center, Houston, Texas*. Repeated studies have proven that garlic stimulates the immune function and also plays a role in the prevention of heart disease by reducing the blood pressure and serum cholesterol. If you do not like garlic because of the odor, try *Kyolic*, an effective, aged, odorless garlic extract. Numerous studies confirm its potential for preventing and healing disease.

Through the *Human Genome Project*, science is discovering in man's genetic code what determines the potential for future disorders. Soon it will be possible to predict if we have the inbred make-up to develop heart disease, diabetes, cancer, and so forth. With this in mind, it is the wise person who uses preventative measures, rather than waiting until illness is inevitable.

You must learn to use what God has created and allow our foods to provide us with the nutrients for health and longevity. *Prescription for Cooking and Dietary Wellness* contains the needed information to guide you in that direction.

This book will show you the way to better health and how to prepare God's foods, so that their healing powers may be known.

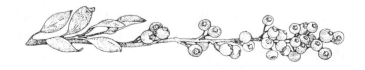

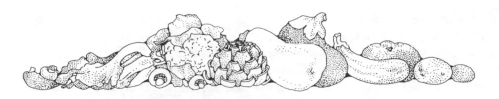

Your Wellness Begins with Your

Immune System

The immune system is truly the Healing Power Within. It is the key to staying healthy no matter what happens to us, from a cut finger to cancer. AIDS (Acquired Immune Deficiency Syndrome) is what happens when the immune system fails. Do all you can to build up and protect your immune system!

Just as our nation spends billions of dollars each year keeping our Army ready for war, so does the body constantly maintain its own defense system. The immune system protects us from invaders in the form of bacteria, viruses and so on, if we only supply the materials. When your immune system is weakened, the invaders soon take over. The results may be disease and premature death.

How do you feel today?

Are you tired most of the time?

Is depression your constant companion?

Do you have frequent visits from the
    "invaders" (colds, flu, etc.)?

Are you living with arthritis, or worse?

If you answered "yes" to any of the questions above, it's time to build up your defense system. This book is designed to take you step-by-step in building and repairing your immune system.

Your immune system consists of white blood cells, called lymphocytes. These are found in the blood, near the intestines, in the thymus gland, in the bone marrow, spleen, and in the lymph nodes in the neck, groin and armpits. All lymphocytes come from a specific ancestral cell, created in the bone marrow. Some lymphocytes become T-cells or B-cells. The "T" stands for thymus, while the "B" stands for bursa. The more important T-cells leave the bone marrow after maturity and go through the thymus gland, the master gland of the immune

system. Here, hormone-like chemicals, called thymosins, program the T-cells so they develop slightly differently from each other, with receptors that enable each T-cell to identify one particular type of invading enemy. The lymphocytes must be in absolutely perfect working order to perform their functions; an imperfect one will self-destruct immediately.

The remaining "quality" T-cells go into the blood stream with blueprints of what is the healthy you and what is an invader. They can also tell the difference between a harmless microbe and a hostile one. These T-cells are so vital to our health, that science will spend many years researching their secrets.

The B-cells stay in the thymus gland and develop "jumping genes" which make particular antibodies (protein molecules) that attack specific antigens (allergenic enemies). Inside the B-cells are seven separate parts, with several different versions of each, that migrate and link up to determine exactly which antibody it will make. These "jumping genes" can produce an astronomical number of molecules that match and seek out the enemy invaders for destruction. It is important for the body to produce these custom-tailored antibodies in order to be able to successfully attack toxins and alien organisms, and thereby destroy all invaders. However, the optimum condition of this army of defenders is totally dependent upon proper diet.

This book is devoted to the idea that you can eat good tasting, healthful food and enjoy all the benefits. Using the guidance and recipes here, you can enhance your Healing Power Within and develop a program that will make you feel, and look better.

Immuno-toxins

An estimated 100,000 chemicals, many brand new each year, are poured into our environment every day--our air, water, earth, and ultimately into the food we eat. Many of these chemicals are "immuno-toxic" (poison to the immune system.) In addition, experts fear these environmental pollutants are a significant threat to longevity. *Al Munson, Ph.D., Professor of Toxicology, Medical College of Virginia*, agrees, "If we do not reduce these environmental toxins, we could have very real problems." An understatement in our opinion! Chemicals have been behind environmental illnesses, allergy problems, and multiple chemical sensitivities (MCS), among other problems. According to clinical ecologists many people with MCS have been misdiagnosed or gone undiagnosed. The *National Academy of Sciences* reported in 1987 that "Fifteen percent of the U.S. population have an increased allergic sensitivity to chemicals commonly found in household products, such as detergents, solvents, pesticides, metals, and rubber, thus placing them at increased risk (of) disease."

Doctors know the potential dangers to the immune-deficient patient, many of whom are purposely immune-suppressed by physicians during organ transplant procedures, to prevent organ rejection. Severe life threatening infections commonly occur in the immune-compromised patient, in spite of the carefully monitored and controlled use of immune-depressing drugs.

The invisible threats of radiation from the sun and harmful electromagnetic waves further contaminate our immuno-toxic environment. Immune cells rely upon micro-electrical fields to communicate with each other. Researchers are concerned that when the invisible waves disrupt communication in the immune system, the loss of communication will leave the system weakened and vulnerable, and a chronic immune deficiency syndrome may develop.

Air pollution, primarily from auto exhaust and factory emissions, increasingly threaten the lungs and immune system. Many air pollutants are known to damage immune function in man. Smog destroys elastin, the connective tissue frame work in the lungs and the supporting immune cells. Most feared, however, is air pollution, a primary carcinogen.

In spite of much talk, little significant environmental action has occurred or is expected in the future. Therefore, a dietary and nutritional supplement program that potentializes and protects our immune function is essential to maintain good health. Since our government does not take pervasive action against environmental immuno-toxins, we must take action and protect ourselves.

Part of this protection comes from buying organic fruit and vegetables. Conventional produce grown on "modern" farms is covered with pesticides and assorted petrochemicals. More than 2.6 billion pounds of pesticides are used on food crops every year, in the U.S. alone. The residue of hundreds of different types of chemicals has contaminated domestic and imported produce. Many of these pesticides are known to cause cancer and genetic damage, and many more have never been tested for safety. The U.S. Congress estimated, in 1972, that up to 93% of all chemicals sprayed on food crops have not been tested for potential harmful effects in humans. When chemicals are shown to be dangerous to humans they may still be allowed to be used, under a policy of "risk assessment." **If the chemical causes no more than one added case of cancer per million people, it is considered an acceptable risk.**

Top 10 Prescription Drugs in the U.S.

Here are the top 10 prescription drugs used in 1991, according to the number of prescriptions written: *Drug Topics magazine 1991.*

1. Amoxil, an antibiotic - 23.4 million.
2. Premarin, given to women who have symptoms of menopause - 22 million.
3. Zantac, used to treat ulcers and related problems - 19.3 million.
4. Lanoxin, for heart disease - 18.9 million.
5. Xanx, an anti-anxiety drug - 17.2 million.
6. Synthroid, for thyroid deficiencies - 16 million.
7. Ceclor, an antibiotic - 16 million.
8. Seldane, an allergy medication - 15.4 million.
9. Procardia, for angina and high blood pressure - 15.3 million.
10. VasoTec, for high blood pressure - 14.9 million.

This clearly points to our problems as a society.

7

Nourishing the Immune System

An underactive immune system leads to an increased risk of cancer and infectious diseases which include viral infections, like Chronic Fatigue Syndrome (EVB), even the common cold is more likely to affect those whose immune systems have been weakened by stress and a lack of basic nutrients.

When our body becomes infected, we use up essential nutrients like **vitamins A, C, and E** and minerals like zinc, potassium, chromium, iron and copper. Unless these nutrients are replaced, the stage is set for more serious disorders. For example, the incidence of **breast cancer** is now the highest in history. A report was released in 1988 by the *National Cancer Institute* stating that the breast cancer rate had been increasing one percent per year since 1973, and the rate continues to escalate. These figures are alarming. It is estimated that approximately one in every eight women will develop breast cancer. We believe the increased rates of cancer are the result of an epidemic of chronic malnutrition leading to chronic immune deficiency. A body cannot defend or heal itself when fed a diet of nutrient-low foods.

A report by the *National Academy of Sciences* entitled "Diet, Nutrition and Cancer," states that cancer prevention requires a diet of foods containing beta-carotene (vitamin A), Vitamin C and E, and selenium. These are the most essential antioxidant nutrients, for lowering the risk of cancer, heart disease and many other diseases, by improving the immune function.

Selenium is also important in preventing heart disease, but is lacking in most of our soils. Therefore, foods that contain this mineral may not contain it in the amounts the body requires. We advise all our patients to take supplements to assure they are getting the required amounts of selenium or garlic and onions in their diet will help to provide the needed amounts of selenium.

The mineral **zinc** is also important in immune function. Recent studies show taking up to 100 mg. a day enhances the immune function, **but over 100 mg. may retard its function.**

Foods High in Vitamins A, C, E and Selenium

Almonds	Kale
Apricots	Red Peppers
Barley	Squash
Broccoli	Sweet Potatoes
Brussels Sprouts	Turnip Greens
Cauliflower	Watercress
Carrots	Wheat Germ
Collards	

Read the section on the Magnificent 12 and Greens & Leafy to help you see how wonderful these plant foods are, and why they are essential in your diet.

Foods High in Zinc

Brewer's yeast	Pecans
Fish	All seeds
Legumes	Soy lecithin
Lima beans	Soybeans
Mushrooms	Whole grains

B vitamins are also found in these foods.

Glutathione

Glutathione (GSH) is a tripeptide (glutamic acid, cysteine and glycine) with antioxident properties which can be manufactured in all cells, although the liver seems to be the major source in the body.

A research group found GSH content in fresh meats to be the highest source, dairy and cereals are poor sources with some vegetables, like asparagus, winter squash and potatoes to be high in GSH. Canning lowers it greatly. Vegetarians take glutathione in tablet form. Glutathione is a tremendous antioxidant.

Immune System Nutrition

The following are some frequently used herbs which reportedly are effective in assisting the function of the immune system.

Astragalus

This herb reportedly acts as a tonic to protect the **immune system**. Enhances the immune response in mice, *K.S. Zaho, C. Mancini, and G. Doria. Immunopharmacology*, 20:225-234, 1990. Recent studies from the *M.D. Anderson Hospital and Tumor Institute*, Houston, Texas have resulted in a stronger focus on the immune strengthening effectiveness of Astragalus Membranaceous.

Echinacea

May be one of the most potent and well researched herbal substances that supports the immune system. Native only to North America, a bitter herb, it is used for **colds, flu, infections**, etc. Echinacea has **antibiotic, antiviral and anti-inflammatory** properties. The active compounds in echinacea are said to increase the ability of white blood cells to surround and destroy **bacterial and viral invaders**.

Golden Seal

This small shade-loving plant is a bitter herb that is reported to strengthen the immune system through its **antibiotic** and **antibacterial** properties. The alkaloids of golden seal, especially *berberine* and *hydrastine*, have been used to fight a wide range of infectious agents. It is considered good for **flus, colds** and **inflammation**, and is also said to help promote **heart** and **respiratory** function, capacity, clean **mucous membranes** and counter infection. This herb works with echinacea, mistletoe and licorice root to support the thymus gland in its role in the **immune system**.

Slymarin

Blocks allergic and **inflammatory reactions**, powerful **liver detoxifier** used to treat **hepatitis** and cirrhosis of the liver. Good **liver function** is crucial for a healthy immune system.

Suma

Described as "Brazilian Ginseng," it is thought to help boost the **immune system** because it contains germanium. There have been several studies reporting the beneficial effects of suma and germanium in treating **cancer**.

Problems Associated with an Underactive Immune System

Breathing disorders	Food allergies	Fluid retention
Frequent colds, flu, infections	Mouth sores	Insomnia
Itchy or watery eyes	Sore muscles	Aching joints
Irritable bowel syndrome	Memory loss	Depression
Excessive urination, bladder spasms	Yeast infections	Fatigue
Diarrhea and/or constipation	Gas & bloating after meals	Colitis
Reactions to chemical fumes, smoke	Crohn's disease	Arthritis
perfume, clothing & cleaning supplies	Quick temper, anxiety & panic attacks	

Your most powerful weapon against disease is your immune system.

ETERNAL YOUTH LAWS

Obey the following rules for wellness to keep your immune system functioning properly and working for you to prevent disease and put life into your years and years into your life.

Dietary Wellness is the foundation for having a healthier, happier, more youthful life, and actually reversing disease. Do you really care enough about yourself to gain optimum health? Eternal Youth is your choice!

1) Healthy diet must be a life long endeavor
2) Digestion starts in the mouth, chew your food well
3) Avoid ice cold beverage and do not drink beverages with meals
4) Do not eat heavy foods upon arising or before retiring
5) Eat only when very hungry, then under-eat
6) Rest on the seventh day
7) Do not consume saturated fats (see Facts on Fats)
8) Consume only natural whole foods, as God intended
9) Avoid highly processed foods which overwork the organs
10) Avoid precooked and processed foods that destroy enzymes and nutrients
11) Consume 50% raw "living" foods and extra fiber
12) Steam, broil or bake your foods and undercook vegetables
13) Omit white flour, white sugar, white rice, white salt and pepper
14) Cleanse your system periodically by fasting with pure, fresh juices
15) Consume foods free of toxic insecticides and chemicals
16) Avoid foods with preservatives and additives
17) Avoid alcohol--cigarettes--caffeine--drugs--stress
18) Take quality multi-vitamin and mineral supplements daily
19) Drink 6-8 glasses of pure mineral or steam-distilled water
20) Enjoy fresh air and sunshine daily
21) Exercise daily--include walking and stretching
22) Keep active mentally and physically
23) Maintain a positive state of mind
24) Pray and be thankful for everything
25) Be grateful for who you are and where you are
26) Do not expect the impossible, set realistic goals and achieve them
27) Love your neighbor as yourself
28) Have faith in God!

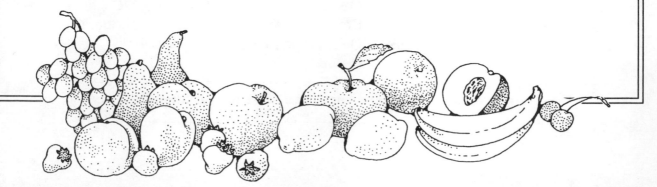

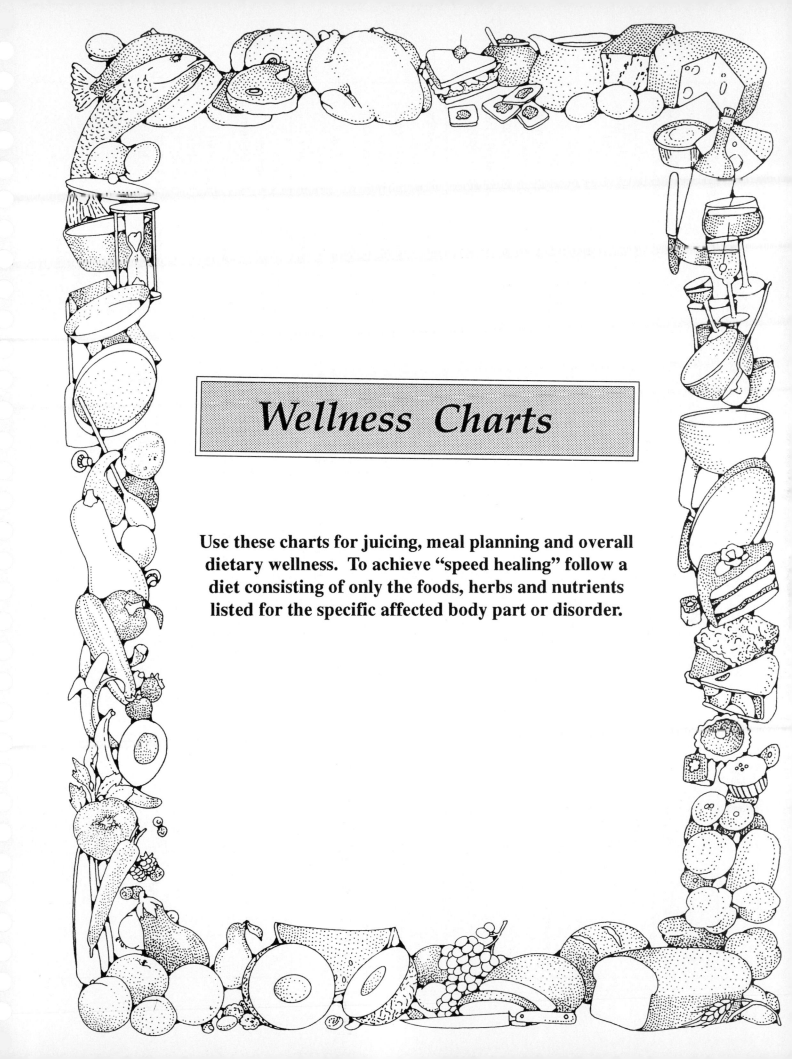

Wellness Charts

Use these charts for juicing, meal planning and overall dietary wellness. To achieve "speed healing" follow a diet consisting of only the foods, herbs and nutrients listed for the specific affected body part or disorder.

Dietary Wellness for Specific Body Parts

Specific Body Part	Vitamins	Minerals	Vegetables	Nuts, Grains & Seeds	Fruits	Herbs
Adrenals	B-complex B-2 B-12 C E Folic acid Pantothenic acid (B-6) Bioflavonoids L-Tyrosine Essential fatty acids	Calcium Chlorine Copper Iron Sodium Magnesium Manganese Phosphorus Potassium Silicon Sulphur Zinc	Asparagus All leafy greens Legumes Lima beans Mushrooms Okra Olive oil Onions Red peppers Sea vegetables Soybeans Sprouts	Almonds Brown rice Cereals Flaxseed Millet Molasses Pumpkin Seeds Whole grains Wheat bran / germ Wild rice	Blueberries Coconut Figs Gooseberries Grapefruit Lemons Oranges Prunes Strawberries	Astragalus Evening primrose oil Ginger Ginseng Juniper Licorice root Lobelia Milk thistle Parsley Royal Jelly
Bladder	A B-complex C D E Pantothenic acid (B-6) Essential fatty acids	Calcium Chlorine Iron Magnesium Manganese Potassium Silicon Zinc	Broccoli Cauliflower Cabbage Green beans Lettuce Parsley Potato skins Red & green peppers Spinach	Almonds Brown rice Flaxseed Molasses Oats Soybeans Sunflower seeds Wheat bran / germ	Acerola cherries Apples Blueberries Cantaloupe Cranberries Grapefruit Lemons Strawberries Watermelon	Buchu leaves Cornsilk Elder flowers Horsetail Juniper berries Nettle Oatstraw Parsley Uva ursi
Bones	B-complex B-12 C D E Pantothenic acid Folic acid	Boron Calcium Chromium Copper Fluorine Magnesium Manganese Molybdenum Phosphorus Potassium Selenium Silicon Sulphur Zinc	All leafy greens Asparagus Broccoli Brussels sprouts Cabbage Cauliflower Kale Lettuce Lima beans Mushrooms Onions Peas Sea vegetables Turnip greens Watercress	Almonds Filberts Flaxseed Molasses Oats Rice Sesame seeds Soybean Sunflower seeds Wheat Wheat germ	Apples Acerola cherries Bananas Blueberries Cantaloupe Figs Kiwi Gooseberries Grapefruit Lemons Oranges Peaches Prunes Red grapes Strawberries	Alfalfa Boneset Dandelion root Garlic Horsetail Nettles Parsley Pokeroot Rose hips

Specific Body Part	Vitamins	Minerals	Vegetables	Nuts, Grains & Seeds	Fruits	Herbs
Brain/Nerves	B-complex B-1, B-2, B-6 B-12, C, D, E Choline Co-Q10, DMG Essential fatty acids Folic acid Inositol L-Glutamine Lecithin Niacin Pantothenic acid	Calcium Chromium Fluorine Iodine Iron Magnesium Manganese Phosphorus Picolenate Potassium Silicon Sulphur Zinc	All leafy greens Avocado, Beans Broccoli, Cabbage Cauliflower Chickpeas Corn, Dry peas Green beans Lentils, Lettuce Potatoes Red & green pepper Reishi mushrooms Soybeans Spinach, Sprouts Tomatoes, Yams	Alfalfa, Almonds Barley Flaxseed Millet Molasses, Oats Peanuts with skins Pecans Rice bran Rye Sesame seeds Sunflower seeds Wheat bran / germ Whole grains Wild rice	Blackberries Black cherries Blueberries Cantaloupe Coconut Figs Gooseberries Grapefruit Oranges Pineapple Prunes Strawberries	Alfalfa Cayenne Ginko Biloba Ginseng Gotu kola Kelp Lobelia Oatstraw Parsley Periwinkle Scullcap St. John's wort Valerian root
Bronchi	Beta-carotene B-complex B-1, B-2 B-6 B-12 C, E Choline Co-Q10 Essential fatty acids Folic acid Inositol Niacin	Calcium Copper Fluorine Manganese Potassium Silicon Iron Selenium	All leafy greens Asparagus, Avocado Broccoli, Cabbage Cauliflower, Corn Dry peas Green beans Green vegetables Lentils, Mushrooms Onions, Potatoes Red & green peppers Rutabaga, Sprouts Tomatoes	Alfalfa, Almonds Barley, Millet Molasses, Oats Peanuts with skins Pecans Rice bran Sesame seeds Soybeans Sunflower seeds Wheat bran / germ Whole grains Wild rice	Apples Blackberries Black cherries Blueberries Cranberries Gooseberries Grapefruit Peaches Prunes Strawberries	Astragalus Black radish Cayenne Eucalyptus Fenugreek Garlic, Ginger Lobelia Mullein, Myrrh Parsley Peppermint Shave grass Yarrow
Ears	A B-complex B-1 B-2 B-6 C D E Niacin Co-Q10 Essential fatty acids	Calcium Manganese (Tinnitis) Phosphorus Potassium	Cabbage Carrot Dry peas Mushrooms Greens (Dandelion, Collard, Mustard, and Spinach) Sweet potatoes Tomatoes	Almonds, Cherries Dried apricot Millet, Oats Peanuts with skins Pecans, Rice bran Sesame seeds Soybeans Sunflower seeds Wheat Wheat bran / germ Whole grains Wild rice	Apricots Blueberries Cranberries Dates Figs Gooseberries Peaches Prunes	Garlic oil Ginko biloba Hyssop Mullein Parsley Yellow dock

Specific Body Part	Vitamins	Minerals	Vegetables	Nuts, Grains & Seeds	Fruits	Herbs
Eyes	A (beta-carotene) B-complex B-1, B-2 B-6, C plus bioflavonoids D, E Choline Inositol L-Glutathione (cataracts) L-Taurine Niacin Pantothenic acid	Calcium Copper Magnesium Manganese Potassium Selenium Silicon Sodium Sulphur Zinc	All dark leafy greens Beans Broccoli Carrots Cauliflower Chickpeas Lettuce Onions Pumpkin Red and green peppers Spinach Squash Sweet potatoes Tomatoes	Almonds Flaxseed Oats Pumpkin seeds Rye Sunflower seeds Wheat bran / germ Whole grains	Apricots Blueberries Canteloupe Cranberries Dates Figs Peaches Prunes Strawberries	Alfalfa Bilberries (night vision) Camomile Elder Flowers Eyebright Garlic Ginko biloba (circulation) Golden seal Horsetail Nettle Oatstraw Yarrow
Female Reproductive Organs	B-complex B-2 B-6 C D E F (essential fatty acids) Lecithin	Calcium Chlorine Copper Iodine Iron Phosphorus Potassium Silicon Sodium Zinc	Asparagus Cabbage Celery Cucumbers Ginger root (increases blood flow to pelvic area) Green vegetables Mushrooms Red peppers Sea vegetables Spinach Watercress	Alfalfa Flaxseed Molasses Nuts Oats Pumpkin seeds Sunflower seeds Wheat Wheat germ	Acerola cherries Apples Cantaloupe Figs Grapefruit Oranges Strawberries	Black cohosh Damiana Dong quai Horsetail Kelp Licorice root Nettle Primrose oil Raspberry Sarsaparilla Saw palmetto Uva ursi White oak bark
Gall Bladder	A B-complex C E L-Glutathione L-Cysteine L-Taurine (prevents gallstones)	Calcium Chlorine Iodine Iron Magnesium Potassium Sodium Sulphur	Broccoli Cauliflower Carrots Lettuce Radishes Red and green peppers Spinach Sweet potato Tomatoes	Flax seed Oats Olive oil Sunflower seeds Wheat Wheat germ	Apples Blackberries Lemons Pears Pineapple	Barberry Burdock Dandelion Fenugreek Gentain root Golden seal Kelp Mandrake White oak bark

Specific Body Part	Vitamins	Minerals	Vegetables	Nuts, Grains & Seeds	Fruits	Herbs
Gums/Teeth	A B-complex B-2 B-6 Bioflavonoids C Essential fatty acids L-Glutathione Niacin	Calcium Fluorine Iron Magnesium Phosphorus Potassium Silicon Sodium Sulphur Zinc	Bok choy Broccoli Cabbage Cauliflower Carrots Kale Lettuce Mushrooms Red and green peppers Spinach Wheatgrass	Almonds Brown rice Flaxseed oil Millet Sesame seeds Wheat bran / germ	Apricots Apples Bananas Cranberries Figs Gooseberries Papaya Prunes	Garlic, Ginger Golden seal (oral and local) Lobelia Myrrh Oatstraw Sage tea Scullcap Tree tea oil (local) Valerian root
Hair/Scalp	A B-complex B-2 Biotin C Choline E Folic acid Niacin, PABA Pantothenic acid L-Cysteine	Copper Iodine Iron Silicon Sulphur Zinc (DMG and Co-Q10 for circulation)	Asparagus Beans, Lentils Broccoli Carrots Cauliflower Dandelion greens Lettuce, Watercress Red and green peppers Sea Vegetables Spinach Sweet potatoes Tomatoes	Alfalfa Almonds Brown rice Flaxseed Millet Mushrooms Nuts, Oats Rye flour Sesame seeds Soy products Sunflower seeds Wheat, Wheat germ	Apples Bananas Cranberries Dates Grapefruit Grapes Gooseberries Oranges Prunes Raisins	Alfalfa Cayenne pepper Chapparral Dandelion Ginko biloba Horsetail Kelp Nettle Oatstraw Primrose oil Sage
Heart	A (beta-carotene) B-complex B-1 B-12 C, E Co-Q10 Bioflavonoids Choline Folic acid Niacin L-Carnitine (amino acid) Essential fatty acids	Calcium Chromium-GTF Cobalt Copper DMG Germanium Iodine Iron Manganese Magnesium Nitrogen Phosphorus Potassium Silicon Zinc	Artichoke Asparagus Avocado Brocolli, Cabbage Carrots Cauliflower Eggplant Kale, Kelp, Lettuce Onions, Parsnips, Peas Potato skins / broth Spinach Sweet Potatoes, Yams Tomatoes Watercress Yellow squash	Almonds Barley Brown rice, Buckwheat Flaxseed Millet Molasses Oats Oat bran Olive oil Psyllium seed Rice bran, Rye Sesame seeds Soybean Sunflower seeds Wheat germ	Apples Apricot Bananas Black cherries Blueberries Dates Figs Kiwi Papaya Peaches Red grapes (lowers cholesterol)	Bilberry Black cohosh Cayenne pepper Garlic Ginko biloba Gotu kola Hawthorne berries Horsetail Linden flowers Shiitake Yarrow --Avoid Ginseng unless supervised

Dietary Wellness

Specific Body Part	Vitamins	Minerals	Vegetables	Nuts, Grains & Seeds	Fruits	Herbs
Intestines	Bioflavonoids B-complex B-1, B-2 B-6, B-12 C, D E, F, K Choline Inositol L-Cysteine L-Glutathione Niacin PABA Pantothenic acid	Calcium Chlorine Iron Magnesium Phosphorus Potassium Sodium Sulphur	Beans, Beets Cabbage, Carrots Celery, Chard Cucumbers Dandelion Kohlrabi Leafy vegetables Lentils Lettuce, Okra Olives, Onions Parsley, Parsnips Peas, Spinach Tomatoes Turnips	Almonds Brown rice Flaxseed Millet Oats bran Rice Rice bran Soybeans Wheat germ	Cantaloupe Figs Gooseberries Grapefruit Papaya Peaches Pineapple Prunes Strawberries	Alfalfa Aloe vera Chamomile Fennel Fenugreek Garlic Golden seal Licorice root Pau D'Arco Psyllium seed
Joints	B-complex B-2 B-6 B-12 C, D, E, F Bioflavonoids Folic acid Niacin Pantothenic acid L-Cysteine (amino acid)	Calcium Fluorine Iodine Iron Magnesium Phosphorus Potassium Silicon Sodium Sulphur Zinc	Beans, Beets Cabbage, Carrots Celery, Collards Cucumbers Dandelion Lentils, Lettuce Olives, Onions Okra Parsnips, Peas Spinach Sea Vegetables Turnips	Alfalfa Almonds Flaxseed Lentils Oats Pumpkin seeds Rice Rice bran Soybeans Wheat Wheat bran / germ	Bananas Blueberries Coconut Figs Gooseberries Grapefruit Lemons Peaches Prunes Strawberries Watermelon	Alfalfa Capsaicin Garlic Horsetail Kelp Nettle Primrose oil Yucca
Kidneys	Beta-carotene A B-complex B-2, B-6 C, E Choline (If you have kidney stones, avoid amino acid-L-Cystine and limit calcium intake)	Calcium Chlorine Chromium-GTF Copper Iron Manganese Magnesium Potassium Zinc	Beans, Beets Cabbage Carrots, Celery Cucumbers Dandelion, Kale Lentils, Lettuce Olives, Onions Parsley Parsnips, Peas Shiitake mushrooms Spinach Turnips	Alfalfa Almonds Brown rice Oats Pumpkin seeds Rice bran Soybeans Wheat Wheat bran / germ	Bananas Blueberries Coconut Cranberries Figs Gooseberries Grapefruit Lemons Peaches Prunes Strawberries Watermelon	Burdock Cornsilk Dandelion root Ginko biloba Juniper berries Parsley leaves and root Slippery elm Shiitake tea Uva ursi White oak bark

Specific Body Part	Vitamins	Minerals	Vegetables	Nuts, Grains & Seeds	Fruits	Herbs
	A B-complex B-12 C D E K Choline Co-Q10 Essential fatty acids Lecithin L-Methionine L-Cysteine L-Glutathione L-Carnitine Niacin Potassium	Chlorine Copper Iodine Iron Magnesium Potassium Sodium Sulfur	All green leafy vegetables Artichoke leaf Asparagus Beets Brussels sprouts Cabbage Carrots Celery Cucumbers Dandelion Endive Green beans Okra, Onions Potato skin Reishi mushrooms Spinach String beans Turnips, Watercress	Almonds Barley Brown rice Corn germ Lentils Oats Oat bran Peanuts Rice Soybeans Sunflower seeds Wheat bran / germ	Apples Blackberries Black cherries Figs Gooseberries Grapefruit Grapes Oranges Papaya Peaches Prunes Strawberries	Astragalus Barberry Black radish Burdock root Cascara sagrada Chaparral Dandelion Echinacea Fennugreek Garlic Milk thistle Suma Red clover Schizandra Thyme Yellow dock
Liver						
	A (beta-carotene) Bioflavonoids B-complex B-1 B-2 B-6 B-12 C, D, E Choline Essential fatty acids Folic acid Inositol Niacin Co-Q10 Pantothenic acid L-methionine	Calcium Copper Fluorine Germanium Iron Magnesium Manganese Potassium Silicon Selenium	All green leafy vegetables Asparagus Beets Cabbage Carrots Celery Cucumbers Dandelion Endive Horseradish Kale Okra Onions Potato skins Spinach String beans Tomatoes Turnips Watercress	Almonds Barley Brown rice Corn germ Flaxseed Lentils Millet Molasses Oats Peanuts Sesame seeds Soybeans Sunflower seeds Wheat germ Whole grain cereals	Apricots Bananas Blackberries Black cherries Blueberries Cantaloupe Coconut Cranberries Figs Grapefruit Gooseberries Oranges Papaya Peaches Prunes Strawberries	Chaparral Coltsfoot Eucalyptus Fenugreek Garlic Licorice root Lungwort Marshmallow Mullein Myrrh Nettle Reishi Rosehips Sage Slippery elm
Lungs Bronchia						

Dietary Wellness

Specific Body Part	Vitamins	Minerals	Vegetables	Nuts, Grains & Seeds	Fruits	Herbs
Lymphatics	A (beta-carotene) B-complex C E Bioflavonoids Co-Q10 Essential fatty acids	Chlorine Copper Potassium Sodium Selenium Zinc	Asparagus, Beets Cabbage, Carrots Celery, Cucumbers Dandelion Dried olives Horseradish, Kohlrabi Okra, Onions Potato skins String beans, Turnips	Almonds Brown rice Flaxseed Oats Oatmeal Pumpkin seeds Sunflower seeds Wheat Wheat germ	Bananas Black figs Blueberries Figs Gooseberries Peaches Prunes Strawberries Watermelon	Black radish Burdock root Chapparral Dandelion Echinacea Garlic Milk thistle Poke root Red clover
Male Reproductive Organs	B-complex C D E Co-Q10 Essential fatty acids	Calcium Iodine Iron Phosphorus Potassium Silicon Zinc	Asparagus, Beets Cabbage Cauliflower Green & red peppers Lettuce, Okra Onions, Parsnips Radishes, Spinach Tomatoes	Almonds, Barley Brown rice Millet Oats, Oatmeal Pumpkin seed Sunflower seeds Wheat Wheat bran / germ	Apricots Black figs Cranberries Dates Gooseberries Prunes Strawberries	Cayenne Chickweed Chlorophyll Ginko biloba Ginseng Kelp Raspberry Saw palmetto
Mammary Glands/ Breasts	A B-complex C D E Essential fatty acids	Calcium Chlorine Iodine Magnesium Potassium Silicon Sodium Zinc	Asparagus Beets, Broccoli Cabbage, Celery Leafy greens Lettuce Okra, Onions Parsnips, Radishes Spinach, Tomatoes	Alfalfa, Almonds Barley, Brown rice Oats, Oatmeal Millet Soybeans (soy products) Sunflower seeds Wheat Wheat bran / germ	Apricots Black figs Cranberries Dates Gooseberries Prunes Strawberries	Black walnut Dong quai Ginko biloba Golden seal Horsetail Kelp Marshmallow Saw palmetto
Muscles	B-complex B-6, B-12 C, D, E Biotin Choline Co-Q10 Essential fatty acids Inositol Lecithin Pantothenic acid Protein	Calcium Chlorine Chromium picolinate Copper Free form amino acids Iron Magnesium Potassium Silicon Zinc	Alfalfa All leafy greens Asparagus Beans Beets Cabbage Lettuce Lentils Onions Parsnips Radishes Reishi mushrooms Spinach, Tomatoes	Almonds Barley Brown rice Flaxseed Millet Mushrooms Oats Oatmeal Sesame seeds Soy beans Sunflower seeds Wheat Wheat bran / germ	Apricots Black figs Cranberries Dates Gooseberries Prunes Strawberries	Horsetail Juniper berries Korean ginseng Mexican yam Nettle Rosemary Sarsaparilla St. John's wort Tansy Valerian root --Apply witch hazel directly to sore muscles

Specific Body Part	Vitamins	Minerals	Vegetables	Nuts, Grains & Seeds	Fruits	Herbs
Nails	A B-complex B-2, B-12 C, D Folic Acid Hydrochloric acid Protein	Calcium Chlorine Iron Magnesium Silicon Zinc	Asparagus Beets, Bok choy Cabbage, Lettuce Onions, Parsnips Radishes Sea vegetables Spinach, Soybeans Tomatoes	Almonds Barley Brown rice Flaxseed Oats Sesame seeds Sunflower seeds Wheat bran / germ	Cherries Coconut Cranberries Dates, Figs Gooseberries Plums Prunes Strawberries	Alfalfa Eucalyptus Horsetail Kelp Mullein Nettle Peppermint
Pancreas	A (beta-carotene) B-complex B-1 B-12 C E L-Glutathione	Chlorine Chromium-GTF Copper Iron Magnesium Potassium Silicon Sodium Zinc	Asparagus, Beets Bok choy, Cabbage Celery root Green beans, Kale Kohlrabi, Okra Onions, Parsnips, Peas Radishes, Spinach Sea vegetables Tomatoes, Turnips Watercress	Almonds Barley Flaxseed oil Oats Oatmeal Pumpkin seeds Sunflower seeds Wheat bran / germ	Apricots Bananas Black figs Cranberries Dates Gooseberries Papaya Pineapple Prunes Strawberries	Alfalfa Dandelion Ginseng Goldenrod Golden seal Horsetail Huckleberry Juniper berry Nettle Red clover
Pituitary Pineal	A C B-complex E L-Glutathione L-Methionine (sulphur containing amino acids)	Copper Iodine Manganese Phosphorus Silicon Sulphur Zinc	Asparagus Beets Cabbage Carrots Legumes, Lettuce Onions, Parsnips Radishes Sea vegetables Soybeans, Sprouts Spinach, Tomatoes Watercress	Barley Flaxseed Oat bran Millet Pumpkin seeds Walnuts Wheat bran / germ Whole grain cereals	Apples Apricots Blackberry Coconut Cranberries Dates, Figs Prunes Gooseberries Grapefruit Pineapple Strawberries	Alfalfa Cayenne Garlic Ginseng Golden seal Kelp Licorice root Nettle Sage Spirulina
Prostate	B-complex B-6 B-12 C D E Essential fatty acids L-Cysteine	Calcium Copper Iron Magnesium Potassium Selenium Silicon Sulphur Zinc	Asparagus Beets Cabbage Lettuce Onions Parsnip Radishes Spinach Tomatoes	Barley Flax seed Oats Pumpkin seeds Sunflower seeds Wheat bran / germ Whole grain cereals	Bananas Coconut Cranberries Dates Figs Gooseberries Kiwi Prunes Strawberries	Alfalfa Bchu Bee pollen Burdock root Golden seal Juniper berries Nettle Saw palmetto berries

Specific Body Part	Vitamins	Minerals	Vegetables	Nuts, Grains & Seeds	Fruits	Herbs
Skin	A B complex B1 B2 B6 B12 Bioflavonoids C, D, E, K PABA Pantothenic acid	Calcium Copper Magnesium Manganese Potassium Selenium Silica (Silicon) Sodium Sulphur Zinc	All leafy greens Avocadoes Beets Broccoli Carrots Celery Cucumbers Kale Kidney beans Lentils Pumpkin Sea vegetables Spinach Squash Sweet Potatoes	Brown rice Leafy seed oil Millet Oat bran Pumpkin seeds Rice bran Soybeans Wheat germ	Apples Apricots Bananas Blueberries Cantaloupe Cherries Figs, Prunes Lemons Papaya Peaches Red grapes Watermelon	Alfalfa Aloe vera Burdock root Dandelion Garlic Horsetail Kelp Nettle Primrose oil Raspberry leaves Yellow dock
Spine	A (beta-carotene) B-complex C D E Essential fatty acids Lecithin	Calcium Copper Magnesium Manganese Molybdenum Selenium Silicon Sodium Sulphur Zinc	Asparagus, Beets Brussels sprouts Cabbage, Carrots Cauliflower, Celery Collards, Cucumbers Dandelions, Dried olives, Kale, Legumes Lima beans Okra, Peas Potato skins, Soybeans String beans, Turnips Yellow corn Watercress	Almonds Barley Brewer's yeast Brown rice Chestnuts Nuts Oatmeal Pignolia nuts Sunflower seeds Walnuts Wheat germ Whole grain cereals	Apricots Blackberries Black cherries Blueberries Coconut Cranberries Dates , Figs Gooseberries Grapefruit Oranges Peaches Prunes, Raisins	Alfalfa Eoneset Dandelion Garlic Horsetail Nettle
Thymus	A B-complex C D E Essential fatty acids Lecithin	Calcium Flourine Iron Magnesium Selenium Silicon Zinc	All leafy greens Beets Brussels sprouts Cabbage Carrots Cauliflower Lettuce, Onions Parsnips Potato peelings Spinach Tomatoes	Barley Brown rice Cereals Corn germ Millet Oats Wheat bran / germ Wheatgrass Whole wheat	Apricots Blackberries Black cherries Cranberries Figs Gooseberries Prunes Strawberries	Angustifolia Echinacea Ginseng Golden seal Licorice Nettle Pokeweed Horsetail Purpurea St. John's wort

Specific Body Part	Vitamins	Minerals	Vegetables	Nuts, Grains & Seeds	Fruits	Herbs
Thyroid	A B-complex Choline E (avoid over 400 IU of vitamin E) Essential fatty acids Inositol L-cysteine	Calcium Chlorine Iodine Iron Magnesium Potassium Sodium Sulphur Zinc	Asparagus Beets Brussels sprouts Cabbage, Carrots Cauliflower, Celery Cucumbers Dandelions Okra, Onions Parsley Potato skins Sea Vegetables Turnips Yellow corn	Almonds Barley Chestnuts Molasses Nuts Oatmeal Pignolia nuts Soybean Sunflower seeds Walnuts Wheat germ Whole grain cereals Yeast	Apricots Blackberries Black cherries Blueberries Coconut Cranberries Dates Figs Gooseberries Grapefruit Oranges Peaches Prunes	Alfalfa Burdock root Dandelion Dulse Garlic Ginseng Golden seal Horsetail Kelp Sage
Uterus	B-complex B12 C E F Essential fatty acids	Calcium Iron Magnesium Silicon Zinc	All leafy greens Beans, Beets Brussels sprouts Cabbage, Carrots Cauliflower, Lettuce Onions, Parsnips Potato peelings Sea vegetables Soybeans, Spinach Sprouts, Tomatoes Watercress	Barley Flax seed Oats Pumpkin seeds Sunflower seeds Wheat bran / germ Whole grain cereals	Apricots Blackberries Black cherries Cranberries Figs Gooseberries Prunes Red raspberries Strawberries	Alfalfa, Bayberry Black and Blue cohosh, Dong quai, False unicorn, Golden seal, Horsetail (unless pregnant) Kelp, Sage Licorice root Primrose oil Squaw vine
Veins and Arteries	A B-complex B-1 B-2, B-6 B-12, C D, E, F, K Bioflavonoids Essential fatty acids Folic Acid Inositol Niacin PABA Rutin	Copper Iodine Iron Magnesium Manganese Potassium Phosphorus Silicon Sulphur Zinc	All green leafy vegetables Asparagus Beets, Cabbage Carrots, Celery Cucumbers Dandelion Dried olives Endive, Legumes Lettuce, Watercress Mushroom Okra, Onions, Parsnips Potato peelings Spinach, Turnips	Almonds Barley Brewer's yeast Buckwheat Chestnuts Flax seed Molasses Oatmeal Pignolia nuts Pumpkin seeds Soybean Sunflower seeds Walnuts Wheat germ	Apricots Blackberries Black cherries Blueberries Cranberries Dates Figs Gooseberries Grapefruit Oranges Peaches Prunes	Alfalfa Buckwheat Butcher's broom Cayenne Green tea Hawthorn berries Kelp Nettle Oat straw Tansy White oak bark Yarrow

Natural Prescriptions

Drugs	Therapeutic Alternatives
Antibiotics	Do not take antibiotics for long periods as they upset the natural intestinal flora. Instead, use Astragalus*, Garlic*, Golden seal, Grapefruit seed extract, Myrrh gum, Red clover, Royal jelly, Saint John's wort*, Pau d'Arco*
Anti-fungal	Acidophilus powder*, Barberry bark, Black walnut hulls, Caprylic acid*, Chaparral, Chlorophyll plants, Garlic*, Grapefruit seed extract, Pau d'Arco*, Tree tea oil
Antihistamines & Decongestants	Anise, Bioflavinoids, Capsicum (Cayenne), Coltsfoot, Echinacea, Ephedra* (Ma Huang), Eucalyptus (as inhalant)*, Garlic, Horehound, Horseradish, Lobelia, Marshmallow, Mullein, Myrrh, Onions, Quercitin-C*, Saint John's wort, Stinging nettle
Anti-inflammatory	Alfalfa, Bromelin (pineapple), Echinacea*, Garlic*, Golden seal*, Horsetail, Licorice, Papaya, Primrose oil, Reishi mushrooms, St. John's wort, Vitamin C (massive doses)
Antioxidants	Astragalus, Chaparral*, Co-Q10, Gamma-Linoleic Acid (GLA), Garlic, Ginko biloba, Kelp*, L-Cysteine* (amino acid to protect cells), L-Glutathione*, Rose Hips, Selenium, Pycnogenal*, Reishi mushrooms, Superoxide Dismutase (SOD), Vitamins A, C, & E*.
Anti-viral	Astragalus*, Cayenne*, Echinacea, Garlic*, Myrrh gum, Pau d'Arco, Saint John's wort*, Shiitake mushrooms
Blood Purifiers	Astragalus, Black radish, Burdock root*, Chaparral*, Dandelion*, Garlic*, Milk thistle*, Oregon grape, Red clover*
Estrogen Blockers	Blocks excess estrogen. Flaxseed*, Buckwheat, Wheat, Wheat bran, ligins found in cruciferous vegetables and flavonoids in citris fruits. Proper liver function importanant.
Estrogen Promoters	Anise, Black Cohosh*, Dong quai*, Fennel, Fenugreek, ginseng, licorice, Primrose oil, Red clover, Sage, Suma, Wild yam. Note: if your physician has you on estrogen blockers, like Tomoxifen for breast cancer, do not use these promoters.
Immune Boosters	Astragalus, Chamomile, Chlorophyll (sources), Echinacea*, Garlic, Ginko biloba, Q-10 Golden seal, schizandra, Reishi & Shiitake mushrooms*, Siberian ginseng, Suma
Muscle Relaxants	Chamomile, Fenugreek, Kudzu root, Peppermint, Saw palmetto, St. John's wort*, Magnesium*, Skullcap, Valerian root*. For muscular pain, apply witch hazel directly.
Steroids (natural)	Beta-sitosterol*, Gotu kola, Liver extract, Mexican yam*, Reishi mushrooms, Sarsaparilla, Saw palmetto berry*
Tranquilizers	Catnip, Chamomile, Hops, Passionflower, Saint John's wort*, Skullcap, Valerian root*
	* Essential

Add Years To Your Life & Life To Your Years

- Astragalus & Reishi Mushrooms to protect the immune system.
- B complex & L-Glutamine for proper brain function & memory.
- Calcium, Magnesium & Vitamin D to protect against bone loss.
- Echinacea & Zinc to protect against colds and flu.
- Ginko biloba to improve brain function and circulation.
- Golden seal & St. John's wort to protect against bacterial/viral infections.
- Hawthorn berries & Garlic to lower cholesterol and protect the heart.
- L-Cystine & essential fatty acids for cell formation, and rebuilding tissue.
- L-Glutathione to protect antioxidants (i.e. vitamins C, E, and Beta-carotene).
- Milk thistle & Dandelion to protect the liver and cleanse the blood.
- Valerian root and Skullcap to induce sleep and calm the nervous system.
- Vitamins A, C, E, and Selenium (antioxidants) to prevent cell damage and cancer.
- Fresh lemon juice added to quality warm water is a great cleanser and healer upon rising.

For Chemotherapy, Toxic Heavy Metal, & Radiation Damage

° Apple pectin
° Chaparral
° Echinacea
° Fiber
° Garlic
° Ginko biloba
° Ginseng
° Kelp
° L-Glutathione

Disease Warning Signs	Possible Cause	Therapeutic Self-Defense
Abdominal Pain	Appendicitis, cancer, colitis, constipation, diarrhea, diverticulitis, food allergies, food poisoning, gas, glandular disorders, hiatal hernia, influenza (flu), irritable bowel syndrome, premenstral syndrome	Aloe vera*, Bee propolis, Cascara sagrada*, Catnip, Chamomile, Charcoal tablets (for food poisoning and bloating), Chlorophyll*, Fennel (for gas), Flaxseed*, Ginger root, Golden seal, High-fiber diet, Kelp, L-Glutamine, Licorice root, Papaya, Pau d'Arco, Peppermint, Psyllium, Rhubarb root, Saint John's wort, Suma, Wheatgrass. Drink plenty of water and juices. Eat a soft-food diet, avoiding sugar and processed foods.
Allergies / Hay Fever	Air pollution, damp places (like moldy basements), inherited depressed immune function, malnutrition, poor diet, "sick buildings", vitamin deficiency	Alfalfa, Barberry bark, Bioflavonoids, Golden seal, Kelp, Lemons, Mullein, Plantain, Quercitin-C*, Red clover, Stinging nettle*. Omit foods, chemicals, and pollutants that cause reactions.
Backache (Lower backache-constipation)	Back strain, bad posture, bladder disorders, disc disease, female disorders, heavy lifting, kidney disorders, lack of exercise, mineral deficiency (calcium), prostate disorders, stress	Alfalfa, Boron, Burdock, Calcium*, Cramp bark & Black hawthorn (for lower back and legs), Horsetail, Magnesium*, Manganese, Nettle, Papaya, Slippery elm, Vitamin C, White willow bark, Zinc. Cleansing enemas relieve pressure and pain.
Breast Soreness (Lumps or cysts may disappear or become smaller after menopause)	Abnormal breast milk production, fibrocystic breast disease, cysts (A cyst is tender and moves freely under the skin, a cancerous lump does not move), excessive estrogen, hormone imbalance, iodine deficiency, trapped fluids	Golden seal, Kelp, Pau d'Arco, Primrose oil, Red clover, Squaw vine, Vitamins A, C, E, B complex, and extra B-6. Avoid caffeine, colas, chocolate, and coffee. Follow a low-fat, high-fiber diet. Check with your doctor to rule out cancer. Apply a poultice of poke root over the breast.
Burning Anus	Acidity, alkalinity, colon disorder, diarrhea, food allergies, hemorrhoids, parasites	Determine food allergies and omit from diet. Do the acid and alkaline self-test in the section on Food Combining. If the body is overly acidic, for quick results, eat two umeboshi plums every 4 hours for 2 days. Try potato skin broth. Also see Parasites in this chart.
Bruise Easily (Bleeding under the skin)	Anemia, excessive use of anti-clotting drugs and/or aspirin, leukemia, malnutrition, obesity, Vitamin C deficiency. An early warning sign of cancer.	Alfalfa, Chaparral, Chlorophyll, Dark leafy greens, Garlic, Kelp, Lemons, Rose-hips*, Vitamin C with bioflavinoids* (8,000 mg. daily in divided doses), Vitamin K. Avoid aspirin.
Canker Sores (Mouth sore spots with white centers, and red borders)	Excessive citrus and acidic foods, fatigue, food allergies, hormonal disturbances, poor dental hygiene, Crohn's disease, stress (causes flare-ups), trauma, viral infections, vitamin deficiencies indicates weakened immune system	Acidophilus, B-12, Black walnut, Burdock, Folic acid, Golden seal, Iron, L-Lysine* (amino acid), Onions & Garlic (sulfur needed), Pau d'Arco, Red clover, Rose hips. See acid test in Food Combining section. Apply golden seal powder/extract* to sore. Avoid acidic fruit, fish, meat, hard-to-chew, and other acidic foods until healed.
Carpal Tunnel Syndrome (Pain, numbness, tingling and weakness in the muscles of the hand)	Repetitive hand motions over an extensive period of time (often afflicts carpenters, computer users, machinists, musicians, painters, typists). Also associated with rheumatoid arthritis, diabetes, and pregnancy. Rotate jobs weekly to keep the same muscles and joints from being overused.	Butcher's broom, Co-Q10*, Capsicum*, Cornsilk, Garlic, Ginko biloba*, Kelp, Parsley, Primrose oil, Vitamins A, B complex, B-6*, C, and E, plus minerals. Adjust the height of your work surface. Find ways to accomplish tasks without bending the wrists. Try to keep your workplace warm and dry, because cool/damp conditions may make CTS worse.

* Essential

21

Disease Warning Signs	Possible Cause	Therapeutic Self-Defense
Childhood Allergies	Inherited lack of enzyme to digest milk, overconsumption of a particular food, too much junk food, weakened immune system	Alfalfa, Aloe vera, Dandelion root, Quercitin-C*, Royal jelly. Omit foods, chemicals, and pollutants that cause reactions.
Circulation (Aching extremities, fatigue, leg & finger cramps, tingling sensations, memory loss)	Arteriosclerosis, lack of elasticity in the walls of the arteries, Buerger's disease, Raynaud's disease high blood pressure, calcium deficiency, hypertension, lack of exercise, smoking, stress	Butcher's broom*, Bilberry*, Calcium & Magnesium*, Capsicum, (increases pulse rate), Chlorophyll, Co-Q10, Garlic*, Ginko biloba*, Ginger root, Hawthorn berries, L-Carnitine, Vitamin C plus bioflavonoids, Vitamin E*. Avoid Black cohosh (slows pulse rate). Exercise will improve circulatory system.
Colds / Flu / Persistent Fever	Bowel disorders, bronchitis, Chronic fatigue syndrome (CFS), chronic infection, Crohn's disease, colitis, depressed immune system, diabetes, Epstein-Barr virus (EBV), inflammation, influenza, Lyme disease, mononucleosis, rheumatic disorders, viral infections	Catnip tea and enemas (good for infants)*, Astragalus, Echinacea, Garlic*, Golden seal*, Hot liquids (including turkey or chicken soup), Mullein, Plaintain leaves, Rose hips*, Saint John's wort, Vitamins A, C, and Zinc. L-Glutamine fights viral infections. Boneset induces sweating to reduce fever. Steam-distilled water every two hours with lemon juice. Consume strawberries for viral infections. No sugar!
Colic in Infants	Allergies, cold food, cold weather, lactose intolerance, mother's diet of gassy foods if breastfeeding, overfeeding, teething, food pieces too large to digest	Chamomile tea, Catnip tea (also as an enema), Fennel seed tea, Ginger tea, Mashed papaya (added to formula), Savory tea, Slippery elm bark tea. Change to soy formula (omit cow's milk).
Colon & Bowel Disorders (Abdominal pain, diarrhea, irritable bowel syndrome, stomach cramps)	Cancer, candidiasis, chemical and/or food allergies, colitis, Crohn's disease, drugs, lack of enzymes, low-fiber and high-fat diet, malabsorption, nutrient deficiency, parasites (worms), poor elimination, stress	Alfalfa (Vitamin K), Aloe vera, Bee propolis, Cascara sagrada, Chamomile*, Ginger root, Golden seal, Ground flaxseed, Kelp, L-Glutamine, Licorice root, Papaya, Pau d'Arco, Peppermint, Psyllium husk*, Saint John's wort, Wheatgrass (green drinks), Yerba Mate' (for Crohn's disease). Avoid meat, fats, dairy products, nuts, seeds, sugar, and grains until healed. Daily bowel movements are important to avoid toxic build-up.
Constipation	Colitis, colon problems, dehydration, drugs, food allergies, high-fat diet, iron supplements, lack of exercise, liver and/or gallbladder malfunction, low-fiber diet	Aloe vera*, Cascara sagrada*, Chlorophyll*, Fennel seed, Flaxseed*, High-fiber diet*, Prunes, Psyllium, Sena Leaves, Suma. Cleansing enemas are helpful. Exercise. Omit caffeine, dairy products, food allergies, fried foods, and yeast products.
Cough (Persistent cough, hoarseness, laryngitis)	Airborne allergies, air pollution, cancer, chemicals, dental work, emphysema, food allergies, lung disorders, mercury toxicity, pneumonia, nervousness, vitamin deficiency	Anise, Barberry*, Bee propolis, Echinacea, Fennel, Licorice root, Lungwort, Marshmallow, Mullein, Myrrh*, Pau d'Arco, Peppermint, Sage, Thyme, Vitamin C* plus bioflavonoids, Beta-carotene*, Zinc

* Essential

Disease Warning Signs	Possible Cause	Therapeutic Self-Defense
Glaucoma (Eye pain, blurred vision, pupil's inability to adjust to light, halos around light)	High pressure within the eye, aging, damaged nerve cells, diabetes, eye injury, high blood pressure, nutritional disorders, stress	Chamomile and Eyebright (alternate teas, apply with eyedropper to relieve pressure). Vitamin C* (2,000 mg. every 3 hours) to relieve eye pressure, up to 10,000 mg. daily. B complex (injections are best), Fennel, Vitamin E (removes particles from the lens of the eye). Avoid alcohol, antihistamines, caffeine, eye strain, niacin (in high doses), licorice herb, tobacco, and tranquilizers.
Grinding Teeth During Sleep	B complex vitamins (especially pantothenic acid deficiencies), excessive stress, lack of calcium, TMJ (teeth out of line)	B complex vitamins & Pantothenic acid* (needed for proper motor coordination), Calcium and Magnesium* (needed to prevent involuntary movement), Horsetail*, Hypoglycemic diet, Kelp*, Nettle, Rose hips. Avoid sugar (in any form) before bedtime.
Gum Disease (Bleeding & sore gums, gingivitis, mouth sores periodontal disease, pyorrhea)	Alcohol consumption, bacterial or viral infections, bad fillings and fittings, improper brushing, blood disease, breathing through the mouth, chronic illness, drugs, glandular disorders, (lack of friendly bacteria), Candidasis, poor diet (including a high-sugar diet, and too may soft foods), tobacco	Calcium (to prevent bone loss), Co-Q10, Vitamins A, E, and C plus bioflavonoids (2,000 mg. 3 times daily), and Myrrh*. Brush teeth with golden seal powder and a soft toothbrush. Use sage tea as a mouthwash to destroy bacteria. At bedtime, rub a dropper full of golden seal extract on gums, and hold in mouth for a few moments.
Headaches (Cluster headaches, migraines)	Alcohol consumption, allergies, asthma, brain tumor, constipation, drugs, excessive toxins, eyestrain, glaucoma, high blood pressure, sinusitis, stress, vitamin deficiency	Catnip, Celery, Feverfew*, Ginko biloba, Rosemary, Scullcap, Valerian root, and Willow bark* Drink an 8 oz. glass of water every 2 hours. Check for allergies (food/chemical/pollution).
Hemorrhoids & Varicose Veins (Blood in stools, itching, pain, pressure, swollen leg veins)	Constipation, food allergies, heavy lifting, lack of exercise, liver disorders, lack of dietary fiber, obesity, pregnancy, prolonged periods of sitting	Alfalfa and Leafy dark greens, Aloe vera, Bilberry, Bioflavonoids*, Buckthorn bark, Butcher's broom, Capsicum, Cascara sagrada, Fiber, Flaxseed oil, Nettle, Psyllium, Sitz baths, Vitamin E (improves circulation), Vitamin K, White oak bark, Witch hazel. Avoid tobacco, fried foods, long periods of sitting or standing, and straining with bowel movements. See Circulation in this chart.
Impotence (Inability to achieve or maintain an erection, premature ejaculation)	Aging, alcohol consumption, arteriosclerotic disease, disorders of the prostate, certain drugs (like hypertensive medications), cigarettes, diabetes mellitis, hormonal imbalance, neurological disorder, peripheral vascular disease, post-surgical, loss of self-esteem	Bee pollen, Borago or Flaxseed oil, Co-Q10, Damiana, Ginko biloba, Mura, Puana, Pumpkin seeds*, Royal jelly, Siberian ginseng*, Uva ursi, Yohimbe*, Vitamins C, E*, Selenium, and Zinc*. Avoid alcohol, sugar, tobacco, yeast, fats, meat and dairy products.
Indigestion (Abdominal pain, belching, gas, heartburn, nausea, vomiting, undigested food in stools)	Acidosis, alkalosis, allergies, Candidiasis, colon disorders, heart disease, junk foods, lack of fiber, lack of enzymes or stomach acid, liver and/or gallbladder problems, pancreas or adrenal disorders, poor diet (including spicy and greasy foods), stress, toxins, ulcers	Alfalfa (Vitamin K), Aloe vera, Acidophilus* Artichoke leaves, Bromelin, Calcium carbonate, Chamomile, Dandelion*, Enzymes, Fennel (tea)* Fenugreek, Fiber, Ginger root, Okra, Papaya (leaf tea), Peppermint, Rosemary. Charcoal tablets (found in health food stores are good for gas and bloating, do not take them on a daily basis), Avoid nuts, seeds, grains, dairy products, meats, fried foods, spicy foods, and fats. Avoid lying on right side after eating.

* Essential

Disease Warning Signs	Possible Cause	Therapeutic Self-Defense
Infertility	Antibodies inactivate partner's sperm, hormone imbalances, infections (like Chlamydia & pelvic inflammatory disease)	Asparagus root, Damiana, Dong Quai, False unicorn root, Kelp, Saw palmetto* berries, Siberian ginseng*, Vitamin E*, Zinc* No fats, sugar, tobacco, or alcohol.
Insomnia (Sleeplessness)	Asthma, Chronic Fatigue Syndrome (CFS), daytime naps, drugs, heavy meals before retiring, hypoglycemia, hypothyroidism, indigestion, lack of certain nutrients, obesity, pain, poor diet, stress, viral infections	Calcium & Magnesium*, Hops, Melatonin (hormone synthesized and released by the pineal gland), Saint John's wort*, Skullcap, Valerian root*. No alcohol, caffeine, fats, cured meats, sugar *(in any form, including sweet fruits), or tobacco. (For CFS 6-10,000 mg. C daily, no sugar in any form, St. John's wort, and rest.)
Memory (Poor memory, brain disorders)	Alcohol, Alzheimer's disease, blood sugar disorders, drugs, food allergies, heavy metals, malfunction of the central nervous system, poor circulation, poor diet, stress, medications, sugar, tobacco	Antioxidants*, B complex*, Extra B-12 and folic acid, Vitamins C & E, Capsicum, Co-Q10, DMG, DMA, Dismutase, L-Glutamine, L-Glutathione, Ginger root, Ginko biloba*, Ginseng, Gotu kola, schizondra, Greens, Kelp, Lecithin, Periwinkle, Superoxide Dismutase, Perosidace, Superoxide Zinc. No alcohol, junk food, fried foods, sugar, or tobacco.
Menopause (Anxiety, confusion, depression, heart palpitations, hot flashes, leg cramps, memory impairment)	Age, animal products, chemical allergies, caffeine, dairy products, estrogen deficiency, fluid retention, food allergies, hormonal imbalance, hypoglycemia, lack of nutrients (including B complex, calcium, & magnesium), stress, sugar, thyroid disorders	Alfalfa, Black cohosh, B complex, Extra B-6, Calcium*, Chaseberry, Damiana, Dong quai*, Horsetail (silica), Kelp, Licorice, Magnesium, Primrose oil*, Raspberry, Sage, Siberian Ginseng, Squaw vine, St. John's wort (relieves anxiety and depression), Uva ursi, Vitamin E and sage tea* (relieves hot flashes), Wild yam*. See Estrogen Promoters in this chart.
Nausea	Chemical/food allergies, colon disorders, drugs, food poisoning, greasy foods, liver and/or gallbladder disorders, pregnancy	Aloe vera, Calcium carbonate, Charcoal tablets, Ginger root*, Licorice root, Peppermint, Vitamin B-6*. Glass of water every hour to help rid the body of toxins.
Nervous Conditions (Anxiety, fear, shaking hands/legs)	Drugs, food allergies, hormonal imbalance, illness, job, loneliness, pain, parasites, sugar (see research findings below), vitamin deficiencies (especially B complex)	B-complex*, Capsicum, Catnip, Chamomile, Genetian root, Hops, Lobelia, Magnesium, Passion flower, Saint John's wort*, Scullcap, Valerian root*. Follow a high-complex carbohydrate diet, with no sugar*! Massage.
Pain (Without pain we would be unaware of any health problems, and the body's need for help to repair itself)	A combination of physical and mental disorders. Side effects from certain drugs can make the problem worse. Note that each person's individual pain tolerance is different. Anticipation of physical pain, when cause is unknown, can heighten the pain. Find the cause!	Angelica (works like aspirin), Black cohosh (for PMS and arthritis), Capsaicin (for cluster headaches), DL-phenylalanine, Feverfew (for migraines)*, Germanium, Hops, Passion flower (for children & elderly), Saint John's wort (good for chronic pain)*, Skullcap, Valerian root*, White willow bark* Glass of quality water every 4 hours. Juice fast (if not diabetic). Latest studies show fresh papaya juice reduced pain in 90% of those treated, and capsicum (cayenne) is good for all types of pain.
Parasites & Worms (Anemia, colon disorders, diarrhea, rectal itching, loss of weight & appetite, poor absorption of nutrients)	Walking barefoot on contaminated soil. Ingestion of eggs or larvae from uncooked fish and meat. Scratching anus will transmit the eggs. Children eating dirt or passing the eggs from one to the other. Eating and drinking food and water in a foreign country.	Heavily salted diet for one week for children with pinworms, and cleansing enemas. Areca nut for tapeworms. Black walnut hulls, Butternut bark (stimulates bowels), Cascara sagrada, Fig juice, Garlic, Papaya seeds, Pau d'Arco, Pinkroot, Raw pumpkin seeds, Wormwood (for all types) and squash seeds for tape and round worms.

* Essential

New research from three studies conducted at the *National Institute of Mental Health* reveals that 75% of patients suffering from panic disorders (severe anxiety), had a dramatic increase in anxiety after eating sugar. *Researcher Dr. Bernard J. Vittone* says, "Millions of Americans who think they have chronic anxiety may actually be having adverse reactions to sugar in their diets" — *Weekly World News, July 7, 1992*

Disease Warning Signs	Possible Cause	Therapeutic Self-Defense
Pneumonia (Bluish nails, chest pains, chills, cough, enlarged lymph nodes in the neck, fatigue, fever, muscle aches, sore throat)	Alcoholism, aspiration under anesthesia, bacteria, chemical irritants, common cold, influenza, kidney failure, malnutrition, sickle cell disease, smoking, stroke, viral infections	Acidophilus*, Alfalfa, B complex*, Bloodroot, Free-form amino acids, Garlic*, Ginger, Golden seal, Lemon juice and distilled water, L-cystine*, Lungwort, Marshmallow, Mullein, Pleurisy root, Protein* (free-form amino acids), Rose hips, Vitamin A (beta carotene*), Vitamin C* (mega dose), Zinc & Selenium.
Poison Ivy or Poison Oak (Blistering, persistent itching, rash, redness, swelling)	Sap from poison ivy/oak plant contacting uncovered skin and producing the symptoms. Do not re-wear contaminated clothing until laundered.	Calamine lotion as directed on label. Poultice of equal parts white oak bark and lime water. Tree tea oil applied directly. Echinacea, Golden seal (also as a poultice), Lobelia, Myrrh, and Vitamin C. Scratching transmits the inflammation. Wash skin immediately with yellow laundry soap, rinse several times in running water.
Skin Rashes	Chemical or food allergies, chicken pox, eczema, Candida (fungus infection), hives, Lupus, Measles, neurodermatitis (back of legs), poison ivy or oak, Psoriasis, shingles, stress	Aloe vera gel, Fenugreek, Vitamins A, C (high amounts throughout the day), and Zinc. Golden seal poultices on affected area. Tree tea oil applied directly. Burdock (may be used as a face wash or tea) for acne & psoriasis. Yeast-free and sugar-free diet.
Stamina & Endurance Low (Tire easily)	Prolonged periods without rest, putting undue stress on the muscles, alcohol consumption, dehydration, eating before lifting, fat, food allergies, heart disorders, illness, improper clothing, improper lifting, improper movements, nutritional deficiencies, poor diet, smoking, sugar	Amino acids, B complex, B-6, B-12, Bee pollen, Beta-carotene, Calcium, Chlorophyll, Chromium picolenate, Co-Q10, Complex carbohydrates for energy, DMG, Dessicated liver, Gamma-Oryzonol, Garlic, Gotu kola, Horsetail, High amounts of Vitamins C & E, Magnesium, Mexican wild yam, Octacosanol, Potassium, Royal jelly, Siberian ginseng, Silicon, Spirulina, Suma, Royal jelly, Zinc. Apply Arnica directly for sprains, and apply witch hazel on sore muscles.
Stress (prolonged stress depresses the immune function and may be at the root of most illnesses)	Can't adapt to change, diet of sugar and junk foods, family relationships, heavy workload, illness, mental or physical strain, trauma, workplace demands and pollutants	Astragalus, B complex, Chamomile, Gotu kola, Horsetail, Saint John's wort, Siberian ginseng*, Skullcap, Spirulina, Suma, Valerian root*, Vitamin C (large doses). Practice breathing slowly & deeply, exercise, massages, enjoy music, reading, and warm baths.
Swallowing Difficulty	Allergies, anxiety, bacterial infection, cancer of esophagus, fear, goiter, hiatal hernia, hormone imbalance, nervous disorder, stress, swollen lymph nodes, thyroid disorder, tonsilitis	Bee propolis, Garlic, Golden seal, Licorice, St. John's wort, Valerian root, Vitamins A (Beta-carotene), B complex, C and Zinc. Gargle with thyme tea. Avoid sugar, stay on a soft-foods diet, and chew food well. Avoid cold beverages.
Sweating Excessively	Cancer, fever, food allergies, heart disease, hormone imbalance, Hodgkin's disease, hypoglycemia, infection, menopause, obesity, pancreas or thyroid disorder, poor diet, stress, sugar, tuberculosis (night sweats)	Alfalfa*, Dandelion root*, Kelp, Garlic, Pomegranates (fruit), Potassium*, Sage*, Spirulina, Uva ursi. Drink 8-10 glasses pure water daily. Juice fast to cleanse the body of toxins (unless diabetic)*. Avoid tobacco, alcohol, dairy products, fat, and sugar (all forms).
Swelling (Abdomen, ankles, feet, hands, legs)	Bladder or kidney disorders, excessive dietary salt, MSG, food allergies, heart disorders, medications, oral contraceptives, steroids	Alfalfa, B complex, B-6*, Cornsilk*, Dandelion root*, Garlic, Horsetail, Kelp*. Avoid alcohol, animal products, dairy products, fat*, salt*, soy sauce* and sugar.

* Essential

Disease Warning Signs	Possible Cause	Therapeutic Self-Defense
Swollen Lymph Nodes	Chronic infection, Hodgkin's disease, lymphoma, toxic metals, toxin build-up	Astragalus, Burdock root*, Chapparral, Dandelion root, Echinacea, Garlic*, Golden seal, Oregon grape*, Red clover*, Selenium, Vitamin A, C, E, and Zinc. Juice fast for 3 days (unless diabetic, pregnant or nursing).
Thirsting Excessively	Diabetes, fever, heavy perspiration, hypoglycemia, infection, excess salt, salty food, junk food, fats, soy sauce, and spicy food.	Astragalus, Echinacea, Golden seal, Milk thistle, Oregon grape. Juice fast for 3 days (unless diabetic, pregnant, or nursing).
Urinary Problems **(Burning, frequent and/or urgent urination, itching)**	Bladder problems (poor emptying of bladder), cancer, food allergies, cystitis (inflammations), diuretics	Celery seed, Cornsilk, Cranberry juice (unsweetened), Golden seal, Hot sitz baths*, Juniper berry, Magnesium, Myrrh, Oatstraw, Parsley*, Psyllium seed, Vitamin C, Rose hips, Uva ursi Drink 8-10 glasses quality water daily.
Vaginal Discharge	Candidiasis (yeast infection), chlamydia, diabetes, genital herpes, gonorrhea, improper douching, pregnancy, trichomoniasis	Acidophilus, Astragalus, B complex, Echinacea, Garlic*, Pau d'Arco tea and/or garlic juice. (may also be used as a douche), Saint John's wort*. Avoid yeast products, sugar, soft drinks and junk foods.
Weight Loss (unexplained)	Anorexia, bulimia, cancer, chronic fatigue syndrome, diabetes, hepatitis, malabsorption syndrome, mononucleosis (EBV), parasitic infection, overactive thyroid, trauma	All nutrients in high amounts, Apples, Blackberries, B complex*, Brewer's yeast, Fenugreek, Floradix formula, Garlic, Spirulina, Wheat germ, Zinc. Follow a high complex carbohydrate and protein diet. Avoid alcohol, coffee, fried food, junk food, soft drinks, and yeast products.

* Essential

NOTE: If you suspect one of these diseases seek a health care professional.

Speed Healing with Nature

The healing powers of plants will be instrumental in major medical breakthroughs in the 90's and the next century. While our pharmacologic technology has advanced at an astounding rate, nature has been reluctant to reveal her secrets. The wellness effects we seek, without the harmful side effects to our bodies, are available to us; however, it takes a willingness to be your own researcher and to work through the healing process to discover that nature's secrets work.

Some of the most powerful healing plants are only found in our rainforests, which are being destroyed at an alarming rate of 50 to 100 acres every minute. While we still have the opportunity, we must uncover ways to achieve wellness, promote speed healing, and delay the effects of aging.

Positive thinking is essential for speed healing, an image in the mind is just as real to the body as the actual event, think health and wellness -- it's mind over matter.

There is only one way to good health, nature's way!

Live Juice & Herbal Therapy

Green Drinks "Healers"	Fruit Juices "Body Cleansers"	Vegetable Juices "Health Restorers"	Herbs "Nature's Medicine"	Herbs & Juices Combined "Speed Healers"
Wonderful energizers!	Powerful antioxidants!	Boosts the immune system, which guards against illness. Removes acid waste from the body and balances the metabolism. Aids in controlling obesity by removing excess fat from the body. Vegetables are the most important of all the foods on our planet, slowing the aging process and preventing degenerative diseases.	Genesis 1:29 - "And God said, Behold I have given you every herb bearing seed."	Promotes speed healing and prevents disease!
Stimulates cells, rejuvenates the body, and builds new red blood cells. Chlorophyll, the blood of plants, promotes fast energy and is an internal disinfectant. It reduces body odor, bad breath, improves blood sugar disorders, anemia, all blood disorders, cleanses the liver, and is excellent for the digestive tract.	Contains high amounts of vitamin C needed for healing and energy. Soft fruits that contain very little water like papayas, bananas, and avocadoes should be pureed in your blender, then added to other juices. Juice fruits with skins on, except for apricots, bananas, citrus fruits, kiwi, melons, mangoes, papaya, peaches, and pineapple.		Try sun tea: Place tea bags in a jar filled with water, place jar in the sun for a few hours. Alternate herbs daily, each has different benefits.	Fresh live juices provide enzymes, vitamins, proteins, trace minerals, carbohydrates, purified water, essential fatty acids, chlorophyll, flavinoids, sulphur, healing chemicals, indols, glucosinolates, sulforaphane, dithiolthiones, carotenoids, caffeis, phenols, isotheocyonates, ferulic, and acetic acid, plus many more that are unidentified. Wow! What could possibly supply more for the body's essential needs?
Always add steam-distilled water to your green drinks. Green drinks cleanse drug and metal deposits from the body and combat toxins.	Remove pits from fruits like apricots, and plums, but leave in small seeds. (One important exception, if you are using more than one apple per drink, remove the seeds because they contain a very small amount of cyanide.)	Rotate colors of vegetables because different colors contain a variety of necessary nutrients for sustaining a harmonious body.	Always use quality, steam-distilled water to prepare your teas, not faucet water. Never heat in aluminum cookware.	
Add carrot or apple juice to your green drinks to sweeten and dilute them. No other fruit should be put in a green drink.		Try using fresh reishi mushrooms. Dip in boiling water to destroy bacteria, then puree mushrooms in your blender before adding to juices.	Summer delight: Freeze melon purees (like canteloupe, honeydew, and watermelon) in ice cube trays, then drop a few cubes in your herb teas. Refreshing and delicious, even in bitter teas!	Remember, fiber is essential to the diet. So, eat at least 2-3 half-cup servings daily of the suggested raw foods, and the rest may be juiced.
Green drinks, including wheatgrass, should be part of cancer treatment (especially radiation therapy). Wheatgrass is full of enzymes and is one of the most potent greens.	Be sure to thoroughly wash vegetables with a small amount of Clorox bleach (1 teaspoon) in one gallon of water, or use a vegetable wash found in most health food stores.	Before juicing, drop garlic into vinegar for one minute to destroy bacteria and mold on the surface. Use only one fresh clove of garlic per two glasses of juice, or you may irritate the lining of the intestinal tract. Be sure to peel waxed cucumbers, and thoroughly wash unpeeled vegetables.	For children, powdered herbs can be mixed with food or made into tea. Do not use pill form. Herb tea mixed with their favorite fruit juice works wonders!	For more information on the power of these foods, refer to the following sections:

* Healing Power of Raw Foods
* Leafy Greens
* Magnificent Twelve
* Raw Juices |
| See the section on Healing Juices for more information on the power of wheatgrass. | Avoid sweet fruits if you have candida or sugar disorders. | | Caution: Do not store herbs in glass. Herbs stored in glass may sweat, and the moisture causes a mold to form. | |

Live Juice & Herbal Therapy

Disorder Condition	Vegetable Juice	Fruit Juice	Herbs	Avoid	Considerations & Precautions
Acne/ All Skin Disorders	Alfalfa All leafy greens* Beet tops Cabbage* Carrots Cauliflower* Cucumber* Green pepper Onions Reishi mushrooms Swiss chard	Apples* Apricots Blackberries Blueberries Kiwi Lemon Raspberries Strawberries (A juice fast is very beneficial)	Alfalfa Basil Chapparral Coltsfoot Dandelion root* Golden seal* Milk thistle Primrose oil* Red clover Yellow dock root	Alcohol Caffeine (chocolate, cocoa) Dairy products (butter, eggs) Fried foods Iodine (salt) Pineapples Saturated fats Sea vegetables Soda pop Sugar* (all forms) Oily cosmetics and shampoos. Medicines that contain bromides or iodides. Drugs to treat epilepsy and tuberculosis. Exposure to industrial chemicals, oils, and grease.	Lavender kills germs and stimulates new cell growth. Use lavender and strawberry leaves as a steam sauna on affected area. Do not use soap on affected area; instead, pat (not rub) on lemon juice 3 times per day. Also helpful to apply a poultice using chaparral, yellow dock root, and golden seal. Zinc gluconate (50 mg. per day) aids in preventing scarring. Cauliflower and cabbage contain sulfur that fights skin infections. Stress can cause an outbreak.
Alzheimer's Disease (All brain disorders, memory loss, personality changes, mood swings, and insomnia)	Alfalfa All leafy greens* Beet tops Cabbage Carrots Dandelion greens Kale* Onions Peppers (red&green) Reishi mushrooms Swiss chard Turnips Watercress*	Apricots Bananas* Cherries Grapes Lemons* Papaya* Peaches* Pineapple Prunes	Borage Oil Blessed thistle Butcher's broom* Cayenne Garlic Ginger Ginko biloba* Gotu kola* Kelp* Primrose oil Seaweed Siberian ginseng* Valerian root (Co-enzyme Q10 and DMG increase oxygen to the brain)	Baking powder Cheese Chocolate Corn Food additives Dairy products Eggs Fried, Junk, & Processed foods Saturated fats Wheat Aluminum canned food and aluminum cookware* Antacids* Antidiarrheal preparations Antiperspirants Buffered aspirin Faucet water Selsun-Blue shampoo	Eating foods one is allergic to results in inflammation of the brain. Brain disorders are also linked to acetyl choline, B-complex vitamins, and thiamine deficiencies. B-complex and B-12 injections are recommended. According to Scrpps Howard News Service, the University of Cincinnati found that some patients are misdiagnosed, and are actually deficient in Vitamin B-12. To improve brain function, consume wheat germ, beans, fish, millet, turkey, sardines, salmon, lecithin, nuts, seeds, and the amino acid glutamic in the diet. Additionally, fiber is important. Ginko biloba (not to exceed 1,000 mg. daily without supervision) protects the brain from free radical damage.

* Essential

Also see Dietary Wellness and Natural Prescription charts for more about specific disorders

Live Juice & Herbal Therapy

Disorder Condition	Vegetable Juice	Fruit Juice	Herbs	Avoid	Considerations & Precautions
Arthritis & Joint Diseases	All leafy greens* Barley grass Beet tops Carrots Celery root* Cucumber Cabbage Dandelion* Green beans Parsley Watercress* Wheatgrass	Apples* Black cherries* Grapes Lemons* Papaya* Pears Pineapple	Alfalfa* Borage Capsicum (cayenne) Dandelion Garlic* Horsetail* Juniper Kelp* Sea vegetables Yucca* Red or Purple Lapacho	Caffeine Citrus fruits (except lemon) Dairy products* Eggs Fried foods* Iron supplements Nightshade vegetables*–see section on "Nightshades" Processed foods Red meat* Saturated fats* Spinach, cooked & juiced Sugar Tobacco	Folic acid, found in dark leafy greens, reduces the harsh side effects of rheumatoid arthritic drugs. A European poultice of mullein leaves may be used for swollen joints. Long term use of horsetail and parsley may deplete potassium in the body. Either take a potassium supplement or rotate horsetail and parsley intake (on for 3 months and off for 3 months). Avoid iron supplements, they are suspected of aggravating pain and swelling in joints. Avoid spinach juice in large amounts, it contains oxalic acid, which promotes joint problems.
Asthma Bronchitis Emphysema (Mucus in bronchial tubes and bronchial spasms caused by bronchial inflammation)	All leafy greens* Barley grass* Broccoli Carrots* Celery Collards Dandelion greens* Horseradish root Onions Parsley Rutabaga* Spinach Turnip & tops* Watercress* Wheatgrass*	Apples* Cranberry* Grapefruit Grapes* Kiwi Lemon* Mangoes* Papaya* Pineapple	Astragalus Bayberry Calendula flower Chickweed* Ephedra/Ma Huang* Eucalyptus leaf Fennel Seed Fenugreek Flax seed oil* Garlic* Ginger root Ginko biloba Horehound Iscaland moss Licorice root Lobelia* Marshmallow Mullein* Peppermint leaf Primrose oil	Animals, animal fats, aspirin, BHA and BHT, caffeine dairy products, F, D, or C yellow #5 dyes, food additives, furs, MSG, pork, poultry, processed foods, red meat, salt, saturated fats, smoke, sugar, tobacco & its smoke, tryptophane, white flour* Gas producing foods: Beans, broccoli, cabbage, cauliflower Ephedra - may elevate blood pressure. Coltsfoot - longterm use may impair liver function. Horseradish (root) - left in contact with the skin may cause blistering.	Use lobelia extract during an attack to soothe and relax the bronchial muscle. Inhale the vapors from eucalyptus leaves to relieve respiratory problems. A hypoglycemia diet should be followed. See Hypoglycemia on chart for guidelines. Also, an allergy-free diet should be followed after identifying which air pollutants and foods should be omitted. Keep a diary (and avoid) whatever provokes attacks. Allergies to pollen, dust mites, pets, and cockroaches may provoke attacks. Also, certain foods containing sulfites (alfalfa, beets, carrots, and cold beverages) may provoke an attack. Colds and flu may trigger an attack as well. Include protein (from vegetable sources) in the diet for tissue repair.

* Essential

Live Juice & Herbal Therapy

Disorder Condition	Vegetable Juice	Fruit Juice	Herbs	Avoid	Considerations & Precautions
Athero-sclerosis (Hardening of the arteries)	All leafy greens* Avocadoes Beet greens Bok choy Carrots Celery Cucumbers Eggplant Kale* Mustard greens* Parsley Swiss chard* Turnip greens	Apples Grapefruit* Grapes Kiwi Lemon* Papya Pineapple Red grapes	Cayenne Chickweed* Garlic* Ginger Ginko biloba Hawthorn berries Lecithin* Borage oil or Flaxseed oil* or Primrose oil Bilberry*	Alcohol All animal fats* Caffeine Colas* Dairy products* Fast and fried foods Red meat* Salt* Saturated fats Sugar products Spiced foods Tobacco White flour	Drink only steam-distilled water. Avoid drinking hard or soft faucet water. Keep your weight down. If taking blood thinning medication, such as aspirin, avoid vitamin K and vitamin K-rich foods, like alfalfa, broccoli, egg yolks, liver, spinach and cauliflower. Eggplant may inhibit the rise of blood cholesterol (induced by fatty foods) by binding it in the intestinal tract. See Cardiovascular Disease for more information.
Cancer & Aids	Cruciferous vegetables--see Magnificent 12* All leafy greens* Asparagus Black radish* Cabbage* Carrot* Dandelion greens* Ginger root Onions Kale Kohlrabi Reishi* & Shiitake mushrooms Spinach (folic acid) Swiss chard Watercress Wheatgrass*	Apples Apricots* Blueberries* (blue pigment is a powerful liver protectant) Cantaloupe Cherries* Papaya* Peaches* Pineapple Plums Red grapes* Strawberries*	Alfalfa Astragalus*, Bilberry* Chaparral Echinacea Garlic* Golden seal Green tea Kelp* Marshmallow Mistletoe Pau de Arco* Red clover* Red or Purple Lapacho Schizandra Seaweed* Suma* Yellow dock*	Alcohol, All fats* Animal protein Caffeine Dairy products Food additives Fried & junk food Hydrogenated oils Peanuts Processed foods Salt-cured, smoked, nitrate-cured meat Salt, Sugar Tobacco & smoke Chemicals, hair sprays, cleaning compounds, paint, garden pesticides, and aerosol products.	Research indicates that folic acid may prevent cervical cancer and when taken before conception, it may reduce spinal defects in newborns. Obesity is a factor linked to cancer. A high-fat, low-fiber diet is linked to cancer. Follow a preventative low-fat, high-fiber diet. Wheatgrass protects against radiation treatment, and should be part of your diet. Add soybean products, beans, millet, and brown rice to your diet. Drink only steam-distilled water. A selenium deficiency is linked to cancer. High amounts of vitamin A, vitamin C, and beta-carotene are essential. If you have breast cancer see Natural Medicine chart on Estrogen promoters to avoid and see Taxol on pg 5.

* Essential

Live Juice & Herbal Therapy

Disorder Condition	Vegetable Juice	Fruit Juice	Herbs	Avoid	Considerations & Precautions
Candidiasis (Yeast-like fungus that can inhabit any and all parts of the body: vaginitis, oral thrush, athlete's foot, toenails, ears, the bloodstream)	All vegetables* All leafy greens* Beet tops Broccoli Cabbage* Carrots* Celery Cholorophyll Kale Onions Rutabagus Turnips Wheatgrass	NO FRUIT JUICES (A high complex carbohydrate, protein and high fiber diet is essential)	Barberry bark Bee propolis Black walnut hulls -- to destroy parasites that normally accompany candida Chaparral Dong quai Garlic* Grapefruit seed extract* Golden seal Lauricidin/Monolaurin Pau de Arco* Primrose oil* Red clover	Alcohol* Butter Cheeses (all forms)* Chocolate Citrus fruits, Dried fruits Mushrooms Fermented foods* Glutens (all forms)* Ham, Honey, Nuts, Pickles Soy/tamari sauces Sugar (all forms)* Yeast products Chemicals, cleaning supplies corticosteroids, oral contraceptives, chlorinated water, damp & moldy places	Candida may be related to allergies and blood sugar disorders. Sugar and yeast products feed the fungus. Sensitivities to the environment and sensitivites to chemicals may develop. Keep the bowels clean with periodic enemas, and follow a high fiber diet. Eating yogurt or some form of acidophilous culture with caprylic acid is very beneficial. Lauricidin (monolaurin) provides antiviral activity and wheatgrass destroys bacteria. Golden seal should not be used for long periods, because it may destroy beneficial bacteria. Avoid golden seal entirely if pain is present in the digestive tract, as it can aggravate the pain by stimulating digestive secretions. Caprylic acid destroys fungus.
Chronic Fatigue Syndrome (All viral infections, i.e. Mononeucleosis, Epstein-Barr Virus, Herpes)	All leafy greens* Beet greens Bok choy Broccoli Cabbage Carrots* Celery Dandelion greens* Onions Parsley Potato with skins Reishi & Shiitake mushrooms Turnips Watercress Wheatgrass*	Apples* Apricots Avacadoes* Bananas Blueberries Cantaloupe Lemons* Papaya* Peaches Red grapes (Keep fruits to a minimum)	Astragalus* Bee propolis Burdock Cayenne* Chaparral Dandelion Echinacea* Garlic* Golden seal Milk thistle Pau de Arco* Primrose oil Saint John's wort* Siberian ginseng Suma*	Alcohol* Animal protein Caffeine Chemicals Dairy products* Faucet water Fried food* Hydrogenated oils* Junk food* MSG Preservatives Processed foods Soft drinks* Sugar (all forms)* Tobacco* STRESS!!!	Rest and stress avoidance are the best treatments. Consume 8+ glasses of quality water per day to rid body of tissue toxins, and aid in avoiding fatigue and muscle aches. Periodic enemas and a high fiber diet are important to keep the bowels clean, and prevent toxic build-up. Vitamin A, free-form amino acids (L-lysine especially), large doses of nutrients, vitamin C, and B complex, St. John's Wort and zinc are needed to keep viruses in check. If using St. John's wort, avoid narcotics, diet pills, asthma inhalants, nasal decongestants, hay fever medications, beer, wine, salami, chocolate, smoked pickled foods and the sun. Reishi mushrooms are used in Japan for debilitating muscle disease.

* Essential

31

Live Juice & Herbal Therapy

Disorder Condition	Vegetable Juice	Fruit Juice	Herbs	Avoid	Considerations & Precautions
Cardio-vascular Disease (Angina, coronary artery disease, heart disorders, high blood pressure, high cholesterol, hypertension, high triglycerides, strokes)	All leafy greens Beet greens Bok choy--high in magnesium* Cabbage Carrots* Celery Garlic Green peppers Kale--for calcium! Onions* Parsley Red peppers Sea vegetables Spinich Swiss chard Turnips Potato skins--high in potassium! (Avoid green potatoes and the eyes, which contain the toxin solanine.) Shiitake mushrooms (lowers level of blood fat and blood pressure)	Apples* Apricots* Avocadoes Bananas* Cantaloupe* Grapefruit Lemons Papaya* Pomegranates Red grapes* Strawberries Watermelon	Alfalfa Apple pectin Butcher's broom* Cayenne* Chlorophyll Fenugreek Garlic* Ginger root Ginko biloba* Hawthorn berries* Horsetail Kelp Mother wort Psyllium* Salmon oil or Flaxseed oil* Suma Valerian root* Yarrow	Alcohol All fats* Baking soda Butter* Caffeine Canned vegetables Dairy products Diet sodas Faucet water Fried foods* Meat tenderizers Milk MSG Mold inhibitors Palm and coconut oil Preservatives Processed foods Red meat Refined foods Salt* Soft drinks Softened water* Spicy foods Sugar Tobacco White flour products Read labels carefully!	Drink only steam-distilled water. Studies show that sugar raises triglyceride levels, and smoking increases the risk of heart attacks. Find a form of exercise you enjoy, walking is good. Substances found in the skins and seeds of red grapes lowers cholesterol. L-Carnitine and CoQ10 will lower risk of heart disorders. Fish oils (omega-3), canola oil, and olive oil lowers risk of heart attacks. Use Chinese and Korean ginseng under medical supervision, since ginseng can affect the use of heart medications like digitalis. If taking anticoagulant therapy (blood-thinning drugs), avoid the supplement vitamin K and alfalfa. To enhance the articoagulant effect include wheat germ, vitamin E, soybeans, lecithin and sunflower seeds to the diet. These foods should be part of the diet for all heart disorders.

* Essential

Live Juice & Herbal Therapy

Disorder Condition	Vegetable Juice	Fruit Juice	Herbs	Avoid	Considerations & Precautions
Depression	Alfalfa* All dark leafy greens* Beet greens Broccoli* Cabbage Carrots Dandelion greens* Green pepper Kale Parsley Spinach	Apples Blueberries Cranberry Lemons Papaya Peaches Pineapple	Aloe vera Flaxseed oil* Garlic* Kelp Siberian ginseng Slippery elm Spirulina* St. John's wort	Alcohol* Allergenic foods Baker's & brewer's yeast Caffeine Cheese Chocolate Dairy products Fried foods* Herring Junk foods* Meat tenderizers Phenylalanine Saturated fats and oils Soy sauce Sugar -- all forms of simple carbohydrates* Yeast extracts	Clinical studies show the amino acid tyrosine and the B vitamins aid in all forms of depression. Caution: If taking MAO inhibitor drugs, avoid L-tyrosine. Food allergies and certain drugs have been linked to depression. Omitting certain foods greatly helps. Insufficient incomplex carbohydrates may cause serotonin depletion and depression. Hypoglycemia, and thyroid disorders, are often causes. Heredity is also a factor. Hormonal imbalances may be behind depression. Melatonin, a helpful brain hormone, is released by bright light and sunlight. Avoid dark rooms.
Diabetes (Elevated blood sugar, insufficient production of insulin by pancreas)	All leafy greens* Broccoli Brussels sprouts* Celery Green beans Green pepper Kale Kohlrabi Parsley* Spinach Turnip greens	NO FRUIT JUICES (A high complex carbohydrate and high-fiber diet is essential)	Buchu leaves Dandelion root* Garlic* Ginger root Ginseng (may lower the blood sugar level) Guar gum Golden seal Huckleberry (helps promote insulin production)* Juniper berry Licorice root Spirulina Uva ursi	Caffeine Canned foods Fats and oils* Fish oil capsules Fried foods* Salt, Sugar (all forms)* Soda pop* Processed foods* White flour Avoid large amounts of PABA and L-cysteine, vitamin B-1 and vitamin C. Pain medication may lower blood sugar too much.	Diet is most important in controlling this disorder. High-fiber, high complex-carbohydrate diet not only reduces the need for insulin, but also lowers fat levels. Weight control is a crucial factor in the treatment of non-insulin dependent diabetics. GTF (chromium) is essential (see chart on Nutrition Deficits for a list of GTF-rich foods). Do not take golden seal for long periods, and avoid it altogether if intestinal pain is present. A low protein diet consisting of less than 40 grams per day is recommended for diabetic nephropathy (kidney disease). Type II diabetics should avoid large amounts of niacin.

* Essential

Live Juice & Herbal Therapy

Disorder Condition	Vegetable Juice	Fruit Juice	Herbs	Avoid	Considerations & Precautions
Diarrhea (Frequent and loose, watery stools)	All leafy greens* Beet greens Cabbage Carrots* Parsley	Apples* Bananas* Blackberries* Papayas* Peaches	Blackberry root* Cayenne, Chamomile Charcoal tabs Garlic, Ginger root Irish moss, Kelp Psyllium seed Raspberry leaves* Slippery elm bark	All glutinous foods* Caffeine, Dairy products Fats*, Nuts* Processed foods Seeds*, Wheat* For fast results, avoid all foods for 24 hours, except brown rice & foods listed.	If persistent or recurring, food allergies may be the cause. You should be tested to determine if a food allergy exists. Charcoal tablets (in most health food stores) will absorb the bacteria that may be causing the loose stools. Add psyllium fiber to your drinks.
Edema (Accumulation of excessive bodily fluids, primarily in the feet, ankles, and hands)	Celery* Chard Cucumbers Leafy greens Parsley* Spinach Watercress*	Apples Bananas* Blueberries Peaches Watermelon*	Alfalfa* Cornsilk* Dandelion root Garlic* Horsetail Juniper berries Kelp	Alcohol Animal proteins & fats* Caffeine Dairy Products* Fried foods* Gravies* Olives, Pickles, Salt* Shellfish Soy sauce* Sugar Tobacco	Food allergies are the main cause of this disorder. To determine which food allergy (ies) exist, eat only the foods listed for two weeks, then add foods back one at a time. Certain drugs cause water retention. Drink quality water, 8 glasses per day is essential. Do not use horsetail for long periods as it may deplete needed potassium in the body.
Gout (Excess uric acid producing arthritis and kidney stones)	Alfalfa All leafy greens* Carrots Celery Kale Parsley Watercress Wheatgrass	Apples Black Cherries* Lemons* Pears Pineapple Strawberries	Alfalfa Burdock root Chaparral Dandelion root* Devil's claw Garlic* Horsetail Juniper Kelp* Psyllium seed Yucca	All meat, Alcohol Asparagus Broths, Cakes Cauliflower, Consomme Desserts, Dried beans Fats, Gravies, Legumes Mushrooms, Oil-rich foods Organ meats*, Peas, Poultry Red meat*, Shellfish, Sardines Herring, Anchovies, Mackerel Mussels Sugar, Sweetbreads Yeast products (in moderation)	See section on Nightshades, and avoid these foods until healed. Diet must be kept simple, 50% raw diet of vegetables, brown rice, millet, etc., and absolutely no highly processed foods. Because chemotherapy treatment causes cellular destruction, it is associated with the release of uric acid into the system. Psyllium seed has been shown to increase the output of uric acid.

* Essential

Live Juice & Herbal Therapy

Disorder Condition	Vegetable Juice	Fruit Juice	Herbs	Avoid	Considerations & Precautions
Hyper-thyroidism (Excessive production of the thyroid hormone)	Alfalfa, Beet tops Broccoli* Brussels sprouts* Cabbage* Carrots, Celery Green peppers Kale*, Mustard greens*, Parsley Spinach*, Turnips* Watercress	Apricots Apples Cranberry Grapefruit Grapes Peaches* Pears* Pineapple	Bayberry Black cohosh Golden seal Skullcap White oak bark	All dairy products All processed and refined foods All stimulants (coffee, nicotine) Antihistamines Chlorine Faucet water, Fluoride, Iodine Salt Soft drinks Sulfa drugs	See section on Magnificent Twelve, and consume these foods often. Do not take golden seal for long periods, and avoid entirely if intestinal pain is present. Eating two servings daily of the following foods may help in reducing thyroid hormones: Brussels sprouts, broccoli, cabbage, kale, mustard greens, spinach, peaches, and pears.
Hypo-glycemia (Low blood sugar and oversecretion of insulin by the pancreas)	Avocado* Beet & tops* Bok choy Cabbage Green pepper Kale* Mustard greens Parsley Spinach Turnip & tops*	Unsweetened Juices Unsweetened: Apples Blueberries Cranberries Grapefruits Kiwi Lemons (Mix with 1/2 water or herb tea)	Alfalfa Bee pollen Dandelion root* Flax seed Garlic Gotu kola* Guar gum* Juniper berries Kelp Licorice root* Royal jelly Spirulina*	Alcohol* Fats* Fried foods* Gravies* Instant rice and potatoes Processed foods Sugar (all forms)* Sweet fruits White flour & its products	Food allergies are linked to low-blood sugar. Diet is extremely important in controlling blood sugar swings. Spirulina between meals aids in controlling blood sugar levels. High fiber, especially in the morning, aids in stabilizing blood sugar levels. It is essential that you eat 5 small meals daily, consisting of complex carbohydrates and protein*.
Hypo-thyroidism (Underproduction of the thyroid hormone)	Alfalfa* All leafy greens* Beet tops Carrots Celery Green peppers Parsley Seaweeds Sprouts Watercress*	Apples* Apricots* Cranberry Grapefruit Grapes* Pineapple	Alfalfa Bayberry Black Cohosh* Ginko Biloba Golden Seal Kelp* Licorice Primrose oil Rose hips Rosemary*	All processed and refined foods Antihistamines Chlorine Faucet water Fluoride Iodine Sulfa drugs	Consume the following in moderation because they may supress the thyroid function: Brussels sprouts, broccoli, cabbage, kale, mustard greens, spinach, peaches, and pears. Do not take golden seal for long periods, and avoid entirely if intestinal pain is present. A deficiency of essential fatty acids causes an imbalance in the thyroid function.

* Essential

Live Juice & Herbal Therapy

Disorder Condition	Vegetable Juice	Fruit Juice	Herbs	Avoid	Considerations & Precautions
Menopausal Symptoms (When women stop ovulating, often referred to as, "the change of life.")	All leafy greens Broccoli* Cabbage Carrots Celery* Collard greens Cucumber* Dandelion greens* Kale* Parsley Spinach Swiss chard	All berries* Apples Bananas Blackberries Grapes Lemon Papaya* Pineapple*	Black Cohosh* Dong quai Garlic* Ginger root Gotu kola Kelp* Licorice* Primrose oil Raspberry* Sarsaparilla* Siberian Ginseng* Squaw vine Valerian root (for sleep)	Caffeine (all forms) Dairy products* Fats Fried foods Junk foods Red meat Soda pop Sugar (all forms)*	Licorice and ginseng aid in relieving menopausal symptoms; however, licorice and ginseng may stimulate estrogen production, so avoid both, if you have a history of breast cancer. See Natural Medicines chart. Symptoms are the result of estrogen production slowing down or stopping altogether. Dairy products, fats and sugars may provoke symptoms. Natural substances that aid the body in producing estrogen are preferred over prescribed chemical estrogen.
Obesity	All leafy greens Broccoli Cabbage Carrots Celery* Cucumber* Green beans Kale* Parsley* Radishes Shiitake (lowers fat in the blood) Tomato Turnips & tops Watercress*	Bromelain (found in pineapple and pill form, is widely used in Europe for weight loss) Cranberry Grapefruit* Lemon* Papaya Strawberry* Tart Apples Watermelon*	Borage oil/ or Primrose oil Cascara sagrada Chickweed* Cornsilk* Dandelion Garlic Ginger root Guar gum* Kelp* Nettle Psyllium seed (fiber) Seawrack* Spirulina*	All forms of animal fats, chocolate, dairy products, fast foods, fats, fatty foods, fried foods, junk foods, nuts, olives, pastries, processed foods, salt, soda pop, sugar, white flour & white flour products. Salty food puts a strain on the thyroid gland. Use moderate amount of natural sweeteners, like rice malt or barley malt. Studies show that substitute sweeteners, such as Nutrasweet and Equal, increase the appetite.	Food allergies are linked to obesity. For fast results, consume only recommended foods and juices. Consume in moderation high calorie foods including: corn, hominy, figs, grapes, green peas, pears, pineapple, sweet potatoes, white rice, bananas, cherries, avocados, coconut, nuts, and seeds. Consume an abundance of raw vegetables and live juices. Important; take psylium half-an-hour before meals. Drink at least eight glasses of quality water daily. Get plenty of exercise, like walking and/or stretching. Cravings for sugar and yeast products may indicate candidiasis, see on chart. Chromium picolinate and L-glutamine are important for glucose metabolism, to reduce cravings for sugar, accelerate fat loss and increase muscle mass.

* Essential

Live Juice & Herbal Therapy

Disorder Condition	Vegetable Juice	Fruit Juice	Herbs	Avoid	Considerations & Precautions

Osteoporosis
 	
(Gradual loss of bone mass, the major cause malabsorption of calcium)
	Bok choy*
	Broccoli*
	Cabbage
	Carrots
	Cauliflower
	Celery
	Collard greens*
	Dandelion greens
	Kale*
	Parsley
	Shiitake mushrooms (rich vitamin D source, found in few foods, vital for calcium absorption)
	Swiss chard
	Turnips & tops*
	Turnip greens
	Watercress*
		Apples*
		Banana
		Blueberries*
		Cherries
		Figs
		Lemons
		Papaya
		Pineapple
		Prunes
		Raisins
		Red Grapes*
		
		(The blue pigment in blueberries is a powerful liver protectant)
			Alfalfa*
			Dulse
			Dandelion
			Garlic
			Horsetail*
			Irish moss
			Kelp*
			Nettle*
			Oatstraw
			Primrose oil*
			Red clover
			Rose hips
			Silica (Silicon)
			Spirulina
				Alcohol
				Animal products*
				Caffeine (chocolate, cocoa)
				Dairy products
				Red meat*
				Salt
				Saturated fats*
				Soft drinks
				Sugar (products with sugar)*
				Tobacco
				
				Citrus fruits and tomatoes may inhibit calcium intake. Limit intake of almonds, beet greens, cashews, chard, rhubarb, and spinach (they contain high amounts of oxlic acid). Avoid diuretics.
					The mineral boron may increase calcium intake by as much as 40%. Do not exceed 3 mg. daily of boron.
					  If taking thyroid supplements, diuretics, or blood thinning drugs, increase your calcium to 2,000 mg. daily.
					  Consume calcium and whole grains at different times. Grains may bind with calcium and prevent absorption. Taking calcium at bedtime is best.
					  The best osteoporosis prevention and maintenance is sunlight, an adequate diet consisting of quality protein, calcium, iron, magnesium, phosphorus, and vitamins A, C, D and F.
					  To make the joints and muscles more flexible, get plenty of exercise, as the oxygen produced by exercising will increase flexibility. Exercise will also enhance calcium absorption.

Pre-Menstrual Syndrome (PMS)	All leafy greens*
	Broccoli
	Cabbage
	Celery root
	Cucumber*
	Kale*
	Parsley* (natural diuretic)
	Turnips & tops
		Cherries
		Kiwi
		Lemon
		Papaya
		Pineapple*
		Raspberry
		Red grapes
		Watermelon*
			Blessed thistle
			Dong quai*
			Garlic
			Ginger root
			Kelp*
			Primrose oil*
			Raspberry leaves
			Sage
			Sarsparilla*
			Squaw vine*
				Alcohol*
				Caffeine
				Dairy products*
				Fried foods and fats
				Highly-processed foods
				Junk foods
				Red meat
				Salt*
				Soft drinks
				Sugar
				Tobacco
					Drink 8 glasses of quality water daily.
					  The B complex (especially B-6) and primrose oil have relieved many symptoms related to this disorder.
					  The avoid list should be entirely eliminated from the diet one week before, and during, the cycle.
					  A hormonal imbalance is one of the causes of PMS. PMS has been linked to candida, food allergies, and hypoglycemia.
					  Sarsparilla balances male/female hormones.
					  Sage contains natural phytoestrogens.

* Essential

Live Juice & Herbal Therapy

Disorder Condition	Vegetable Juice	Fruit Juice	Herbs	Avoid	Precautions
Tuberculosis TB (Primarily affects the lungs, but can spread to the bones, kidneys, intestines, spleen, and liver. Caused by a bacteria, myco-bacterium)	Alfalfa All leafy greens* Barley grass* Beets & tops Broccoli Carrots* Celery Collards* Green pepper Kale* Onions Reishi mushrooms Watercress Wheatgrass*	All berries Apples* Canteloupe* Cranberry Grapefruit Grapes Lemon* Pineapple Papaya* Rose hips	Astragalus Bayberry Echinacea* Garlic* Germanium Golden Seal* Horsetail Kelp* Mullein Myrrh Pau d'Arco Primrose oil Rose hips St. John's wort Wheat germ	Alcohol All processed foods Animal products Caffeine Dairy products Fried foods Junk foods Red meat Salt Saturated fats Soda pop Sugar (all forms) Tobacco & smoke White flour products Faucet water, consume steam-distilled water only. Avoid polluted areas.	Rest, sunshine, and fresh air are vital. Diet should essentially consist of 50% raw live juices and raw foods. Free-form amino acids are important for tissue repair. Kefir milk, yogurt and acidophilus should be added to the diet. Massive amounts of vitamin C, beta-carotene, L-cystine, vitamin E, and selenium are needed. Reishi mushrooms must be dipped into boiling water to kill bacteria before using. Germanium works best when used for two months, and then off one month.
Ulcers	Cabbage* Carrots Celery Kale Leafy greens* Okra* Parsley Potatoes Red pepper Rutabaga* Watercress*	Bananas Blue grapes* Cantelope Papayas	Aloe vera* Chamomile Ginger root Golden seal Peppermint* Psyllium seed	Alcohol* Caffeine/Decaffeinated coffee Carbonated drinks* Chocolate Dairy products Fried foods Salt Saturated fats* Spicy foods* Tobacco*	Aspirin and vitamin C may create more acid. Aspirin taken for long periods may promote ulcers. Studies show fresh cabbage juice heals ulcers. If symptoms are severe, juice fasting may alleviate symptoms. Fiber and plenty of quality water are important! Consume small, frequent meals.

* Essential

Nutritional Deficiency

Vitamin	Sources	Symptoms of Deficiency
A **Beta Carotene**	Fish liver oil, Spirulina, Watercress, Kale, Garlic, Dandelion greens, Carrots, Beets, Cantaloupe, Parsley, Spinach, Peaches, Swiss chard, Sweet potatoes, Pumpkin, Yellow squash, Broccoli, Alfalfa, Apricots, Mustard, Turnip greens, Papaya	Eye disorders, Lung disorders, Sterility, Dry-Scaly skin, Night blindness, Cancer, Frequent infections, Nerve deterioration, Stunted growth, Glandular malfunctions, Premature aging, Over-active mucus membranes, Inhibited healing processes
D	Sunshine, Egg yolks, Butter, Milk, Halibut, Cod liver oil, Salmon, Tuna, Oatmeal, Sweet potatoes, Alfalfa, Vegetable oils	Bone diseases, Rickets, Cataracts, Calcium malabsorption, Gum disease, Hair loss, Muscle weakness, Tooth decay, Retarded growth, Osteoporosis
C **Plus** **Bioflavonoids**	Collards, Onions, Turnip greens, Broccoli, Mustard greens, Kale, Sweet peppers, Parsley, Rose hips, Watercress, Turnips, Strawberries, Grapefruit, Persimmons, Papaya, Currants, Lemons, Oranges, Beet greens, Asparagus, Spinich, Mangoes, Brussels sprouts, Cantaloupes, Pineapple, Swiss chard, Green peas, tomatoes, Radishes, Avocados	Bruises easily, Scurvy, Mouth/Gum disease, Fragile bones and joints, Gastric ulcers, Frequent colds and flus, Cancer, Anemia, Adrenal malfunction, Stiff joints, Low resistance to infections, Lung disorders, Deficient lactation, Impaired cardiac function, Asthma, Bronchitis
P **Bioflavonoids**	Lemons, Oranges, Grapefruit, Cherries, Grapes, Buckwheat, Apricots, Prunes, Rose hips	Varicose veins, Hemophilia, Alkalosis Heel and bone spurs, Hemorrhoids Infection, Colitis, Bronchitis Bruises easily, Immune deficiency
F	Salmon, Fish, Vegetable oils, Wheat germ, Primrose oil, Linseed oil, Olives & oil, Flaxseed oil, Soy oil, Seeds, Safflower oil	Heart disorders, High cholesterol, Female disorders, Yeast infections, All skin disorders, Low fertility, Hypertension, Cystic fibrosis, Celiac disease, Liver disorders, Maformation of tissue, Intestional disorders
K	Green leafy vegetables, Egg yolks, Blackstrap molasses, Oatmeal, Wheat, Rye, Cauliflower, Safflower oil, Liver, Soybeans, Alfalfa	Hemorrhoids, Bruising, Hemorrhaging, Delayed blood clotting, Colon disorders, Multiple sclerosis, Liver disorders, Leg ulcers, Diverticulitis, Colitis, Intestinal disorders, Hemophilia
B **Vitamins**	Wheat germ, Brewer's yeast, Brown rice, Nuts, Seeds, Oats, Whole grains, Lentils, Lima beans, Kidney beans, Egg yolk, Buckwheat flour, Fresh peas (legumes), Asparagus, Brussel sprouts, Alfalfa, Soy Products	Beriberi, Pellagra, Digestive disorders, Poor appetite, Tongue-cracks/shiny/purple, Memory loss, Confusion, Canker sores, Cardiovascular disorders, Weight loss, Nervous disorders, Glandular disorders, Hair loss/shine, Skin disorders, Fatigue, Depression, Itchy/burning eyes, Eczema, Brittle or rigid nails
E	Wheat germ, Cold-pressed oils, Dry beans, All green-leafy vegetables, Brown rice, Nuts, Milk, Eggs, Cornmeal, Oatmeal	Cardiovascular/circulatory disorders, Premature aging, Hot flashes, Fertility, Female problems, Impotence problems, Nervous system imbalance, Heart disorders, Weakened immune system

Vital Minerals

Mineral	Deficiency Symptoms	Food Sources
Calcium	Muscle spasms, Softening of bone, Insomnia, Susceptibility to bone fractures, Hypertension, Menopause, Colitis, Rheumatism, Rickets	Yogurt, Goat milk, Collards, Carob, Asparagus Green and leafy vegetables, Almonds, Kale, Tofu, Brewer's yeast, Oats, Broccoli, Kelp
Chromium	Depresses growth rate, Glucose intolerence in diabetics, Atherosclerosis, Hypoglycemia, Fatigue, Memory/Muscle loss	Corn oil, Clams, Whole grain cereals, Meats, Brewers yeast, Dried beans, Cheese, Corn oil, Potatoes, Brown rice
Chloride	Hypochloremic alkalosis (pernicious vomiting)	Animal foods, Table salt
Copper	Anemia, Aneurysms, Arthritis, Loss of hair, Heart disorders, Constipation, Ulcers, Leukemia, Difficulty breathing	Liver, Kidney, Egg yolk, Legumes, Whole grains, Soybeans, Seafood, Avocados, Raisins, Oats, Nuts, Almonds, Pecans
Iodine	Low vitality, Hypothyroidism, Goiter, Obesity Nervousness, Dry hair/skin, Irritability	Seafoods (fish, shellfish, plants), Table salt, Sea vegetables, Onions, Garlic, Spinach, Carrots, Tomatoes, Pineapple, Cod liver oil
Iron	Headaches, Listlesness and fatigue, Irritability, Heart palpitations during exertion, Dizziness, Susceptibility to infections, Reduced white blood cell count, Impaired antibody production, Anemia , Pale color	Meat (liver), Poultry, Fish, Eggs, Breads and cereals (whole grain or enriched with iron), Leafy vegetables, Potatoes, Fruit, Milk
Magnesium	Tremors, Convulsions, Muscle contractions, Confusion, Delirium, Irritability, Behavioral disturbances, Heart disorders, Insomnia, Hypertension, Menopause, Rapid pulse, Nervousness, Tooth grinding, Hyperactivity	Fresh green vegetables, Milk and dairy, Figs, products, Meat, Fish and seafood,Nuts, Tofu, Peanuts, Blackstrap molasses, Apples, Kelp, Soybeans, Seeds, Wheat germ, Figs, Oatmeal, Cornmeal, Rice, Apricots, Brewer's yeast
Manganese	Skeletal, Inner-ear imbalance, Possible convulsions, Ringing in ears, Dizziness, Epilepsy, Nerve disorders, Memory loss	Whole grain cereals, Egg yolks, Green vegetables, Nuts and seeds (hazlenuts, pecans), Avocados, Seaweed, Blueberries, Spinach
Molybdenum	Decreased growth and food consumption	Liver, Kidney, Whole grains, Legumes and green vegetables
Phosphorus	Weakness, Weight loss/gain, Nervous disorders, Appetite loss, Memory loss, SLowed hair, nails and bone growth	Sesame, Milk and dairy products, Meat, Fish, Sunflower/pumpkin seeds, Garlic, Asparagus, Brewer's yeast, Nuts, Whole grains,
Potassium	Nervous disorders, Insomnia, Headaches, Constipation, Fluctuations in heartbeat, Nausea and vomiting, Muscle weakness, Spasms and cramps, Water retention, Edema, Irritability, Sunburn, Diarrhea, Dry skin	All vegetables (green leafy), Bananas, Oranges, Whole grains, Sunflower seeds, Mint leaves, Potatoes, Dairy products (cheese), Meats, Poultry, Fish, Legumes, Nuts, Garlic, Brewer's yeast, Avocados, Raisins,
Selenium	Premature aging, Impaired growth, Heart Disorders, Cancer, Immune deficiency, Hypertension, Menopause, Allergies	Bran and germ cereals, Broccoli, Onions, Tomatoes, Tuna, Brewer's yeast, Garlic, Brown rice, Brazil nuts, Chicken, Turkey
Zinc	Impaired ability to heal, Loss of appetite, Impaired night vision, Impaired acuity of taste and smell, Impaired growth, Impotence, Colds and Flu, Stunted growth, Fatigue, Hair loss	Meats, Poultry (dark meat), Fish and seafood (oysters), Liver, Eggs, Legumes (peanuts), Whole grains, Brewer's yeast, Mushrooms, Wheat germ, Pumpkin seeds, Soybeans

Diet Guidelines

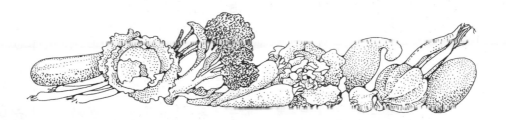

Eat a variety of foods to minimize repeated exposure to food toxins, sprays, etc. All foods are handled differently in different parts of the country.

Eat organic foods if you can. Certain foods are laced with dangerous pesticides. Wash all fresh foods thoroughly especially melons, as there have been several cases of salmonella poisoning found from cutting into the melons before washing them. Grow your own if possible.

Eat more fiber to speed dangerous toxins through the intestinal tract and to bind and neutralize them before they can do any harm. Fiber should be part of every meal. It is found in whole grains, beans, legumes, vegetables, and fruits. Processed foods lack fiber, be sure and add fresh food to every meal. Fiber also cuts down on food reactions and blood sugar fluctuations, in addition to preventing constipation.

Reduce fat consumption since toxins are concentrated in the fat of an animal and saturated fats used in commercial cooking. These products are potentially dangerous toxins.

Avoid old nuts, grains and seeds that are not nitrogen sealed or kept under refrigeration. Aflatoxin, a mold that grows on these foods has been linked to cancer.

Refrigerate all fresh foods or cooked foods quickly so bacteria cannot form.

Avoid highly processed foods like ketchup, beef jerky, hot dogs and tomato based sauces, these have concentrated toxins.

Avoid burned foods because they contain carcinogens that are cancer causing substances.

Buy only frozen fish, ''fresh fish'' in a grocer's case may have been around many days. Do not eat raw fish. See Fats and Fish section.

Do not consume liver. Toxins from the body of the animal are left in the tissues of the liver after it has cleaned them out of the blood supply. Avoid all organ meats.

Avoid foreign-made dinnerware, glassware, etc. It could contain leaded glasses and glazes that may leach into tour food. Also, avoid antique crystal dishes and other dinnerware made before the law was passed in the States against the use of lead in dinnerware.

Do not use plastic wrap in microwave ovens, plastic containers, etc. Use only glass for food storage. Plastic leaches petro chemicals into food.

Fat and spicy foods put stress on the gall bladder and the liver, resulting in heartburn and indigestion, so avoid fried food, gravies, and dairy products.

Overeating overloads the stomach, pressure forces acid back up into the esophagus, leading to heartburn, gas, and bloating. The end result is obesity.

Last but most important---**eat all natural foods.** Additives aren't good for you, avoid them.

President Jimmy Carter and his family ran a peanut plantation in Georgia and several of the family members died of pancreatic cancer. Is there a link between pancreatic cancer and dangerous aflatoxins found on peanuts?

FOR WELLNESS

	Avoid	Enjoy
Beverages	Alcohol, coffee, cocoa, sodas, pasteurized and sweetened juices, fruit drinks, black tea	Herb teas, fresh vegetable and fruit juices, coffee substitutes, cereal grains from health food stores, mineral or distilled water, bottled juices (without anything added)
Dairy Products	All soft cheeses, ice cream, all pasteurized cheese products with orange coloring, milk, sour cream, cream cheese (Avoid all dairy products to promote the healing process.)	Raw goat or soy cheeses, nonfat cottage cheese, kiefer, unsweetened plain yogurt
Eggs	Fried, pickled or raw	Boiled or poached (limit to 3 per week)
Soups	Canned with salt, preservatives, MSG, high-fat stock or creamed	Homemade (salt-free and fat-free) bean, lentil, pea, vegetable, barley, brown rice, onion, mushroom, potato, tomato
Sweets	White, brown or raw sugar, corn syrups, chocolate, sugar candy, fructose, all syrups, all sugar substitutes, jams and jellies with sugar	Barley malt syrup or powdered (preferred), rice syrup, small amounts of raw honey, pure maple syrup, unsulphured molasses, blackstrap molasses
Fruits	Canned, bottled, or frozen with sweeteners added	All fresh, frozen, stewed and dried without sweeteners, and unsulphured
Vegetables	All canned and frozen with salt or additives	All raw, fresh, frozen or home-canned, steamed, broiled, or baked (undercook slightly)
Sprouts & Seeds	Seeds cooked in oil and salted	All sprouts, slightly cooked (except alfalfa), wheat grass, all raw seeds

FOR WELLNESS

	Avoid	Enjoy
Seasonings	Black or white pepper, salt, white vinegar, all artificial vinegar	Garlic, onions, dried parsley, Spike, all herbs, chives, dried vegetables, apple cider vinegar, tamari, miso, seaweed, dulse, all sea vegetables, vegetable bouillon
Fish	All fried fish, all shellfish, raw fish, salted fish, anchovies, herring, fish canned in oil	All white fish from deep, fresh cold waters, salmon, broiled or baked fish, water-packed tuna--eat 3 to 4 times per week (see Fat & Fish section)
Meats	Beef, all forms of pork, sausage, bacon, lunchmeats, hot dogs, smoked, pickled, all processed meats, corned beef, duck, goose, short ribs, organ meats, gravies	Skinless turkey or chicken--limit meat to only 2 times per week
Grains	All white flour products, including spaghetti and macaroni, crackers, white rice, overly processed oatmeal and cereals	All whole grain products using unprocessed grains: cereals, breads, muffins, crackers, cream of wheat/rye/rice, buckwheat, millet, oats, brown rice, wild rice--limit yeast breads to 3 times per week.
Oils	All saturated fats, hydrogenated margarine, refined processed oils, shortenings, hardened oils, saturated oil in mayonnaise, dressings	All cold-pressed or expeller pressed oils: safflower, canola, rice bran, flaxseed, sesame, olive, corn, sunflower, margarine, and salad dressing from these oils, eggless mayonnaise
Nuts	Peanuts, all salted or roasted nuts	All raw, fresh nuts (except peanuts)--be sure they aren't rancid and have been kept refrigerated or tightly sealed--cashews only sparingly
Beans	Canned pork and beans, canned beans with salt or preservatives, frozen beans with added salt, etc.	All beans and legumes cooked without animal fat, salt or preservatives

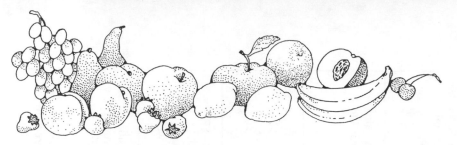

Nutrition for Children

The average childhood diet today consists of high-fat and high calorie foods. The fast food chains have helped to make our children overweight, hyperactive, and deficient in nutrients. High cholesterol levels are also a serious problem. The *American Heart Association* suggests that children as young as two years of age limit their fat intake to stave off clogged arteries in adulthood. The average American child starts the day with a high-sugar breakfast of highly processed cereals, and a lunch of french fries, hot dogs, hamburgers, or pizza. They have a soda in their hands from breakfast to dinner.

From 1963 to 1980, the *American Heart Association* found that obesity increased 54% in children aged 6 to 11 and 39% in ages 12 to 17. *The Journal of the American Dietetic Association* states that day care centers frequently include high-fat and high-sugar foods in children's meals and snacks. A recent study conducted by the *Journal of School Health* shows that 39% of the calories in an average school lunch are from fat. In the meantime, nutritional guidelines recommend limiting fat to 30% of daily calorie intake. School lunches also are loaded with salt, with the average lunch containing 1,244 mg. of sodium. The *Food and Nutrition Board of the National Academy of Sciences* recommends a total daily sodium intake of 600 to 1,800 mg. for children 7 to 10 years old. A connection between sodium and high blood pressure has been observed, and nearly 3 million children between ages 6 and 17 suffer from this condition. These high sodium levels are unhealthy and unwise, *Vegetarian Times,* Sept. 1990.

Children two years and older should have a diet containing no more than 30% of calories from fat, no more than 10% of calories from saturated fat, and no more than 300 mgs. of cholesterol daily. This means that a child of 6 should have about 60 gms. of fat, and 67 gms. of fat for a 7 year old. Children need some fat in their diet to supply calories so they will grow normally. Do not completely eliminate fat. Just check and be sure they are getting no more than the recommended 30% of their calories from fat. Be sure to choose good fats, not saturated fats from animal products.

The *Child Nutrition Advisory Council* states, "It has long been recognized that eating patterns and the foods to which children are exposed in the early years of life are among the most influential factors determining their nutritional health as adults. **"A child's capacity to learn is directly related to food intake and good nutritional habits."** *Clint Eastwood* told those at the Carmel Youth Center, in California, "If you stay active physically and mentally, you build respect for yourself. We can't leave the physical education of our youth to chance. You have to provide them with opportunities." *Arnold Schwarzenegger* also supports this view, "Our youth need to build strong minds and healthy bodies so they can be the leaders of the future."

Recently, a clue to one of the causes of childhood earaches has come to light. *Talal Nsouli, an Allergist at Georgetown University, Washington, D.C.,* wanted

---

CALCIUM AND HYPERTENSION

Besides building bones and teeth, adequate calcium in childhood may help ward off hypertension in youngsters, a study at *Boston University Medical School* suggests.

Kids should get their Recommended Dietary Allowances of calcium: 800 mg. a day until age 11, and 1,200 mg. a day from 11 to 18.

Source: *American Health,* May 1992, pg. 9

to learn if allergies might be a contributing factor in **ear infections**. After examining more than 100 children, *Nsouli* found that 78% were sensitive to foods, including milk, wheat, peanuts and corn-- standard childhood fare. When the foods were eliminated from their diets, ear infections in 70 of the 81 children were eliminated. Were that not persuasive enough, when the children were put back on their diets (milk, wheat, peanuts, etc.), **66 of the 70 that had been cured, suffered a return of their ear infection.** We must also look for soy-related problems. Soy is found in nearly all processed foods. We have found soy and chicken a problem for children also.

Because both parents work outside the home, there are fewer meals cooked at home. Family schedules are busy, meals are prepared based on convenience and not nutrition. Kids don't think about eating what's good for them, only what tastes good.

We see more and more clinically **depressed** children. Research is now beginning to recognize that neurological function is very sensitive to nutritional requirements. It is often the first system to be adversely affected by nutritional imbalances. Sugar, high-fat, and low-nutrient foods are the cause. Calories are present, but even marginal nutrition is missing.

Children especially need a well-balanced diet to develop properly. An example is a deficiency of biotin (a B-vitamin) which is linked to seborrheic **dermatitis**, a dry scaling of the scalp and face. Seizures and acidosis may also result from biotin deficiency. A zinc deficiency has been linked to **hyperactivity**.

COMMON DEFICIENCIES IN CHILDREN

One in six are seriously deficient in calcium
One-third of children are deficient in iron
About 50% lack sufficient zinc
Over 90% are deficient in magnesium
One in six lack vitamin A
Nearly half are seriously deficient in vitamin C
Nearly one-third are deficient in vitamin B-6
One in seven are deficient in vitamin B-12
One in five are deficient in folate
Nearly 3 million between 6 and 17 years suffer from high blood pressure

Vitamin Supplement Journal

Giving your child reasonable amounts of vitamin supplements will ensure they are receiving their needed amounts of nutrients. There are studies that show this could increase your child's intelligence. If nothing else, vitamin supplements ensure your child gets the vital nutrients essential for well-being. The cost of supplements is a small price to pay for a healthy child. Since iron is not easily absorbed and needed by children we recommend *Floradix* from West Germany, found in health food stores. **Do not give your child iron supplements unless they have been prescribed by your doctor**. There is also *Floradix Children's Liquid Multi-vitamin.*

Because of nutrient-deficient diets and other problems, we see children turning to alcohol, drugs, and seeking other activities to make them feel better. Junk foods are behind our nation's problem children, causing depression and fatigue.

We must guide our children in their eating habits. Set a good example for your children. Don't tell them not to eat sugary junk foods and then polish off a quart of ice cream yourself. Keep more fresh fruits for them to snack on such as grapes, bananas, peaches, melons, apples, and any other favorites. Children must learn there are good sweets. Have convenient foods to eat in a hurry that offer nutrients such as skinless turkey or chicken breast, water-packed tuna, and salads prepared ahead of time like bean, potato, coleslaw, homemade fruit Jello, yogurt with fruit, nut butters and whole wheat bread or crackers. Have sliced, raw vegetables ready for snacks. Keep juice, iced tea, and lemonade handy so the children will not grab a soft drink. Keep a supply of raw seeds and nuts on hand. Avoid nuts from heated showcases or bulk bins. Always purchase sealed raw nuts and seeds.

Cow's milk has been suspected of causing **colic** in babies (although breast-fed babies may also suffer from inconsolable crying). Research from the *Washington University School of Medicine in St. Louis* suggests that the colic-causing substance found in cow's milk can make its way into breast milk after the mother eats dairy products. A study of 59 women found that there was a 31% higher level of a specific antibody, present in cow's milk, found in the mother's milk of the colicky babies, compared to the mother's milk of the non-colicky babies. *Anthony* the study, suggests that **breast-feeding** mothers should stop consuming dairy products for seven to ten days to determine if the child's colic is triggered by the cow's antibody. Parents of a formula-fed baby should switch to a hydrolyzed, casein-based formula, which is made from milk curd and is anti-body free.

Observe your child, if s/he is crying and sulking a lot, you had better change the diet. If s/he's content and laughing a lot, you are probably giving your child a good start in life nutritionally.

If you are nursing and your baby has **colic,** avoid eating the brassica family (brussels sprouts, cauliflower, cabbage, etc.), yeast breads, and dairy products. Chamomile, catnip, or fennel are good in a tea to relieve colic symptoms. Place the tea in a baby bottle with apple juice as a sweetener.

For **teething**, catnip and chamomile are soothing. In teething solutions look for garlic oils and clove to apply topically to the gums. You can make your own with 5 drops each of clove, anise oil, and Kyolic (garlic) oil, mixed with 2 tablespoons olive oil. Rub the gums every four hours. Store this mixture in a cool place.

Diaper rashes occur from either the diet of the mother or the baby being overly acidic. Both the child and the nursing mother should avoid citrus fruits, tomatoes, and sugar products. When washing the diapers, add 1/4 cup pure apple cider vinegar to the rinse water. Calendula cream and Tree Tea oil applied locally, are good for healing and soothing. Also, homemade plain yogurt promotes healing, if applied directly where there is a persistent problem.

For **cold relief**, peppermint and catnip teas are good for fever, ginger tea aids in loosening up mucus, and echinacea stimulates the immune function in children and nursing mothers. Try alcohol-free extracts taken in small, but frequent doses.

See the *Garlic* section for ear infections and other problems.

For **vegetarian babies**, the first form of milk should be either breast milk or soy formula. The infant receives many benefits from breast milk including: protection against infection, enhancement of the immune system, and a lower risk of developing allergies. Nursing mothers should be particularly careful that they are getting enough B-12, and that their babies receive at least 2 hours total of indirect exposure to the sun a week. Vitamin D supplements are recommended for nursing mothers, who have limited exposure to the sun. A deficiency of vitamin

---

Since infants brains are so easily damaged by lead, doctors warn that you check the water used to prepare formula. The first tap water of the day or water boiled in a lead-based kettle may contain high amounts of lead. Run your cold water for 2 minutes in the morning to flush the lead from the pipes. It is best to use distilled remineralized water, *Children's Hospital of Boston*

D can lead to rickets, which causes soft, improperly mineralized bones.

Some baby formulas include iron, because as the baby grows the iron received from the mother at birth is depleted. Supplementing iron in the baby's diet may lead to **stomachaches** and **constipation**. Iron drops are difficult to digest. Iron fumerate can be easily absorbed and does not irritate the intestines as much. **Iron should only be given to a baby when prescribed by a physician.**

Soy milk should not be substituted for soy formula for infants. It does not contain the correct amounts of protein, carbohydrate, fat, minerals, and vitamins. Mashed papaya, a 1/4 teaspoon of brewer's yeast, 1/2 teaspoon pure black strap molasses added to 1 quart plain soy milk is a good alternative to soy formula. It is also good when weaning the child and provides iron.

When babies begin to eat **solid food**, introduce one new food at a time to reduce the risk of allergic reactions. The first food often recommended is an iron-fortified rice cereal. This can be mixed to a thin consistency with expressed breast milk or soy formula. Barley, corn, and oats may be ground to a fine consistency and made into cereal. Be sure to introduce these to your child one at a time. After the baby is eating the cereals regularly, fruits, fruit juices, and vegetables can be started. Once again, introduce these foods one at a time, after the child is 6-8 months old. Try making your own baby food from fresh vegetables, fruits, and whole grains; all you need is a blender. Add tofu to the foods, for protein. There are many organic baby foods to choose from at a health food store, including several varieties by *Earth's Best* and *Simply Pure*.

Australian researchers have found that babies of women who smoked during their pregnancies are more likely to develop asthma as they grow older. This does not mean that smokers' children will all grow up with asthma, but a higher percentage will be asthmatics, *New England Journal of Medicine*, No. 17/1991, pg. 324.

Two recent studies showed that there was a significant reduction in complications from **measles** when children were given vitamin A.

The first study, published in the *Journal of the American Medical Association,* Vol. 323, July 1990 and the second study published in the *Journal of Alternative and Complementary Medicine,* March 1991, was of 15, 000 preschool children in India. It showed that giving as little as 8,333 I.U.s of vitamin A weekly reduced mortality from measles by more than one half. The Recommended Dietary Allowance of vitamin A is 5,000 I.U.s. Parents who choose to avoid the measles vaccination can help protect their child's health in other ways.

Rotavirus is the most common viral cause of **diarrhea.** Last year in this country alone, some 500,000 children visited a doctor and 70,000 were hospitalized for this kind of diarrhea. According to researchers at the *Johns Hopkins Children's Center,* it would be less common if day-care centers weren't so popular. The rotavirus is found in the feces of an infected child and easily spread. But even the researchers were taken aback when they found it on the surface of 44% of the toy balls, 26% of the diaper-changing areas and 16% of the floor samples.

"Protecting your children from this virus is difficult, but it helps if the day-care center you take them to is kept as clean as possible," said *James Wilde, Johns Hopkins University, Baltimore, Maryland.*

Many children have a **cow milk allergy** and may even be **allergic to soy products**, so be a dectective. Substitute different milks in your child's diet like Rice Dream milk, nut milks and soy milk when the cow milk allergy is a problem. Pay close attention to the child's behavior shortly after they consume each item.

Trace amounts of pesticide residue have been found in lanolin, a common ingredient in lipsticks,

lipglosses, and nipple creams, *John Bailey, Ph.D., Acting Director, FDA's Colors and Cosmetics Division,* urges nursing mothers to avoid lanolin-containing nipple creams, since they are ingested by breast-fed infants, *Self Magazine,* April 1991.

Children and teens who have flu or chickenpox symptoms should not take products containing salicylates (aspirin), as they increase the risk of **Reye's Syndrome.** Some of these products are:

- Alka-Seltzer Effervescent Antacid and Pain Relievers
- Alka-Seltzer Plus Night-Time Cold Medicine
- Anacin Maximum Strength Analgesic Coated Tablets
- Ascriptin A/D Caplets
- BC Powder
- BC Cold Powders
- Bayer Children's Cold Tablets
- Bufferin - all forms
- Excedrin Extra-Strength Analgesic Tablets and Caplets
- Pepto-Bismol
- Ursinus Inlay-Tabs
- Vanquish Analgesic Caplets
- Some arthritis products

Teenage girls should be particularly cautious of an acne product called Accutane (isotretinoin). A vitamin-A derivative used for treating cystic acne, it poses an extremely high risk of birth deformities should pregnancy occur.

HOW MUCH IRON IS TOO MUCH?

Too much iron may be cause for greater concern than too little. The *British Medical Journal* reported on a study indicating that the practice of routinely feeding babies iron to prevent anemia may increase the risk of sudden infant death syndrome (SIDS) or crib death.

If the child tests anemic, then give iron supplements, if not, do not give iron to the child. The best way to provide iron is through diet, include these iron-rich foods: raisins, prunes, figs, leafy greens, sea vegetables, winter squash, tofu, grains, kidney beans, millet, rice and blackstrap molasses. To assure absorption, add a food source of vitamin C or a supplement.

Carob- Peanut Butter Cheesecake

No cooking required. Kids and grown-ups will love this.

1/2 cup carob powder

8 oz. low-fat cottage cheese or cream cheese or yogurt cheese (see recipe)

16 oz. tofu (for dairy-free cheesecake use all tofu increase to 24 oz. drained and patted dry)

2/3 cup honey or sweetener of your choice

8 oz. peanut butter (can use any type nut butter, almond, sunflower, etc.)

1/2 teaspoon vanilla

1 small banana

Blend well in processor or by hand until smooth. Pour into your favorite pie crust and chill. Whole grain, sugar-free crumbled cookies makes a nice crust. Top with whole nuts if desired.

Frozen Yogurt Pops

3 cups plain yogurt with fruit or add fresh fruit of your choice

1 cup any kind fruit juice concentrate (apple is good)

Pour into ice cube trays and put wooden popsicle sticks in each and freeze.

Kids Graham Treats

Adults will love these too!

Peanut, almond, or cashew butter

Graham crackers or cookies

Carob chips

Bananas

Crushed nuts

Spread crackers or cookies on cookie sheet and top with nut butter of choice, sliced bananas, carob chips, and crushed nuts. Can use only peanut butter and carob chips on crackers if desired.

Bake in 300 degree oven just until chips melt.

Fruit-Nut Bars

1 cup date pieces

1 cup soft raisins (soak for a few minutes in warm water to soften, if needed)

1/4 cup honey or your choice of sweetener

1 cup ground almonds (or any type nuts desired)

1 cup ground cashews

3 teaspoons lemon juice or orange

1 cup chopped dried apricots

1 cup dried pineapple, chopped

1 cup fine ground coconut

Put all ingredients through food processor or chop finely and make certain all the dried fruit is in small pieces, add honey, juice and mix well. (Can put all in food processor and blend with bits and pieces of the dried fruits). Form into balls and coat with melted carob chips, grated coconut, chopped nuts, etc. Wrap in wax paper and store in refrigerator.

Frozen Popsicles

Freeze any unsweetened fruit juice in ice cube trays with a stick in each. Use watermelon for **weight loss**. *Very delicious!*

See the Sweet Treats recipes for more things children will enjoy.

Crispy Bars

3 cups puffed or crispy rice cereal

3/4 cup pecan or other nut butter

1/3 cup honey or brown rice syrup

1/3 cup crushed pecans or other nuts (optional)

Add extra fructose if you need it softer or sweeter.

Mix ingredients together with oiled hands and press into 6x10" greased pan and refrigerate until firm. Cut and serve.

HYPERACTIVITY

Hyperactivity in children decreases dramatically when sugar, artificial colors and flavors, chocolate, MSG (monosodium glutamate), caffeine (in soft drinks, etc.), and preservatives, are eliminated from their diets.

Chili Pie

3 cups chili or Hain's or Health Valley Chili
1/2 cup chopped onion
1 tablespoon taco seasoning *(optional)* added to
    cornbread mixture
1/2 cup shredded cheese, your choice
1/4 cup chopped green pepper

Make your favorite cornbread or use *Arrowhead Mills* "Multigrain Corn Bread" mix, and add 1/4 cup melted margarine to the recipe. When using this mix just for cornbread, add 1/4 cup honey and 1/2 cup corn germ (corn germ has more nutrients than wheat germ).

Pour batter into a greased 8" x 8" x 2" pan, or any baking dish. Spoon chili into center of cornbread batter, sprinkle onion and cheese over the chili. Bake at 450 degrees for 25-30 minutes, until cornbread is done. Do not overcook and dry out. This freezes well for later use. Put into single serving dishes, if freezing. Top with fresh avocado and tomatoes before serving.

Soda Pop

Make your own soda pop that's good for the kids too! See recipe in Healthy Drink section.

The following sandwishes will keep longer than those made with meat and eggs.

Banana-Nut Spread

1/2 ripe banana
2 tablespoons almond or sesame butter
2 teaspoons tofu mayonnaise
1 tablespoon soft raisins

Blend all together, serve in a pita pocket, on bread or with crackers.

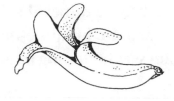

Date-Pecan Spread

1 cup yogurt cream cheese (see Yogurt section)
2 tablespoons chopped dates
2 tablespoons chopped pecans
1 tablespoon tofu mayonnaise

Gently mix all together. Refrigerate until ready to use.

Veggie-Tahini Spread

1 tablespoon tamari sauce
3 tablespoons tahini
1 tablespoon minced onion
1 tablespoon chopped green pepper
1 tablespoon grated carrot
1 teaspoon miso

Blend altogether and serve.

Chick-Pea Spread

4 cups chick-peas, cooked until tender
3/4 cups brown rice
2-1/2 tablespoons Dijon mustard
Sprinkle of garlic granules
1/2 chopped green or red pepper
Dash of sea salt
1 teaspoon grated horseradish

Mix all the ingredients together until smooth. Refrigerate. Try spread in a pita pocket with sliced cucumbers, tomatoes, and alfalfa sprouts.

SIDS

Susceptibility to botulism-related sudden death syndrome may be caused by bottle-feeding. None of the unfortunate cases in a 1981 study had been breast-fed. Current speculations as to the cause of susceptibility to these air- and food-borne bacteria, include limited experimental support for the theory that the altered bacterial ecology of the infant gut may be a major factor, *Doctor's UPDATE*, 1989, Natren, Inc.

AIDS and Pancreatic Cancer on the Rise

Since the death of TV star Michael Landon, a shocked public realizes that cancer of the pancreas, once thought to be rare, is a disease of grave proportions and increasing frequency. Film star Rock Hudson's death from AIDS, in a like manner, increased our awareness.

Although HIV is considered by the experts to be the sole cause of AIDS, while the underlying cause of pancreatic cancer remains unknown, many nutritionists and health care practitioners are convinced that environmental and dietary factors (poor nutrition habits) are deeply involved co-factors.

Both diseases are manifestations of an "Acquired Immune Deficiency." Both diseases are killers resulting in premature death, with a high financial cost, and untold suffering and pain.

Recently, there has been a drastic and dangerous change in the American Diet. Highly processed foods from supermarkets, many with toxic preservatives and chemicals added, fast-foods, and numerous imitation foods created in laboratories, that rapidly result in destruction of the immune system have become our staple foods. All lack freshness and nutrients. Today most of the so-called food consumed by people lack sufficient nutrients to sustain life.

Consider how our foods are prepared often cooked in microwave ovens. These potent and dangerous electromagnetic waves adversely alter the food. Further, day and night our bodies are exposed to these lethal waves through television, electrical appliances, radio, computer screens, and many other modern high-technology miracles of man. Even the kitchen, with its electrical appliances, once safe and sacred, must be considered a danger area.

We are convinced that if a nationwide survey were conducted, millions in our nation would be found to exist on prepared foods that do not supply even sub-optimal amounts of vitamins A, C, E and the essential trace mineral selenium necessary for immunity to disease. No wonder we are an immune-deficient society, unprotected and vulnerable to a plethora of illnesses including pancreatic cancer and AIDS.

50

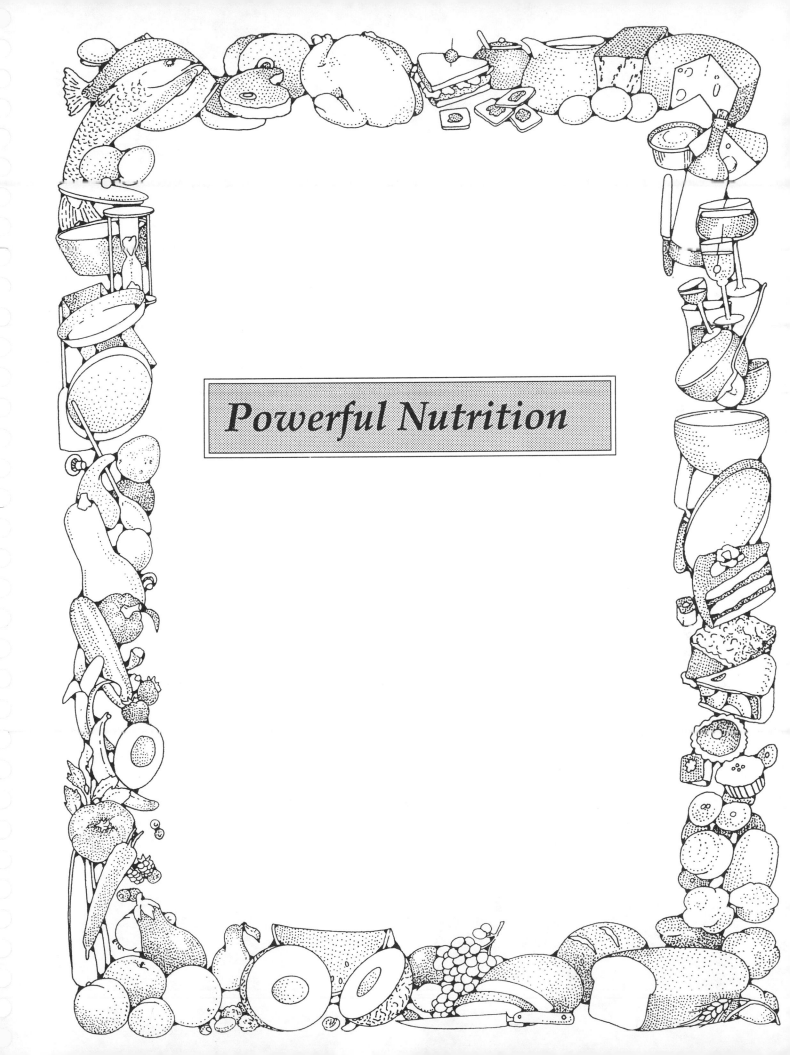

Powerful Nutrition

The Importance of the
Bountiful Bean

Beans are an excellent addition to the diet. They are one of nature's near perfect foods, containing an abundance of B-vitamins and iron. They are low in calories, sodium, and fat containing calcium, zinc, potassium, magnesium, and copper. A wealthy supply of most protein-building amino acids, beans also contain more fiber per serving than oat bran. One cup of kidney beans provides 5.8 grams of total fiber and oat bran has four 4 grams of fiber. A report published in the *American Journal of Clinical Nutrition* states that, "beans significantly lower cholesterol levels even in high fat diets."

If you do not eat beans very often, it's more likely you will bloat after eating beans. You need to build up a tolerance for beans by eating small amounts at first and then slowly increasing your intake, so that the body can adjust. Try adding 1/2 cup of uncooked brown rice or 1 teaspoon of fennel seeds to beans while cooking. This helps reduce intestinal gas and bloating. Some people soak the beans overnight, rinse, and then cook in fresh water. It is believed that soaking and rinsing the beans will rinse some of the gas-causing carbohydrates off. However, soaking the beans will cause some of the nutrients to be depleted. Baking soda also will help reduce gas, but we prefer not to use

it, because it also depletes the body of certain nutrients. Try the brown-rice method (rice and beans are a complete protein) and eat only a 1/2 cup serving the first few times, then gradually increase your consumption.

If you do overeat at times, take four charcoal tablets after your meal. This will stop the gas and bloating. It is fine to take charcoal tablets occasionally, but do not take them often because they will also absorb good nutrients.

Anti-nutrients are edible-plant ingredients that take minerals and proteins from foods and push them undigested through the body. Anti-nutrients are a diverse group including *lectins, phytates, tannins*, and *enzyme inhibitors*. They are most concentrated in beans, lentils, and peas. But they are also found in nuts, whole-grain cereals, whole grain flour (bread, pasta), and oilseeds like sunflower and sesame.

Anti-nutrients bind directly to minerals, proteins, and starches in foods, they also inactivate the digestive enzymes which break down starches and proteins. The enzyme-blocking action, in turn, inhibits nutrient absorption. If the body is already low in mineral reserves, a diet loaded with anti-nutrient foods may

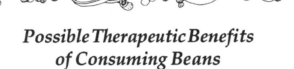

Possible Therapeutic Benefits of Consuming Beans

* *Reduces blood cholesterol*

* *Contains chemicals that inhibit cancer*

* *Controls insulin and blood sugar*

* *Lowers blood pressure*

* *High fiber for colon disorders*

* *Aids hemorrhoids and bowel disorders*

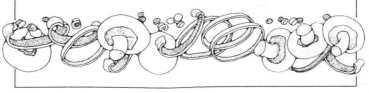

only add to a mineral deficiency. Cooking and processing, which slow anti-nutrient activity, are factors to be considered, *Lilian U. Thompson, Professor of Nutritional Science, University of Toronto.*

Foods high in fiber keep blood-sugar on an even level. People who are attempting to control their cholesterol level and diabetics should eat a high fiber, high carbohydrate diet. In testing, legumes were found to produce the lowest blood sugar response.

Navy beans contain the anti-nutrients *phytic acid* and *lectin.* However, a new report has found that in addition to their possible uses in preventing cancer, they also help slow the increase of blood sugar in diabetics. The higher the anti-nutrient level, the lower the blood sugar in both normal and diabetic subjects.

Beans, peas and lentils, should be consumed frequently, but in moderation, one or two servings a week is recommended. It is important to cook legumes to break down anti-nutrients and avoid intestinal distress.

The primary cause of fecal odor or gas, is sulfur-containing compounds. Not the skatoles (nitrogen compounds found in feces) or indoles (crystalline compounds also found in feces), according to researchers at *Utah's Salt Lake VA Medical Center.* Some studies have found that more gas is produced by the body after consuming beans, brussels sprouts, apple juice, prune juice, and raisins. Gas is the result of sugars, starches, and fiber that reach the large intestine without being digested or absorbed. When these undigested particles reach the bowel, the harmless bacteria that reside there eat them, giving off gas by-products. A very common source of gas is found in the sugar lactose, a natural component of milk products. The body needs lactase, an enzyme, to digest lactose. Another source of gas is found in the soluble fiber in fruits and oat bran. Oats, wheat, potatoes, and corn, in fact almost all starchy foods except rice, have been found to cause flatulence.

Oats increase the excretion of bile acids, which contain cholesterol, through the feces. The fiber found in beans is fermented in the colon into a short chain of fatty acids, which is then re-absorbed by the body, possibly inhibiting the body from making cholesterol.

"Gassy foods also contain *oligosaccharides*, complex sugars that can not be broken down in the stomach. When these sugars reach the large intestine, they are digested by bacteria, and one of the bacteria's by-products is gas", *Leonard J. Newman, M.D. Director of Pediatric Gastroenterology and Nutrition, New York Medical College.*

Lactaid, Inc. has introduced Beano, that contains a sugar-digesting enzyme all humans lack. This enzyme, *alpha-galactosidase*, is derived from the fungus pergillus niger, and should prevent gas by breaking down *oligosaccharides* in the stomach. Four studies regarding Beano's claims are being planned at *John Hopkins, McGill University, New York Medical College*, and *UCLA*. Undigested protein is a contributing factor to the odiferous compounds of the body's gas. Beano may break down raffinose sugars in foods, which may decrease the gas producing bacteria in the bowels. This reduces the bloating and distension that causes discomfort in many gas-sufferers, though not necessarily the odor. A free sample of Beano can be obtained by calling *Akpharma* at 800-257-8650 weekdays from 8:30 to 5:30 Eastern time, *Nutrition Action Healthletter, March 1991.*

Most beans are cooked according to their size. For instance, because they are larger, soybeans and chick peas (garbanzo beans) typically take longer to cook. Use four parts water to one part beans. Cook beans slowly to retain their shape. If you forget to presoak overnight, bring them to a rolling boil, remove from the heat and cover. Allow to sit for a couple of hours.

Add more beans to your diet--combined with rice, wheat or corn they make a complete protein. Just one cup contains fifteen grams of protein.

A Note of Caution

Australian researchers noted that canned baked beans caused higher levels of blood sugar and should be avoided by diabetics. All canned goods should be avoided.

Preventing Constipation

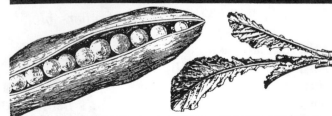

A fiber-rich diet can help prevent constipation, which is important because the strain caused by constipation is how many hemorrhoid problems begin. Good sources of fiber include:
- potatoes
- beans—kidney, navy, lima, pinto
- whole-grain breads
- bran
- fresh fruits
- vegetables, especially asparagus, brussels sprouts, cabbage, carrots, cauliflower, corn, peas, kale, and parsnips.

It will also help to limit these low- or no-fiber foods: ice cream, soft drinks, cheese, white bread, and meat. ■

Bean Types

Adzuki

Small tender red beans from China and Japan often added to brown rice dishes. They are delicious in barley soup (and many other soups), casseroles, and loaves. Adzuki beans cook faster than most beans because they are small and very tender. They have less calories per cup than any other bean, but are the highest in nutrients of most brands. They are popular in the macrobiotic diet. This diet consists mostly of grains, beans, vegetables, seaweed, sea vegetables, soups, cereal grain coffee or bancha tea, umeboshi plums, seeds, sesame salt and sesame butter. Small amounts of fish and fruit are permitted, but no dairy products, red meat or sugar in any form. Some have claimed a cure from cancer on this diet.

Anasazi

Anasazi is a superior source of protein, iron, phosphorus, thiamine, and contain many other essential nutrients. They have an unusual flavor and are generally sweeter and meatier than other types of beans. The name means ''The Ancient Ones'' in the Navajo language.

Black Turtle

They are good in Spanish-style foods, with seasonings of garlic, bay leaves, cumin and tomato sauces. Also good cooked and then put through a food processor and blended with seasoning and served as a soup.

Fava

Fava beans are lima-shaped beans rich in B-vitamins, calcium, protein and iron. They are good by themselves or added to soups. Soak fava beans overnight and cook with three parts water.

Great Northern

They are large white beans useful for soups and vegetable chowders. Mix with other beans.

Lentils

The lentil is a member of the pea family. High in calcium and magnesium, phosphorus, sulfur, and vitamin A. Lentils are a good source of proteins, and are a nutritional power food. These beans do not need to be presoaked. Garlic is a good addition when cooking lentils.

Lima

Lima beans have a distinctive flavor and are rich in potassium, minerals, vitamins and fiber.

Navy

Navy is the second most popular type of bean in our country after kidney beans. These are used primarily for soups and stews or as a main course with corn bread.

Pinto

These are not a complete protein and they are high in calories. The light brown beans lose their black spots when cooked. They are often used to make refried beans, and in burritos and stews.

Red Kidney

Red kidney beans are very popular for chili, salads and soups. They are rich in all nutrients, protein and fiber. These are the richest in fiber of all beans.

Soybeans

Soybeans have the highest protein content of the bean family, with 50% more usable protein than steak. They require longer cooking than other types. This bean is extremely popular in the health food industry and is used in tempeh, tofu, tamari sauces, miso, flour, cheese, grits, milk powder, liquid milk and much more.

Chick Peas or Garbanzos

They are used in salads for their nut-like flavor. Chick peas or garbanzo beans are great in dips and vegetable burgers. They take longer to cook and should be cooked slowly so they keep their shape. These beans have high concentrations of calcium, iron, potassium and vitamin A.

Protein Rich Lentil Burgers

2 cups of lentils
1 green or red pepper, finely choped
1/2 pound mushrooms, finely choped
1 onion, finely choped
1 carrot, shredded
1/4 cup oat bran or quick-cooking rolled oats or
    1 cup cooked sweet, short grain rice
1/4 cup catsup or tomato paste

Wash and cook lentils in 1-1/2 quarts of water for 1-1/2 to 2 hours and saute pepper, mushrooms and onion lightly in olive oil. Add carrot and season with Spike seasoning or sea salt.

When the lentils are soft, drain and mash or put through a blender adding sauteed vegetables until mixed but not mushy.

Add bran, oats or rice. Add to this mix, catsup or paste.

If too soft add more oats until mixture is the consistency of hamburger. Form into patties and broil or saute until golden brown.

Serve in a sandwich or place on top of veggies and rice or pasta. *Hain's* Dry Gravy Mix is delicious prepared and placed over the patties. Serve with mashed potatoes and a vegetables.

Dr. Ann Kennedy, Harvard School of Public Health, found that *protease inhibitors* (found in beans) can <u>reverse</u> the initial cancer-causing damage to cells in studies done on tissue cultures. This was once considered impossible by scientists. *Dr. Kennedy* believes that *protease inhibitors* may combat all forms of cancer, except stomach cancer.

Other experiments have shown *protease inhibitors* to retard the growth of human colon and breast-cancer cells. This may account for the reduced rate of cancer in Japan, where one of their main staple food products is derived from soybeans.

Dr. James Anderson, University of Kentucky, believes a cup of cooked pinto or navy beans per day will lower blood cholesterol.

Beans may also aid in fighting viruses. Unlike bacteria, a virus cannot produce on its own, therefore, it penetrates a healthy cell. At the *John Hopkins University School of Medicine,* researchers did a study mixing human rotaviruses with *protease inhibitors*, the inhibitors kept the viruses subdued.

Soybeans and garbanzo (chick-peas) beans have the highest concentrations of *protease inhibitors* but all legumes contain high amounts. Other sources rich in the inhibitors include tofu, all seeds, nuts, sweet potatoes, most grains and sweet corn. These *protease inhibitors* survive heat and processing.

Double Pea Soup

1 carton *Taste Adventure* instant Split Pea soup
2 cups boiling water
1 red bell pepper, chopped
1 cup fresh or frozen peas

In pan combine water, pepper, and peas and boil. When vegetables are tender, stir in split pea soup flakes, remove from heat, cover, and let stand for 5 minutes. Serve.

Quick Guide to Cooking Beans

Do not overcook beans or allow the water to boil for more than 10 minutes. Beans should be tender, but firm and simmering will bring the best results. Although beans come in a wide variety of shapes and sizes, the cooking directions below apply to all the beans listed in this book.
    (1) 1 cup of beans to 5 cups of water.
    (2) Bring water to a boil and simmer for 2-3 hours (or until tender).
The only exception to these steps is with garbanzo and Great Northern beans which must be simmered for at least two hours (or three hours for the larger varieties of Great Northerns).

Beans are rich in fiber. Dietary fiber is believed to protect against cancer, mainly colon cancer which is on the rise, *Science News*, Aug. 4, 1990. Fiber binds the carcinogens and estrogen in the bowel and they are removed from the body. Also, fiber passes more quickly through the intestinal tract so the toxins cannot build up in the colon. Fiber is more effective when consumed as a natural part of whole food rather than as added fiber in the diet.

Taste Adventure is a pre-cooked, instant bean soup product, found in health food stores. Fast and nutritious meals can be made using pre-cooked beans.

Lentil Salad

1 carton *Taste Adventure* instant curry lentil soup or *Hain's* Lentil Soup Mix
    1-1/2 cups boiling water
    1 cup diced cucumber
    1 cup diced tomatoes
    1 tablespoon capers
    1/4 cup chopped walnuts
    1/2 cup chopped red cabbage
    3 tablespoons chopped fresh parsley
    1 tablespoon freshly squeezed lemon juice
    1 tablespoon red wine vinegar
    1 tablespoon olive oil
    1/4 teaspoon mustard
    Pepper to taste

Combine instant lentil soup with boiling water, stir. Cover 5 minutes, allow lentils to cool. Add remaining ingredients, stir. Chill and serve.

> **Soybeans have the highest concentrations of *protease inhibitors* of any food. For this reason consuming soybeans (and other types of beans) will help cells in a pre-cancerous stage revert to normal.**

Black Bean Dip

1 tablespoon vegetable oil
1 stalk chopped celery
1 large clove of garlic, minced
1/4 red bell pepper, chopped
1-1/2 cup boiling water
1-1/2 cup *Taste Adventure* instant black
   bean soup or black bean flakes, or cook
   and blend your own
1 tablespoon lemon juice
1-2 grated radishes
1 tablespoon salsa

In a pan saute celery, garlic, and pepper in oil. Add water and boil. Stir in beans, remove from heat and add lemon juice, radishes, and salsa. Serve hot or cold.

Tostada Pizza

Pizza dough for 1 large pizza
   1-1/2 cups *Taste Adventure* Pinto BeanFlakes
or cooked mashed beans
   1-1/4 cup boiling water
   1/2 cup enchilada sauce
   3/4 cup monterey jack cheese
   3/4 cup cheddar cheese
   1 cup mozzarella cheese
   1 cup chopped olives
   3-4 cups shredded lettuce
   1/4 cup chopped green onions

Add boiling water to *Taste Adventure* bean flakes to make instant refried beans. Layer beans on pizza dough, cover with enchilada sauce, add cheese and chopped olives. Bake at 450 degrees about 20 minutes. Mix lettuce, tomato, and onions together, add to pizza when it is done cooking. Serve with salsa or guacamole.

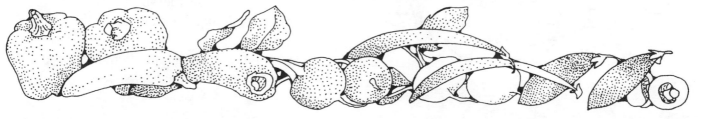

Bean Burritos with Sweet Potatoes

1 tablespoon expeller-pressed olive
  or canola oil
1 large onion, finely chopped
4 cloves of garlic, finely minced
6 cups cooked adzuki, kidney, or
  garbanzo beans or a mixture
2 cups of the bean liquid, drained and
  set aside after cooking the beans
1/2 green pepper, chopped
2 tablespoons chili powder
2 teaspoons ground cumin
Dash of cayenne pepper *(optional)*
2-3 tablespoons tamari sauce
3 cups cooked, mashed sweet potatoes
8 large whole wheat tortillas

Thinly slice avocado, chop lettuce, dice tomato and mix with the salsa and plain yogurt.

Preheat oven to 375°. Saute onion until almost transparent, add garlic, and green pepper. Mix in beans, bean cooking liquid, chili powder, cumin, mustard, and cayenne. Bring to a boil, then cover and simmer 20 minutes. Stir in tamari. Mash the drained beans in the cooking pot. Simmer and cook uncovered, until excess liquid is gone.

Spread approximately 2/3 cup of the bean mixture down the middle of each tortilla and top with approximately 1/2 cup of the sweet potatoes. Roll, place seam side down in a casserole dish, keeping them close together. Bake 5-10 minutes.

Top with lettuce, tomato, avocado, salsa, sprouts, green onion, and yogurt.

Variation: Try cooked brown rice instead of sweet potatoes.

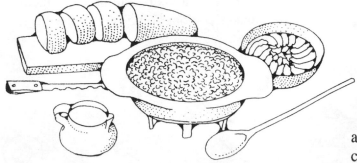

Lentil Stew with Pumpkin and Greens

High in all needed nutrients, excellent for cancer, heart disorders, and anyone in need of a highly nutritious meal.

2 tablespoons olive or canola oil
1 large minced onion
1 tablespoon minced fresh ginger
1 tablespoon whole cumin seeds
3/4 teaspoon ground cinnamon
1/2 teaspoon ground coriander
1/4 teaspoon ground cardamom
4-1/2 cups water
1-1/4 cups lentils, rinsed
2 pounds pumpkin, peeled and cut
  into 1 inch cubes (or sweet potatoes)
1/2 cup golden raisins
1 cup diced apples
1/2 pound fresh cooking greens
  (see *Leafy & Green* section)

Heat oil in a large saucepan. Saute onion and fresh ginger about 5 minutes. Stir in cumin seeds and spices, 2 -1/2 cups of the water and the lentils. Bring to a boil, cover, and reduce heat and simmer for 30 minutes. Add pumpkin, raisins, diced apples, and the remaining water. Cover and simmer over medium heat until the lentils are barely tender, about 10 minutes. Stir in the greens, cover, cook a few more minutes. Serve with cooked brown rice.

Fiesta Bean Dip

1-1/2 cups *Taste Adventure* Pinto Bean Flakes, or cooked, mashed beans of your choice.
1/2 cup plain yogurt or sour cream mixed with taco seasonings or dash of cayenne pepper *(optional)*
1/2 cup chopped olives
1/4 cup chopped green onions
1/2 cup guacamole or fresh, mashed avocado
1/2 cup grated soy cheese
1/2 cup fresh diced tomatoes
3 tablespoons salsa

On a plate layer each ingredient in the order it appears, beginning with the beans. Serve with corn chips.

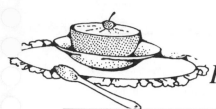

Breakfast
Healthy Ways to Start Your Day

Our busy lives make a traditional breakfast of eggs and bacon too time consuming to prepare, and we know fat-loaded foods should not be consumed at any meal. Fats cause the blood to become sticky and as a result it circulates slowly through the brain.

Instead of eggs and bacon or other fatty foods, we need complex carbohydrates and protein. Protein for better brain function and complex carbohydrates for a steady release of glucose into the bloodstream maintain stable blood-sugar levels. A high-sugar breakfast will cause a drop in the blood sugar, resulting in a tired feeling all morning.

Children especially need a sound breakfast to help them think clearly and function better all day in school. Soy milk, almond milk are good on cereals and if you use fruit juice no additional sweetener is needed. Whole-grain cereals are the best to provide the steady energy we need each morning.

Healthy Breakfast Choices

U.S. Mill's - 100% organic cereals - Stroodles and Poppets (for children)
Uncle Sam's Raisin Bran Cereal
Nature's Warehouse Pastry Poppers
Erewhon - Crispy Raisin Bran
Right Start - Organic Wheat Bran, sprouted barley & raisin juice (fat free)
Fruit & Wheat
Wheat Flakes
Hot Cereals - oatmeal, barley plus, brown rice cream cereals
Golden Temple Swiss-Style Muesli
Granola Grizzly's Papa Porridge
Sunrise Granola, New England's Organic Products
Country Grown cereals without honey or any type of sweetener added
Golden Kamut for wheat sensitive people
Knudsen - has fresh fruit and sugar-free syrups
Arrowhead Mills, Firn Natural Foods and *Heartland Mills* - biscuit and pancake mixes
New Morning Oatios
New Morning Fruit-e-O's
Erewhon's Crispy Bran Flakes
Breadshop - Health Crunch (no oil) and Puffs 'N Honey (93% fat free, corn, rice, and millet cereal
          with honey)
Rhine Harvest muesli cereals - 6 varieties, no added fats or oils
American Prairie Creamy Rye & Rice
Lumberg - Rice Cereal, Creamy Cinnamon-Raisin
Arrowhead - Seven-Grain Hot Cereal
Elams - Steel Cut Hot Oats

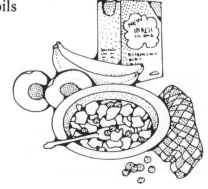

Breakfast Ideas

- Try a baked sweet potato topped with cinnamon, a sweetener, and sprinkled with wheat germ.
- Top a rice cake with nut butters and sliced bananas, sesame, or sunflower seeds.
- Children of all ages will love to spread nut butters on a apple slices.
- Spread left-over hot cereal in a shallow pan and chill overnight, you can cut it into squares in the morning. Cook it in a nonstick pan with a small amount of *Hain's* margarine and sprinkle with cinnamon and maple syrup or honey. Hot millet cereal is an excellent choice because of it's high protein and carbohydrates.
- For more fiber add a tablespoon of oat bran, rice bran, apple bran or corn bran mixed into your hot cereal before serving.
- Use high-fiber dry cereals with skim milk or fruit juice or a sliced banana or dried fruit for a fast start. Do not load your cereal with sugar and whole milk, because milk is high in fat and sugar gives a jolt to the system with a big let down. Before lunch you may not be able to concentrate clearly and will feel tired.
- Raisins will also sweeten a cereal. It is better to add your own raisins that have been soaked in water for few minutes, than to buy packaged cereals that contain raisins.
- A glass of a sweet fruit juice like grape juice, may also cause a fast rise in blood sugar and a fast drop, so consume the whole fruit. The fiber will slow down the blood sugar reaction. Juice on a high fiber cereal will slow down a reaction, because of the fiber content. *Knudsen* has a line of organic, sugar-free juices. Try them on your cereals. They're good and healthy.
- If you have been having **colon** disorders, drink or add 1/4 cup of aloe vera juice to your fruit juice.

Seven-Grain Meal

2 cups 7-Grain Cereal by *Arrowhead Mills*
4 cups of water
1/2 cup nutritional yeast or wheat germ
1 cup fresh or frozen blueberries, strawberries,
   or peaches

Mix ingredients (except for fruit) together in a crock pot, cook on the lowest setting for 6-8 hours, longer may make the cereal dry, so use more water if needed. Let set overnight and in the morning cook over medium heat for about 20 minutes until done. Stir occasionally while cooking and bring to a boil. Then cover and simmer for 20-30 minutes on lowest setting. Do not lift the lid, the steam will soften the grain preserving the nutrients.

This is good any time of the day. You can also use *Roman Meal Cereal*, a combination of oats, wheat, rye, bran, and flax.

Cooking the fruit with the cereal will give a nice sweet taste without added sweetener. Add 1/2 cup powdered soy milk if desired, for extra protein and taste. Chopped fresh apple and a little cinnamon is also good when added while cooking any cereal.

No-Egg French Fruit Toast

A child's delight and a vegetarian goody, great for breakfast, at lunch, as a dessert or a snack.

1 mashed banana
1/2 fresh mashed papaya
1/3 cup frozen apple juice or concentrate
1/4 cup soy milk or Rice Dream milk
1/2 teaspoon cinnamon
6 slices whole grain bread or English muffins

Blend together all ingredients except the bread. Pour the mixture over the bread and let it stand 2-5 minutes. Cook on both sides on lightly oiled skillet or under a broiler, until lightly browned.

Variation: Use other fruits like peaches, blueberries or strawberries or a combination in place of papaya. Top with a fresh piece of fruit and serve. Pure maple syrup drizzled on top makes a delicious, good for you dessert.

Nutritional Oatmeal

1 cup rolled or steel cut oats
2 cups water
1/2 cup wheat germ
1 cup Rice Dream milk

Place in a crock pot and stir. Simmer on lowest setting all night up to 8 hours, if longer use an extra 1/2 cup water. Top with fresh fruit and enjoy. A complete protein breakfast loaded with nutrients.

Variation: Add raisins or other dried fruit

Cruciferous Vegetables

The Magnificent 12

Everything that grows out of the ground contains proteins, especially our vegetables. Contrary to past beliefs, vegetarians can receive all the needed proteins from vegetables. Combining two or three per meal will assure you of sufficient protein intake. Vegetables also contain the needed essential fatty acids, vitamins, minerals, trace minerals, and many unidentified nutrients.

The Magnificent 12, Cruciferous Vegetables

Eating more vegetables will dramatically reduce and prevent disease. These twelve vegetables are the power fighters against cancer and heart disease, the two top killers in our country. They all have flowers with four petals that botanical historians describe as resembling the crucifix or Cross, thus they are called cruciferous.

Consume three, one cup servings from this list, each day. Eat one cup raw and two cups slightly steamed, except for horseradish. Use horseradish grated fresh in sauces, spreads. Alternate the vegetables daily.

Broccoli	**Kale**	**Rutabaga**	**Brussels sprouts**
Kohlrabi	**Turnip**	**Cabbage**	**Mustard greens**
Cauliflower	**Radishes**	**Watercress**	**Horseradish**

Broccoli

Lowers the risk of cancer, primarily **cancer of the colon, esophagus, larynx, lung, prostrate, oral cavity, pharynx, and stomach.**

Experiments using broccoli reveal the *sulforaphane* it contains to be the most powerful natural chemical for **stopping the growth of tumors**. It is high in cancer antidotes like *indoles, glucosinolates,* and *dithiolthiones*. It also contains *carotenoids* (vitamin A). It **blocks cell mutations** which foreshadow cancer, possibly due to the abundance of chlorophyll. A study by *Dr. Saxon Graham, Buffalo, NY,* found that people who ate more broccoli, cabbage, and brussels sprouts had a lower risk of **colon and rectal cancer**. Experiments in the 1950's discovered broccoli helped protect guinea pigs from lethal doses of **radiation**. Cabbage also worked but broccoli was found to be more effective. *Dr. James R. Marshall,* working with *Dr. Graham, Roswell Park Memorial Institute, Buffalo, NY* found that women who ate more broccoli were less prone to **cancer of the cervix**. It is believed that green vegetables, along with dark orange vegetables, act as **antidotes to the cancer process** that continues for years after exposure to carcinogens.

Always buy green broccoli to ensure freshness, never when it is yellow. Steam broccoli lightly to keep its nutrients intact.

Brussels Sprouts

Inhibit cancer, particularly malignancy of the **colon** and **stomach.**

Countries where brussels sprouts are frequently consumed have a low incidence of **gastro-intestinal cancer**. Researchers have found there are specific substances in brussels sprouts that **retard cancer**. These include chlorophyll, *dithiolthiones, carotenoids, indoles,* and *glucosinolates*. Studies revealed they detoxified aflatoxin, a fungal mold linked to cancer, particularly **liver cancer. Aflatoxin often contaminates peanuts, corn, and rice, and is a serious threat in third world countries.**

From experiments done on rats, it was found that those fed high levels of brussels sprouts or *glucosinolates* (the ingredient in brussels sprouts that disarms aflatoxin), remained almost free of malignant **liver tumors** when infected with aflatoxin. High concentrations of *glucosinolates* neutralized the cancer potential of the aflatoxin.

A juice made of brussels sprouts, string beans, lettuce, and carrots provide the needed elements to regenerate and improve the insulin-producing capacity of the **pancreas**. Brussels sprouts are rich in vitamins A, C, riboflavin, iron, potassium and fiber.

Cruciferous vegetables, including brussels sprouts, are thought to **depress thyroid function** because of a certain substances they contain. Researchers have concluded that cooking neutralized the thyroid-depressing substances.

Lee Wattenberg, M.D., Professor, University of Minnesota School of Medicine, found those whose diet was rich in brussels sprouts and cabbage improved the functioning of their **metabolic system aiding in cancer prevention.**

Cabbage

Kills bacteria and **viruses**, prevents **cancer**, particularly of colon, prevents and **heals ulcers** and the juice **stimulates the immune system.**

Eating cabbage once a week may reduce your chances of **colon cancer** by 60%. Eating it more frequently is even more likely to boost its anti-cancer potency. "Cabbage is therapeutically effective in conditions of **scurvy, diseases of the eyes, gout, rheumatism, pyorrhea, asthma, tuberculosis, cancer,** and **gangrene.** It is excellent as a **vitalizing agent,** and a **blood purifier,**" according to the *American Medicine Journal,* January 1927.

A study conducted in Japan in 1986, discovered that those who consumed the most cabbage had the lowest death rate from **all cancers.** This puts cabbage in the same category as yogurt and olive oil, as potential **life extenders.** Within cabbage are chemicals called *indoles,* that block cancer formation. Also there are *dithiolthiones,* which suppress the activation of cancer-causing (carcinogenic) substances. These include: *chlorophyll,* certain *flavonoids, isothiocyanates, phenols* like caffeic, *ferulic, acetic acid,* and vitamins E and C.

Dr. Garnett Cheney, Professor, Stanford University School of Medicine, believes fresh cabbage to be a natural **anti-ulcer** food. He found that guinea pigs given fresh cabbage juice did not develop **stomach ulcers** when ulcer-causing substances were

fed to the guinea pigs. From this *Dr. Cheney* determined that one quart of cabbage juice daily for the average ulcer sufferer should cure the **ulcer.** When the theory was tested on 55 ulcer sufferers, all but three felt better. The cabbage juice reduced the healing time for the ulcer by 83%.

The healing factors in cabbage are present only when taken raw, usually as a juice. The best cabbage to use is fresh spring and summer cabbage. Fall cabbage is less effective, winter ones are the least effective. To make a suitable drink, add three quarters cabbage juice to one quarter celery juice. Celery also contains an **anti-ulcer** factor. For extra flavor add pineapple juice to the cabbage juice. Drink a quart a day if you are suffering from an ulcer. Within three weeks, if not less, you should feel some results. The chlorophyll in raw cabbage also helps to prevent **anemia.** The high levels of vitamin A in cabbage aid in **tissue rejuvenation.** The sulphur content helps fight **infection** and protects the skin from **eczema** and other **rashes.**

Different types of cabbage to consume include Napa (Chinese cabbage), bok choy, and celery cabbage. All are from the cruciferous family and contain **anti-cancer** chemicals. A number of studies have determined that raw cabbage and cole slaw give protection against **stomach cancer.**

A study conducted by *Saxon-Graham, Ph.D.,* and his colleagues in Buffalo, New York, found people who never consumed cabbage were three-times more likely to develop **colon cancer.**

Cauliflower

Reduces risk of **cancer,** particularly of the **colon, rectum,** and **stomach,** and possibly the **prostate** and **bladder.**

Cauliflower contains compounds, like *indoles,* which stimulate the **natural defenses** to neutralize carcinogens. It is high in essential sulphur compounds. It is not as high in carotenes or chlorophyll, so it is less likely to inhibit **lung and other smoking-related cancers.** However, cauliflower is rich in vitamin C, potassium and fiber. This vegetable is better for **diabetic** people than cabbage.

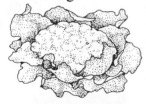

Horseradish

Benefits **asthma, bronchitis,** and **lung disorders, lymphatic congestion** and a **digestive** stimulant.

Horseradish belongs to the mustard family. The root of the plant is used to flavor meats, seafood, and sauces.

Fresh horseradish left in contact with the skin will cause blistering. Avoid contact with the eyes after getting it on the hands.

Kale

Kale is one of the best **cancer** fighting vegetables we have on our planet. Unfortunately, we do not usually have it to our diets. Kale is the richest of all leafy greens in *carotenoids,* powerful anti-cancer agents. All leafy greens lead the list of cancer preventives.

Kale is rich in vitamin A, C, riboflavin, niacin, calcium, magnesium, iron, sulfur, sodium, potassium, phosphorus, and chlorophyll. This leafy green is excellent in protecting smokers against **lung cancer.** All members of the cruciferous family protect against **cancer of the stomach, esophageal, colon, oral, throat,** and **gastrointestinal cancer.** Lower rates of cancer have been reported in the areas of the **breast, bowel, bladder,** and **prostate** as well. Kale's calcium is easily assimilated, making it a wonder food for **arthritis, osteoporosis,** and **bone loss** disorders.

Heat destroys some of the *carotenoids* but the resulting balance is more available to the body, and the chlorophyll content does not seem to be affected. It is wise to consume kale both in the raw and cooked forms.

Kohlrabi

Good for **indigestion, jaundice, diabetes,** the **lymph system,** and **alcoholism.** The fresh juice has been used in China to stop **nosebleeds.**

Kohlrabi seed powder is also used in China to improve **urination after childbirth** and to improve **eyesight.** This vegetable contains high amounts of vitamin C, calcium, and potassium. It is also a good source of fiber. The taste is like a mild turnip. Try it raw or cooked.

Mustard Greens

Mustard greens have the same nutrient content as other green, leafy vegetables and should be included in the optimum diet. They contain high amounts of calcium, iron, vitamin A and niacin. It is superior to spinach, because of the lower oxalic acid content, so the benefit of the calcium content is not lost.

In Russia, they use mustard seed oil in place of olive oil.

Radish

Stimulates the appetite, a **diuretic,** good for **colds** and **flu,** helps **respiratory infections** and cleanses **gall bladder** and **liver.**

In Chinese medicine the radish is used to promote **digestion,** remove **mucus,** soothe **headaches,** and heal **laryngitis.** The juice is mixed with ginger juice to cure laryngitis. For **sinusitis,** drink the juice of 6 radishes, one cucumber, and one apple. This is also a very beneficial drink for the **liver** and the **gallbladder.** A mustard oil, derived from the radish, is especially good for **gall stones.** Contains vitamin A, B-complex, and C.

Daikon is a long, white radish with a sweet-pungent flavor. Eat it raw, cooked or pickled.

Rutabaga

Clears up **mucus** and **congestion,** has an **alkalizing** effect on the body and contains **anti-cancer** qualities.

The rutabaga is a member of the turnip family, producing a large yellow root. Because the roots grow in the dark, deeply connected with the earth, they draw in many nutrients.

Rutabagas should not be consumed by anyone who has **kidney** problems. They contain mustard oil and may cause gas in some people.

The most nutritious root plants include: carrots, parsnips, turnips, celery root, radishes, onions, garlic, daikon, ginger, horseradish, and rutabaga.

Turnip

Balances the calcium in the body, reduces **mucus**, helps **asthma** and **bronchitis** and relieves **sore throats.**

Turnips are good raw or shredded for salads. Cook the green tops like any green or steam lightly or add to soups and stews. Being a cruciferous vegetable, they have cancer-fighting compounds plus high amounts of antioxidants, mainly vitamins A and C. High in calcium, iron and niacin.

> Researchers theorize that antioxidants, particularly vitamin C and carotenoids like beta-carotene in fruits and vegetables, retard oxidation damage to the lens of the eye. Oxidation is primarily responsible for age-related cataract formation.
> *American Journal of Clinical Nutrition*, Supplement to Vol. 53, January 1991.

Watercress

A wonderful food for **anemia, calcium deficiencies, blood** purification, **catarrhal** conditions, **liver** and **pancreas** problems, **appetite** stimulation, **thyroid** problems, **arthritis** and **emotional** problems.

Watercress is another member of the mustard family, the last of the **Magnificent 12**. The Brazilians have used a syrup from watercress as a remedy for **tuberculosis.** It is high in potassium, sulfur, vitamin A, calcium, and iron. It also contains copper, magnesium, sodium, potassium and iodine. Add it to juices and chop fresh for salads. Excellent added to bulgur wheat salads.

Anyone who is **ill** should chew on a few stalks of watercress daily.

Healing Properties of Other Vegetables

Alfalfa

The Arabs called it "Al Falfa," which means the "Father of all foods."

Arthritis

Hair growth

Congestion and **respiratory disorders**

Alfalfa contains vitamins A, B, C, D, E, K, and U. The only known land plants that contain vitamin B12 are alfalfa and comfrey. It is rich in magnesium, trace elements, biotin, essential fatty acids, pantothenic acid, pyroxidine, phosphorous, magnesium, iron, selenium, zinc and is also a source of eight enzymes and *steroidal saponins*. Alfalfa is one of the richest chlorophyll foods. It is high in nutrients because alfalfa roots travel down as deep as 250 feet into the clean deep earth. It contains natural fluoride that prevents **tooth decay** and is used in the treatment of **arthritis, mineral deficiencies** and most **illnesses.**

Taken daily, one pint of alfalfa sprout juice combined with lettuce juice stimulates **hair growth.**

> **Orange, yellow and dark-green vegetables and fruits are the best sources of beta-carotene,** *American Journal of Epidemiology*, April 1991.

Asparagus

Protects against **cancer**

Builds healthy **capillaries**

Builds red **blood cells**

Stimulates **kidney** and **liver function**

A potent **diuretic**

Asparagus contains high amounts of vitamins A, B-complex, and C, as well as potassium, manganese, and iron. It contains rutin which contributes to a **strong capillary system**. Another important element in asparagus is asparagine, which **stimulates the kidneys**, resulting in diuresis. World wide cancer clinics use 3 tablespoons of pureed asparagus in their therapies. The high amounts of carotene, vitamin C and selenium, make this vegetable excellent for **cancer** treatment.

In preparation, do not cut off the tips until after cooking, this preserves nutrients. Keep the highly nutritious liquid after cooking and drink it.

Fresh asparagus contains high amounts of *histones, folic, and nucleic aids* that stimulate the **immune function**. *Methyl mercaptan*, a substance excreted in the urine after eating asparagus, is also anti-carcinogenic.

Avocado

Reduces risk of **heart attack**

Aids in **blood** and **tissue regeneration**

The avocado is high in protein. The oil contains vitamins A, D, and E, and contains 14 minerals especially copper and iron. Also, avocados are rich in phosphorus, magnesium, calcium, sodium, and manganese. They contain more potassium than bananas, and the potassium is balanced in a ratio with sodium, making it an excellent food for **heart disorders**.

Avocados are very good for **hypoglycemics** because they stabilize the blood sugar. In addition they contain high quantities of protein and beneficial fats, thereby stimulating **tissue growth and healing**.

Another advantage is that avocados are rarely sprayed by growers. Interestingly, the avocado is actually a fruit, although we normally use it as a vegetable.

Green Beans

Helps **gout** and **rheumatism**

Increases **urinary** output

Energizes

Green beans contain: vitamins A, B-complex, and C, chlorophyll, carbohydrates, calcium and phosphorus, copper and cobalt. They are a rare source of inositol, found most in the string bean variety. Green beans have been found to promote the normal function of the **liver** and **pancreas**.

Beets

Aid **lymphatic** function

Aid **gall bladder** and **liver function**

Aid **digestion**

Aid **anemia**, builds **red blood cells**

Since ancient times, beets have been used for **medicinal** purposes.

Beets are full of calcium, phosphorus, sodium potassium, iron and magnesium. Cooking concentrates the minerals. However, vitamins A, B-complex, and C are lost when the beet is cooked. They also contain high amounts of amino acids.

The leaves and roots should be used also, especially for juice. Beet and carrot juices provide a wealth of phosphorus, sulphur, potassium, as well as vitamin A.

Carrots

Powerful **anti-oxidant**

Build healthy **skin** and **tissue**

Good for **heart disease**

Reduce risk of **cancer** (especially lung)

Help stop **diarrhea**

Stimulate **appetite**

Help build healthy **teeth**

Improve **eyesight**

Prevent **eye** and **mucus membrane** infection

Aid **diuresis**

Carrot juice is very important in the treatment of **severe illness**, especially **cancer**. Raw carrots are high in *beta-carotene*, vitamin B-complex, C, D, E, K, iron, calcium, phosphorus, sodium, potassium, magnesium, manganese, sulphur, and copper. Wash them and add them to salads, and soups. Before juicing, wash but do not peel the carrot. It is best to use organic carrots.

Carrot soup is excellent for the treatment of **infantile diarrhea**, even in newborns, premature infants, and in all children suffering from acute **colitis** or **diarrhea**. Adults with acute **enterocolitis**, diarrhea, and all **colon disorders** are helped by using carrot soup and/or fresh juice. Carrot soup also prevents **dehydration** from diarrhea by supplying water and the essential minerals that have been lost.

Although carrots do not contain vitamin A, they do contain *beta-carotene* which the body can convert to vitamin A. *Carotenoids* have been linked to the prevention of certain types of **cancer**, particularly **lung cancer**. Vitamin A may be taken as a supplement in the form of either *beta-carotene*, *retinols*, or a combination of the two.

Dr. J. Michael Gaziana, Cardiologist, Harvard's Brigham and Women's Hospitals, conducted a five year study that revealed a 50% reduction in **heart attack, stroke,** and **cardiovascular** deaths for those who took 50 mg. beta-carotene supplement every day. "It provides a compelling reason for people to include foods rich in *beta-carotene* as part of a balanced diet."

Carrot Soup

3 or 4 large carrots

Scrub carrots well, chop finely, and steam for a few minutes, until the pieces are soft. As an alternative method, cook in one cup of water in a pan fo 15 minutes or until done. Strain through a fine strainer and add enough steam distilled water to make a quart. Add 1/8 teaspoon sea salt. For infants and very young children put in a nursing bottle and eliminate salt.

Celery

Aids **digestion**
Lowers **blood pressure**
Aids **kidney** and **liver function**
A **diuretic**
Controls **dizziness** and **headaches**

Celery contains vitamins A, B-complex, and C, and choline, as well as magnesium, manganese, iron, iodine, copper, potassium, calcium, sulphur, sodium, and phosphorus. It is also rich in pectin. The components in celery help regulate the **nervous system**, by having a calming effect. Celery is also helpful in diseases of **chemical imbalance** and in **arthritis**. Celery is good for **water retention**, **weight loss**, **cancer** and for stimulating the **sexual drive**. In experiments, celery lowered **blood pressure** in rats. It is good for **diabetes**. Celery helps to balance **acidity** in the body. Celery is excellent added to other vegetables as a juice. Use it chopped in soups or with other vegetables to avoid the strong flavor.

It is obvious, celery is good for you!

Chard

Corrects **calcium deficiency**
Improves **digestive** function
A **diuretic**

Chard, often called Swiss chard, is a white rooted beet. It contains vitamins A, and C, potassium, sodium, calcium, and iron. It is used to build **energy**, and as a **diuretic** and a **laxative**. When the juice of chard is mixed with carrot juice it helps control **urinary tract infections, hemorrhoids, constipation**, and **skin diseases**.

Don't overcook! Steam lightly to preserve nutrients.

Chili Peppers

Medicinal for the **lungs**
An expectorant and **decongestant**
Eases chronic **bronchitis** and **emphysema**

Helps dissolve **blood clots**
Kills **pain**

Chili pepper contains *capsaicin*, which causes the mouth to burn when it is consumed. This component has a **soothing effect** on the **bronchial passages and lungs**, producing a secretion that thins the mucus in the respiratory system. Chili peppers are an irritant to the stomach and signal the bronchial cells to pour out fluids, making the lung and throat secretions less thick and sticky. They are good for those suffering from **asthma** and **hypersensitive airways**. The capsaicin has been found to reduce the **swelling of the tracheal and bronchial cells** caused by cigarette smoke and other irritants.

Capsaicin is also a **pain killer**. It causes a reduction in nerve cells of substance P, that relays pain sensations to the central nervous system. Experiments confirm that applying *capsaicin* to an **aching tooth**, drains the dental pulp of substance P, reducing the sensation of pain.

Chili peppers are good, as a fibrinolytic stimulant, meaning that the hot peppers are good at preventing and dissolving **blood clots**. Although the effect of chili peppers only lasts a short while, their frequent consumption reduces the possibility of **circulatory blockage**.

Collards

Improves **nervous system**
Respiratory system
Skeletal system
Urinary system and all glands
Osteoporosis
Helps **colon disorders**
Arthritis
Cancer

A close cousin to kale and an excellent source of calcium and vitamins A and C. Use as you would cabbage, raw in salad, cooked in soups and stews, and with grains or steamed slightly.

If consuming cruciferous vegetables gives you an upset stomach or causes bloating and gas, you may lack Alaphagactrosidase, an enzyme that breaks down certain complex sugars.

Add these vegetables gradually so your system can tolerate them. Start with half a cup two times a week and increase. Beano, a product that provides the missing enzyme may also help. It is found in health food stores.

American Health, June 1992, pg. 44

Corn

A **brain** food
Good for the **nervous system**
A **bone and muscle builder**
Good for **weight gain**
May **lower cholesterol** and aid in preventing **hardening of the arteries.**

Corn provides vitamins, A, B, and C, potassium, phosphorus, iron, zinc, potassium, magnesium, and is also high in fiber. Research at the *University of Nebraska* reports the quality of protein in corn is better than nutritionists once believed. Yellow corn is the best, containing the most nutrients. Corn for many is an allergy-producing food and should be avoided if you have **digestive disorders** or are on a **weight loss** diet. Cornmeal that is enriched with *lysine* makes a complete protein.

Eggplant

Prevents **atherosclerosis**
Enhances **immunity**
Prevents **convulsions**

Eggplant contains a substance that inhibits the rise of **blood cholesterol** induced by fatty foods such as cheese. It binds up the cholesterol in the intestinal tract, so it is not absorbed into the bloodstream. It works best when it is not eaten alone, but with essential fatty acids and cholesterol containing foods.

Compounds called *acopoletin* and *scoparone* block **convulsions**. Using eggplant to prevent **epilepsy** and other causes of convulsions is logical.

Traditionally, the Chinese used eggplant to aid the function of the large intestines, spleen and stomach.

Eggplant, a nightshade vegetable, should be avoided by those who suffer from arthritis.

Mushrooms

Thin the **blood**
Lower **blood cholesterol**
Prevent **cancer**
Stimulate the **immune system**
Inactivate **viruses**

Few medicinal benefits have been linked to the button mushroom, most commonly consumed in the United States. A raw button mushroom contains cancer causing *hydrazides*. *Hydrazides* are killed by cooking. As with all mushrooms, the protein content is high. However, Oriental mushrooms contain elements that stimulate the **immune system**, hindering **blood clotting**, and slowing the development of **cancer**.

There are five types with proven benefits: Enoki, Oyster, Reishi, Shiitake, and Tree ear.

Enoki is a white stringy mushroom, usually used in soups or eaten raw. They have a delicate flavor. It stimulates the **immune system** and helps fight **viruses** and **tumors**.

The oyster mushroom is a white lily-like fungus, with a oysterlike flavor, used primarily in sauces, vegetable sautes or stuffings. In animal studies it has been found to be effective against **cancer**.

The shiitake mushroom is a large brown beefy mushroom, good for soup stock, remember to remove the woody stems before serving. Shitakes are tough and need a longer cooking time than other mushrooms. They contain the **antiviral** substance, *lentinan,* that stimulates the **immune system**. Japanese experiments have found *lentinan* to be more powerful than the prescription antiviral drug Amantadine hydrochloride. The shiitake stimulates the immune system to produce more *interferon,* a natural compound that fights *viruses and cancer.*

Tree-ear mushrooms can prevent **blood platelets** from sticking together, this anticoagulant activity may aid in preventing **heart attacks**. Tree-ears have also been **found to slow cancer** in animals.

Mushrooms found in the Produce Department

Cepe mushrooms have flat tops and large caps, a rich meaty flavor good in soup stocks and baked squash and with other veggies, as well as stuffing. Rinse them well before cooking.

Chanterelle mushrooms are golden and trumpet shaped, they have a light flavor, good in soups and sauces. They are often used in gourmet cooking to make rich cream sauces. Use soon after buying.

Morel mushrooms resemble brown sponges on a thick stem. Wash carefully to remove insects. They have a rich flavor, good in omelets and sauces and with broiled tempeh or tofu.

Porcini mushrooms have large caps with fat, beige stems and a flavor similar to hazelnuts. They are good in soups and sauces.

Okra

Helps many **intestinal disorders** including:
Colitis
Inflammation of the colon and spastic colon
Diverticulitis

Stomach **ulcers**

An excellent demulient food which protects the internal membranes and relieves irritations of the linings of the **digestive tract**.

Dr. J. Meyer, Chicago did a study using a dry powdered form of okra to treat ulcers of the stomach and **inflammation of the intestine** with good results.

Onions

Known to benefit in:
Hay fever and **asthma**
Colds and **fever**
Bronchitis and **croup**
Lung infection
Heart disease
High blood pressure
Blood cleansing

A very important vegetable from the same family as garlic. The Egyptians regarded the onion as a symbol of the universe because of its sheaths (the layers that encircle the bulb).

Contains an acrid, volatile oil, calcium, magnesium, phosphorus, sulphur, potassium, sodium, iron, vitamins A, B, and C, traces of zinc, iodine, silicon, phosphoric acids, and citrate of lime. Onions are potent **antioxidants.**

Effective as a **poultice**, applied to the chest for **colds, congestions** and **bronchitis** and on the ear for **ear infections**. Also as a syrup for **coughs** and **bronchitis**. For croup - slice into thin slices and place in a small amount of honey and let stand for about two hours. Makes a syrup for relief of **asthma, colds, sore throat,** and **bronchitis**. For colds, place a slice in hot water for a few minutes and sip throughout the day. Place a slice by your beside to get relief from **congestion.**

Parsley

Improves function of:
Kidneys, bladder and **prostate**
Adrenal and **thyroid gland**
A **diuretic**
A solvent for uric acid
Corrects **vitamin deficiency**
Assists **digestion**

Parsley is extremely high in nutrients. Only a small amount of juice is needed. Very rich in vitamins A, B1, B-complex, C, potassium, manganese, phosphorus, calcium, and iron. Parsley contains *mucilage, volatile oil and apiol.*

For **urinary tract disorders** drink as a tea, dry the fresh leaves or purchase as a tea in a health food store. An excellent **cleanser and potentiator of all bodily functions.**

Parsnips

Colon disorders
Constipation
Heart problems
High blood pressure

Parsnips contain more fiber than any common vegetable. They are rich in potassium, and sweet and delicious. They are also powerful **cancer** fighters, by helping to keep the digestive tract free of cancer causing substances.

Prepare the same as potatoes; steam, bake, in soups, stews and grated in salads.

Combine with other vegetables for a side dish.

Don't choose larger parsnips as small to medium ones are more tender.

Peas

Prevent **appendicitis** and **ulcers**
High in **anti-fertility** agents
Lowers **blood cholesterol**
Controls **blood sugar**
Lowers **blood pressure**

Studies in Wales and England have found a connection between pea consumption and low rates of **acute appendicitis**. The vegetable is thought to contain a chemical that suppresses organisms which cause infection in the appendicular wall.

Peas contain high amounts of fiber, carotene, plus vitamin C, and no fat, making them a good **cancer** fighter. **Don't buy canned peas.**

Puree the peas when used as a treatment for **ulcers**. Peas contain an **anti-fertility** chemical, *m-xylohydroquinone*. This compound meddles with the reproductive hormones estrogen and progesterone, reducing fertility. Rats fed a diet containing 30% peas stopped having litters. The pea's chemical has not been produced as a contraceptive because the performance is not as predictable as the Pill.

The pea is high in soluble fiber, this reduces the level of the harmful *LDL cholesterol.* Green peas contain the same amount of soluble fiber as kidney beans, 2.7 grams per half cup. Lentils and split peas are also high in soluble fiber, with 1.7 grams per half cup. They help control **blood sugar level** and may **lower blood pressure.**

Peppers, Green & Red

These sweet peppers contain more vitamin C than citrus fruits. Because of their extra high vitamin C content they are good for all types of **illnesses**.

Cancer and most **degenerative diseases** thrive in an acid environment as a result sweet peppers are a good substitute for citrus fruits.

Potatoes

Contain **anti-cancer** substances
Aid in **lowering blood pressure**
Balance **alkalinity** and **acidity** in body

The potato is an almost perfect food. Good for **alkaline** body conditions and rich in vitamins, minerals and protein. Very high in vitamins A, B, and C, and potassium.

When consumed raw white potatoes have high concentrations of *protease inhibitors*, compounds known to block carcinogens. The chemicals in potatoes protect against **viruses** even better than soybean inhibitors. The skin of the potato is particularly rich in *chlorogenic acid* that prevents **cell mutations**, the precursor to **cancer**. The skins have antioxidant activity which gives them the ability to neutralize free radicals that damage cells.

The consumption of potatoes could be detrimental to **diabetics**, as they raise insulin and blood sugar levels quickly.

A baked potato, eaten with the skin, has about 220 calories, is high in vitamins B, and C, iron, potassium, and has a small amount of protein and fiber.

When you add fat to the potato it reduces the nutritional qualities. Unfortunately much of America's potatoes are eaten fried, dehydrated, or frozen. French fries and hash browns are soaked in fat. Mashed potatoes and scalloped potatoes are made with butter and milk, or cream. Baked potatoes are often served with butter and sour cream. Potato salad is mostly fat, because of the mayonnaise content.

Alternatives for baked potato toppings include mashed avocado, nonfat plain yogurt, low fat cottage cheese, herbs, or even steamed vegetables. Mix mashed potatoes with yogurt or low fat milk, and omit the butter.

To give the taste of fried potatoes without the calories of the fat, preheat your oven to 400 degrees, slice a potato thin, lightly coat a cookie tray with oil, arrange potatoes in a thin layer and bake for 30 minutes. Turn once while cooking.

Eat the potato skin to get the greatest amount of nutrients from your potato. **Do not eat the skin if it is green, it may make you ill, if eaten in large quantities.** So peel away the green area and any sprouts. To keep potatoes fresh buy them in small quantities. When exposed to light potatoes produce solanine, a toxic chemical, this is the reason they turn green. If you see green or partially green potatoes, they have been exposed to some light.

Raw potato juice is an excellent source of potassium and good for all **heart disorders**. Cut out the very center and juice the well-scrubbed skins with about one inch of potato. When boiling potatoes, drink the broth that is left over, as most of the potassium content is lost in the water. Steam potatoes instead of boiling to avoid losing the potassium. **Potatoes should be avoided if you are suffering from arthritis.**

Tomatoes

Lower risk of **cancer**
Neutralize uric acid found in animal products
Aid in **cleansing of toxins**
Prevent **appendicitis** and **digestive disorders**

A study of 14,000 American men and 3,000 Norwegian men showed that eating tomatoes more than fourteen times a month cut the chances of **lung cancer**. The tomato is not high in *beta-carotene*, but has a high concentrate of *lycopene*, another type of *carotene*, which possibly gives the tomato its cancer-protecting qualities. A study done in Wales (the United Kingdom) showed tomatoes to be a protection against **acute appendicitis** and other **digestive disorders**. Fresh, vine ripened tomatoes are the best. **Tomatoes should be avoided by those suffering from arthritis.**

What is the Healthiest Vegetable ?

Recent studies at the Center for Science in the Public Interest have found sweet potatoes to be the healthiest of all vegetables.

The study was based on the percentage of the Recommended Daily Allowance for six nutrients: vitamin A, vitamin C, calcium, iron, folate and copper in each vegetable.

Raw carrot was second followed by collard greens, red peppers, kale, dandelion greens, spinach and broccoli.

Yams

A variety of sweet potato that:

Lowers risk of **cancer**

May lower **blood cholesterol**

Studies reveal that sweet potatoes, winter squash, and carrots are **particularly helpful in forestalling lung cancer, even for ex-smokers**. *The National Cancer Institute* found that men who ate half a cup of sweet potatoes, carrots or winter squash every day were half as likely to develop **lung cancer** than men who ate almost none.

Dark orange vegetables somehow interfere with the processes that lead to lung cancer. Smokers who have quit within the last five years are those most likely to benefit from these vegetables. Even those who have quit years ago can reduce their chances by eating these vegetables.

Non-smokers, who are afraid of developing **cancer** from passive smoke, should eat yams. These deep orange vegetables protect nonsmokers, particularly women.

The main cancer fighter found in yams is *beta-carotene*, though they are also rich in *protease inhibitors*, which have been found to stop cancer in animals. The *protease inhibitors* also protect the body against **viruses.**

The darker orange coloring of the yam indicates a higher concentration of disease fighting carotenoids.

The Bottom Line

Vegetables contain many **cancer** fighting substances. *Indoles* (cancer inhibitors) are found in cabbage and related vegetables like broccoli, brussels sprouts, cauliflower, kale, and mustard greens, all members of **The Magnificent Twelve.** *Sterols* are found in cucumbers, *terpines* in citrus fruits. *Polyacetylenes* are in parsley, *sulphur* compounds in garlic, and *osoflavones* are found in peanuts, beans, and peas. *Lignins* come from flaxseeds, *quinones* from rosemary, and *triterpenoids* from licorice root.

All plant life has built-in protection against insects. These "protective pesticides" are usually in micro amounts and safe for human consumption. *Dr. Bruce Ames*, a biochemist, has devised the *Ames Test*, designed to measure the levels of these plant "pesticides," and other potential lethal substances in ordinary foods, including foreign herbicides and other pollutants, *Business Week Science and Technology, Oct. 1990.* How amazing, the vegetable kingdom has their "defense system" too.

Science News, Aug. 12, 1989, reported that **obese people** and **heavy alcohol drinkers** have a far greater incidence of **cancer** than those whose diets are high in fresh vegetables and fruits. There are many other reports, confirming our contention, that whole fresh vegetables and fruits were designed by The Creator of all things, to nourish and protect us. You can be truly blessed with good health by regularly consuming the **Magnificent 12**, and other vegetables.

"**Two-thirds of all deaths in 1987 in this country could be attributed to diet,**" **says the** *Surgeon General of the U.S.* **Heart disease** is still the number one killer in the United States. Since 1985, more than one million Americans have a **heart attack** every year that's two heart attacks occuring each minute. **Cancer** is our number two health offender, and one out of every four Americans will die of cancer. According to the American Cancer Society, as reported in *East West Journal, March 1981,* "cancer takes a life every 60 seconds in this country. Over 765,000 Americans are told they have cancer each year and over 1 million cases are treated each year."

Dr. William Castelli, director of the Federal government's *Framingham Heart Study in Massachusetts*, remarked in reference to a group of macrobiotic vegetarians in Boston that, "the vegans have cholesterol levels so low, they'd never get a heart attack."

"By eating more beans, whole grains, vegetables, fruit, fiber, vitamins A and C, and other substances (such as *indoles* and cruciferous vegetables or *protease inhibitors* in legumes) in their foods, vegetarians might prevent the development of cancer," says *Drs. Phillips and Snowden.* They have monitored the health of 25,000 Seventh Day Adventists for over 20 years at *Loma Linda University.*

Chemical fertilizers adversely affect the quality of crops, according to *Sharon Hornick, Ph.D.*, a USDA researcher. In addition to nutritional losses, chemically fertilized crops have decreases in the following areas:

taste, storage ability, insect resistance, and disease resistance

Chemically grown Kale, for example was found to have only one-half the vitamin C content of organically-grown kale.

PRODUCE NUTRITION INFORMATION CHART

■ VEGETABLES (RAW)

	Total Calories	Protein	Carbohydrate	Total Fat	Dietary Fiber	Sodium	Vitamin A	Vitamin C	Calcium	Iron
	kcal	g	g	g	g	mg	\% U.S. RDA			
Asparagus, 5 spears (3.5oz/93g)	18	2	2	0	0	0	10	10	*	*
Bell Pepper, 1 medium (5.5oz/148g)	25	1	5	1	2	0	2	130	*	*
Broccoli, 1 medium stalk (5.5oz/148g)	40	5	4	1	5	75	10	240	6	4
Cabbage, Green, 1/12 medium head (3oz/84g)	18	1	3	0	2	30	*	70	4	*
Carrot, 1 medium (7" long, 1½" diameter), (3oz/78g)	40	1	8	1	1	40	330	8	2	*
Cauliflower, 1/6 medium head (3oz/99g)	18	2	3	0	2	45	*	110	2	2
Celery, 2 medium stalks (4oz/110g)	20	1	4	0	2	140	*	15	4	*
Corn, Sweet, kernels from 1 medium ear (3oz/90g)	75	3	17	1	1	15	5	10	*	3
Cucumber, 1/3 medium (3.5oz/99g)	18	1	3	0	0	0	4	6	2	2
Green Bean, (snap), ¾ cup cut (3oz/83g)	14	1	2	0	3	0	2	8	4	*
Green Onion, ¼ cup chopped (1oz/25g)	7	0	1	0	0	0	3	20	*	5
Lettuce, Iceberg, 1/6 medium head (3oz/89g)	20	1	4	0	1	10	2	4	*	*
Lettuce, Leaf, 1½ cups shredded (3oz/85g)	12	1	1	0	1	40	20	4	4	*
Mushroom, 5 medium (3oz/84g)	25	3	3	0	0	0	*	2	*	*
Onion, 1 medium (5.5oz/148g)	60	1	14	0	3	10	*	20	4	*
Potato, 1 medium (5.5oz/148g)	110	3	23	0	3	10	*	50	*	8
Radish, 7 radishes (3oz/85g)	20	0	3	0	0	35	*	30	*	*
Squash, Summer, ½ medium (3.5oz/98g)	20	1	3	0	1	0	4	25	2	2
Sweet Potato, 1 medium (5"long, 2"diameter), (4.5oz/130g)	140	2	32	0	3	15	520	50	3	4
Tomato, 1 medium (5.5oz/148g)	35	1	6	1	1	10	20	40	*	2

(Data source: FDA)

* Contains less than 2% of U.S. RDA

Ways to Eat 6 Vegetables & Fruits a Day

Does eating six servings of fruits and vegetables a day sound like a lot? If so, try these ideas.
- *Serve soup*--use vegetables and legumes as a base for soups or as added ingredients.
- *Thicken sauces without fat*--substitute cooked and pureed vegetables for cream or whole milk.
- *Be creative*--pasta and stir-fry dishes are ideal ways to serve lots of different vegetables and small portions of meat.
- *Enhance old standbys*--add fruit to your breakfast cereal and raw, grated vegetables or fruit to muffins and cookies.
- *Don't let lettuce limit salads*--choose a wider variety of greens, including arugula, chicory, collards, dandelion greens, kale, mustard greens, spinach and watercress.
- *Steam them and serve over rice*

Mayo Clinic Health Letter, July 1992, pg.2

Vegetarian Varieties

The *Institute of Food Technologists*, in the July 1991 issue of *Food Technology*, describes six types of vegetarians.

semi-vegetarian--dairy foods, eggs, chicken, and fish, no other animal flesh
pesco-vegetarian--dairy foods, eggs, and fish, no other animal flesh
lacto-ovo-vegetarian--dairy foods and eggs, no animal flesh
ovo-vegetarian--eggs, but no dairy foods or animal flesh
vegan--no animal food of any type

Buying Guide for Dried Fruit

- All dried fruits should be dipped or soaked in boiling water to remove bacteria that forms during the drying and storing process
- Boil water and remove it from the stove
- Drop in dried fruit for a few seconds, remove it from the water
- Store them in the refrigerator until used

Dried fruit is good chopped and added to cereals, in baking and mashed into a puree to use as a sweetener or to flavor yogurt.

Additives

Sulphur

Used in products to preserve them, specifically so they will retain their light color during and after drying. Products that are not sulphured will turn a dark brown or black after drying. Sulphur will turn an alkaline fruit acidic. It is considered by most health-oriented people to be a harmful substance. However, most consumers prefer the appearance of sulphured dried fruits.

Potassium Sorbate

A preservative added to high-moisture dried fruits, such as figs and pitted prunes. Without this preservative, the fruits with a high-moisture content would become moldy a few days after being dried. Preservatives do not have to be labeled on bulk packs of dried fruits and generally are not. Beware of suppliers who claim their fruits do not have preservatives. If it is true, you will have disastrous mold problems. And if not, why not buy from an honest supplier who will tell you up front exactly what you are buying?

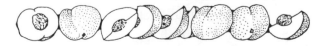

Organically Grown

Products grown without the use of harmful pesticides or chemical fertilizers are called organically grown. Considered better by most people, they are generally 20 - 40% higher in price. Therefore many shoppers avoid buying them.

Following are some clues that will help you determine what types of chemical additives might be in dried fruits. The best dried fruits to buy are those without additives, like suphur. You want to purchase dried fruit that is only fresh fruit with the water removed.

FOOD IRRADIATION

Food Irradiation is a controversial subject. It is supposed to kill organisms that damage foods and/or make people ill, so it cuts down on spoilage. Opponents say it is costly, adds another step to food processing, may pose a danger to human health and is a clear threat to the environment.

Irradiation is the process of treating foods with gamma radiation from radioactive cobalt or cesium or other sources of x-rays.

Current choices for irradiation are fresh produce like strawberries, potatoes and other perishable items like poultry, seafood and pork. These have already been approved by the FDA for irradiation, though few of these items and no meats have been offered for sale.

University of California at Berkley Wellness Letter, May 1992

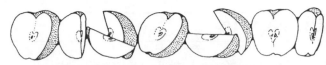

Apples

Varieties - Many kinds
Sulphured - White in color
Unsulphured - Off white in color

Figs

Varieties

California calimyrna - a big, brown, sweet fig from Turkey grown in California.

Black Mission - a black fig
White fig - chewy, gray fig
Adriatic - dark brown fig, strong flavored
Turkish Smyrna - gray, very sweet fig
Greek string - gray, very chewy fig

Fig Processing

Pulled - The hard tip of the stem has been pulled off.
Retorted - Hydrated to make softer and remove the natural sugar coating on the outside of the figs.

Papaya

Unsweetened

It is uncommon to find unsweetened papaya. The unsweetened variety would taste very bland, and cost five times that of regularly sweetened papaya. It is very thin and chewy, like shoe leather.

Honey Dipped

After papaya is sweetened in a sugar concentrate, it is dipped in a honey water. This product has the same amount of sugar as the sweetened product and also has a coating of honey.

Regular Sweetened

A product with sugar which Americans love.

Low Sugar

Has high amounts of sugar, though not quite as high as regular sweetened papaya.

Color

Primary - Red to orange to yellow but varies with variety of papaya.
Minor - Small amounts of color are sometimes added.

Secondary Darkness
Varies due to the amount of sulphur used. An unsulphured papaya would be dark brown, it is unlikely that you could get anyone to buy it.
Minor Darkness
Varies due to how ripe the papaya is when picked.

Peaches

Sulphured - Yellow in color
Unsulphured - Dark brown in color

Pears

Sulphured - Yellow in color
Unsulphured - Dark brown in color

Prunes

Varieties

Italian - naturally tart, very distinctive flavor
Brooks - slightly tart yet sweet prune
French/Date - very sweet, fancy store quality
Moyer/Perfection - sweet, large and meaty

Pitted

Ashlock Process - Pit is punched through a hole leaving the prune whole and unblemished.
Ellliot Process - Prune is pushed by a rubber roller into a spiked roller that catches the pit.
Sunsweet Process - Usually they pit in their own retail pack, the process is highly secret, but probably similar to the Ashlock Process.

Pineapple

Most are from Taiwan and Thailand

Regular   Sweetened
Another sugar-coated product that Americans love.

Low   Sugar
Sweetened less than the regular sweetened pineapple, but still contains high amounts of sugar.

Honey-Dipped
Regular sweetened pineapple that is dipped in a honey water solution.

Unsweetened   Pineapple
No sugar and a a very chewy product. Generally it has a bitter, sharp, tart taste.
(If it tastes sweet, it 's sweetened pineapple.)
Unsweetened pineapple is generally high in *bromelain*, a good enzyme, but if you eat several pieces of this type of pineapple, the tongue will feel slightly burned as the brom-elain eats away at the surface.
Timber Crest Farms' (Sonoma Brand) dricd pineapple is an organically grown product. It does **not** contain sugar, and is just fresh pineapple with the water removed.

Raisins

Varieties
Thompson - made from the light green Thompson seedless grapes
Monukka - *big,* black, and high in nutrition, sometimes chewy and seedy
Ruby Red - uncommon store item.
Other Varieties
Unsulphured - black in color
Sulphured - yellow in color
A darker suphured raisin occurs when a riper grape is picked.
Grades
Fancy - very light greenish yellow
Extra Choice - dark yellow
Choice - yellow brown
Sun dried - black raisin
Tunnel dried - dark brown, less oxidation when drying

The USDA's Dietary Guidelines

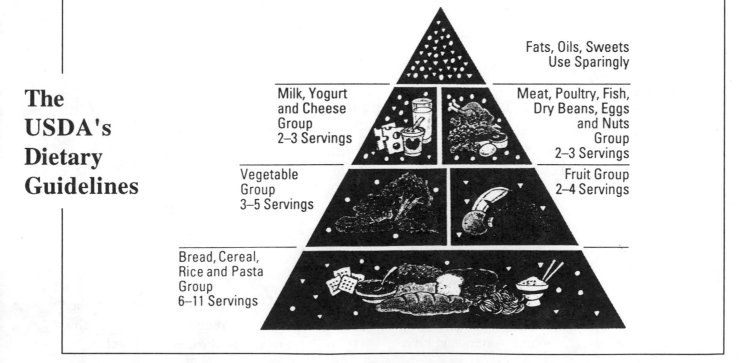

The USDA's dietary guidelines recommend that you eat four to six servings of fatty milk, meat and eggs everyday, even though research shows these foods promote cancer and heart disease. For wellness eat more vegetables, fruit, beans, whole grains, seeds and nuts in place of these fatty foods.

Facts on Fat & Fish

The Fat Story

There are good and "bad" fats -- some toxic, some neutral, and some essential to good health. All animal and plant fats, can be broken down into fatty acids, glycerin, and water. Fats and lipids are better energy sources than protein or carbohydrates. We need to add fats to our diets because they carry the fat-soluble vitamins A, D, E, and K. Vitamin K is easily destroyed by the use of mineral oil, Heparin and Dicumarol (blood thinners), drugs or aspirin. Most people overlook the need for vitamin K, but it has recently been linked to intestinal disorders. It is important in the treatment of arthritis. One rich source of vitamin K is alfalfa.

Fats have the highest calorie density of all foods 9 calories per gram, for both protein and carbohydrates, it's 4 calories per gram. One tablespoon of oil contains 120 calories, all pure fat and energy. Fats act as an intestinal lubricant and combine with phosphorous to form a substance that helps build tissues and body cells. Fats stay in the digestive tract for longer periods, giving us a full, satisfied feeling after a meal. They also generate body heat. Fats soothe the nerves and coat them with a protective shield. Fat is found in all body cells in combination with other nutrients. Essential fatty acids are a most important link in our health chain.

The right kind of fat is essential for good health. Most people consume too much of the wrong kind. Excess fat is stored in the liver, in arteries around the heart and in all tissue. Cancer of the breast, prostate, and colon, not to mention obesity and an increased risk of heart attack, are linked to a high fat consumption. The typical American diet consists of 40-50% fat, a primary reason for the rise in the disorders mentioned above.

SATURATED FATS

Saturated fat is found in all animal products and many vegetable oils:

Butter/lard	Milk/cream
Poultry (mainly skin)	Processed cheeses
Beef	Cheese
Chocolate desserts	Bacon/pork
Palm kernel oils	Palm
Coconut	Coconut oils

Saturated fats are behind many health problems and should be omitted from your diet. They are behind heart disorders and arteriosclerosis (hardening of the arteries). High intake of saturated fats have been shown to elevate serum cholesterol and contribute to heart disease and cancer. Do not consume saturated fats! They slow the liver's ability to remove artery-clogging LDL (low density lipo proteins) from the blood. **However, the monounsaturated and polyunsaturated fats aid in removing LDL (bad fats) from the blood stream.**

Beware of labels stating no cholesterol. Saturated fats can elevate cholesterol in the blood stream and damage coronary arteries. The worst fat to consume is coconut oil, and the next is palm oil. These are called "vegetable oils" on labels and contain almost as much "bad" fat as lard (pure saturated animal fat).

Saturated fat is the culprit behind elevated cholesterol. Experiments suggest that the body has trouble changing the molecules of this fat when it has been exposed to extremely high heat, like in the hydrogenating process--it can be carcinogenic (cancer-causing). Hydrogenated fats are excessive in margarine or any oil that is firm at room temperature.

Hydrogenated or hardened oils are almost impossible for the system to assimilate. Foods fried in oil, like those from fast-food chains and many restaurants, cause a vitamin F ("good" polyunsaturated fat) deficiency.

When you hydrogenate (harden) fat, it destroys the essential fatty acids, a process used to prolong shelf life. Most foods on the grocer's shelf have many chemicals added for this purpose.

Soybean oil is most commonly hydrogenated. In 1988, the average American consumed 5 gallons of soybean oil. This is more than all other fats and oils combined. Half of that amount was partially hydrogenated. Soybean oil is fast becoming a prevalent allergy-producing food. Liquid soybean oil is only 15% saturated, along with safflower, corn, and olive oils. Both saturated and unsaturated fatty acids are present in all vegetable and animal fats. But partially-hydrogenated soybean oil, which is processed to make shortening like Crisco, increases the fat to 25%. This is still much better than palm oil, which is 52% saturated fat, and coconut oil which is 92% fat.

There are 3 types of fats found in oils: *monounsaturated fats, polyunsaturated fats,* and *saturated fats.* Polyunsaturated fats and their near relation monounsaturates, are the good fats. The information below should help you understand different fats, and the nature of the different oils you can purchase.

Polyunsaturated Fats

Polyunsaturated fats are liquid and remain that way--ready for use. *Linoleic* and *linolenic acid,* essential fatty acids also known as Vitamin F, are found primarily in:

Nuts	Seeds
Vegetables	Fish
Walnut oil	Soybeans

Highest in polyunsaturated fats are:

Safflower oil	Primrose oil
Wheat germ oil	Cod liver oil
Pine nuts	Corn oil
Cottonseed oil	Sesame oil
Sunflower seeds	Flax oil
Some soft margarines	Pecans
Soy oil	

usually from health food stores

Remember, when these are over processed, many benefits are lost. <u>Use only cold- or expeller-pressed oils.</u>

Polyunsaturates are essential for good health. Fish are the best source of polyunsaturated fats. Fish from cold, deep waters have the highest content of these oils. Atlantic mackerel, Atlantic herring, salmon and albacore tuna are the highest in the *omega 3* fatty acids (polyunsaturated). These help to keep blood clots from forming in the arteries and lower cholesterol levels, reducing the chance of heart problems. They are also known to reduce joint inflammation in arthritis, and are good for female disorders and breast disease, and beneficial attributes would fill a book by

themselves. Frozen fish is better than fresh fish because by the time you purchase fresh fish at the market, it is 7-10 days old. Fish are normally frozen within 4 hours after a catch and the freezing kills bacteria. Fish should not smell "fishy," but like a fresh-grated cucumber. When a fish smells, the fatty acids have started to break down becoming rancid.

Monounsaturated Fats

Monounsaturated fats are found in several foods, but not in red meats. This form is desirable because it doesn't effect the blood-cholesterol level. It is acceptable in the diets of those with cholesterol problems.

Monosaturated fats are found in:

Olive oil	Peanut
Avocado	Cashews
Pecans	Almonds
Canola oil	Hazelnuts
Olive oil in soft or solid form	

Diets high in monounsaturated fats lower *"bad"*, LDL cholesterol without lowering *"good"* HDL. *New England Journal of Medicine,* March 20, 1986. These oils, *especially olive oil* are better than polyunsaturated fats like corn oil.

Virgin olive oil is the best and the hardest to find. Olive oil has cholesterol-lowering benefits and helps control blood pressure and diabetes. It will not become rancid like most oils do without refrigeration. The unrefined olive oil should be kept refrigerated. Olive oil is especially good for salad dressing. It is not good for frying.

Canola is one of the oils with the least amount of saturated fat and highest in monounsaturates. Some authorities believe these are superior to polyunsaturates for lowering cholesterol.

Canola has 10% linolenic acid, a polyunsaturate and essential fatty acid, and is also rich in *Omega-3's.* Canola is 6% saturated, 36% polyunsaturated (26% of which is linolenic acid), and high in monounsaturates (58%). Linolenic acid is important in membrane structures and in the synthesis of metabolically active substances like *prostaglandins.*

A study has shown that olive oil lowered LDL even more than a low-fat diet, without changing the IIDL, *the American Journal of Clinical Nutrition*, June 1988.

A tablespoon of olive oil averages almost 10 grams of monounsaturated fat.

You can get the same amount from these nutritious alternatives:

4 teaspoons unrefined canola oil
1-1/2 tablespoons raw almond butter
1/2 fresh avocado
1/4 cup raw almonds
3 tablespoons raw hazelnuts
2 tablespoons raw macadamia nuts
1/4 cup raw pecans
1/4 cup raw pistachios

The body uses only arachidonic acid. The linolenic and linoleic acids of the monosaturated fats can be converted to arachidonic acid in the liver.

In a study conducted at the *University of Manitoba*, young men were fed a diet with canola products. These men experienced a lowering in serum-cholesterol levels. Canola oil supplied nearly all the fat in the diet and 38% of all the energy requirements.

Toxic Substances in Oils

There are many toxic substances in some oils, even canola contains erucic acid. This acid can effect many organs. During the 1960's, canola oil was marketed containing 40% erucic acid. Now with improved government standards, canola oil contains only 5%. This oil is a good choice with the new standard. Even castor oil contains 80% ricinoleic acid. This is why the body throws off this oil and everything else in the intestines quickly.

Peanut oil may contain carcinogenic substances because peanuts are grown in damp places and contaminated by fungus. Aflatoxins are found primarily in peanuts and corn, but traces are in many other grains. Aflatoxins may cause liver cancer.

Peanut oil, even though it is a monounsaturated oil and is only 17% saturated, appears to promote arteriosclerosis - hardening of the arteries. *Pathology Professor Vesselinovitch, University of Chicago*.

Cottonseed oil contains up to 1.2% of a cyclopropene fatty acid that has a toxic effect on the liver and gall bladder. It also interferes with the functioning of the needed essential fatty acids. This oil enhances the potential of the cancer-causing aflatoxins in the body. Cottonseed also contains gossypol, a substance containing benzene rings, which may irritate the digestive tract. This oil may also cause shortness of breath and water retention in the lungs. Cottonseed also has the highest content of pesticide residues. Cotton and rape seed oils contain toxic ingredients also, even though they may be natural.

One must be very careful not to use rancid oils. Heating oils to high temperatures produces free radicals which damage the body. **All oils should be refrigerated**. Oils should be marketed in dark containers to protecting them from light and heat.

VITAMIN E-THE PROTECTOR

Vitamin E will protect the body's cell membranes from free radical damage that takes place when oils are heated or rancid ones are ingested.

Pesticides, herbicides, chemicals, and other foreign substances are stored in the fatty tissues of animals. The more animal and dairy products you consume, the more chemical toxins you ingest. You can't avoid eating carcinogenic substances, if you consistently consume the wrong foods, and animal fat is one of the worst!

HIGHEST IN MONOUNSATURATED FATS

Monounsaturated fats lower "bad" LDL cholesterol without lowering "good" HDL.

OIL	%MONO	%POLY	%SAT	COMMENTS
OLIVE	11	9	14	Virgin olive oil is best and also hard to find. Olive oil has cholesterol-lowering benefits and may help control blood pressure and diabetes. It will not become rancid like most oils without refrigeration. Good for salad dressings, etc.
AVOCADO	74	14	12	These oils can contribute to a healthy monounsaturated intake. The high price, required refrigeration and strong taste make these less popular oils. They are good rubbed on the skin as a moisturizers.
ALMOND	73	18	9	
APRICOT	63	31	6	
CANOLA	58	36	6	Canola oil has a high percent of monounsaturates. The fatty acids in canola may have the same blood-fat and blood pressure-lowering benefits as fish oil. Canola oil is next best to olive oil, with a milker flavor.
PEANUT	48	34	18	
SESAME	42	43	15	Unrefined types do not withstand high cooking temperatures well, but refined types do. This is still a good oil to use for salad dressings, etc.

HIGHEST IN POLYUNSATURATED FATS

Polyunsaturated fats reduce both "bad" LDL and "good" HDL.

OIL	%MONO	%POLY	%SAT	COMMENTS
SAFFLOWER	13	78	9	Both contain immune-boosting vitamin-E.
SUNFLOWER	20	69	11	
WALNUT	24	66	10	Not good for frying. Rich in omega-3 fatty acids. Rich in vitamin E
WHEAT GERM				
CORN	25	62	13	A good all-purpose oil, but should be avoided by those with corn allergies.
SOYBEAN	24	61	15	Contains linoleic acid which is converted to the same fatty acids found in fish oil. High vitamin-E content also.
COTTONSEED	19	54	27	This is a cotton by-product found in most commercially baked goods.

HIGHEST IN SATURATED FATS

Do Not Consume - Linked to elevated serum cholesterol and contributes to heart disease and cancer.

OIL	%MONO	%POLY	%SAT	COMMENTS
COCONUT	6	2	92	Contains lauric acid which is linked to clogged arteries.
PALM KERNEL	12	2	86	
BUTTER	30	4	51	Relatively high percentage of monounsaturated fats.
PALM	39	10	52	

How Oils are Processed

Expeller-pressing

A screw or expeller-type press is used to crush the seeds. The seeds are pushed against a metal press head in a continually rotating movement and a spiral shaped auger moves the seeds forward similar to a meat grinder. The oil is squeezed out of the seed by force of pressure. This pressed oil may be filtered then bottled as "cold-pressed", natural, crude, or unrefined oil. This pressing process takes only a few minutes at 85-95 degrees. **This pressed oil is the best type to purchase.**

Refining

This process involves mixing the oil with caustic soda (-sodium hydroxide - NaOH), which is a very corrosive base). A mixture of NaOH and sodium carbonate (Na_2CO_3) may be used, agitated, and then separated, removing the free fatty acids from the oil. Phospholipids, protein-like substances, and minerals are also removed in this process. The oil still contains pigments, usually yellow or red. The refining temperature is around 75 degrees.

Degumming

Degumming involves the removal of protein-like compounds, complex carbohydrates, and true gums from the oil. Lecithin is isolated and sold separately in health food stores. Degumming also removes chlorophyll, calcium, magnesium, iron, and copper from the oil. Degumming is carried out at 60 degrees.

People who eat a high-meat diet and less fish have higher cancer rates, *Science News,* June 24, 1989. Obese people and those who smoke, and drink heavily are at a high risk for cancer, but diets high in raw vegetables may be preventative, *Science News,*   August 12, 1989.

Solvent extraction

The oil is removed from the seed by dissolving it out of the seed meal using a solvent (such as hexane), at temperatures of 55-65 degrees. Traces of the solvent remain in these oils. The oils from expeller-pressed and solvent extracted problems may be combined and sold as "unrefined" oil. Unrefined oil is treated by several processes (degumming, bleaching, refining, and deodorizing).

Bleaching

Chlorophyll, beta-carotene, and traces of soap are removed by the use of filters, acid-treated activated clay, and/or Fuller's earth. Natural polycyclic and aromatic substances are removed, taking place at 110 degrees for 15-30 minutes.

Supermarket process

Refined oils found in supermarkets have several synthetic antioxidants added to them to replace the natural vitamin E and beta-carotene, which are removed during refining. This list of substances includes: butylated hydroxytoluene (BHT), butylated hydroxyanisole (BHA), propyl gallate, tertiary butyhydroquinone (TBHQ), citric acid, and methylsilicone. A defoamer is added, and the oil is then bottled and sold.

Deodorization

Aromatic oils and free-fatty acids are removed by steam distillation and the exclusion of air during this process. Pungent odors and unpleasant tastes not present in the natural seed before processing are also removed. Deodorization takes place at extreme temperatures of 240-270 degrees for 30-60 minutes. The oil then becomes tasteless and cannot be distinguished from oils derived from other sources treated in a similar manner.

Vitamin-and-mineral-deficient oils are the result of this treatment. The oil can still be sold as "cold-pressed" because no external heat was applied during the pressing of the oil. Understanding the difference between true "cold-pressed" oil and the other processed oils is very important.

LOOKING AT THE REFINERY

Be aware of how oils are processed, the ingredients they contain and what has been removed. A product may be advertised as unsaturate but manufacturers don't have to list the trans-fatty content. These act like saturated fats in the body.

Margarine and shortening are hydrogenated oils and tend to act like saturated fats in the body. They are bad for your health and raise cholesterol levels.

Purchase margarines with less hydrogenated oil from a health food store. Look carefully at the ingredients listed first. The first ingredient listed is the one found in the greatest amount. If the label states "liquid oil," it is the best to use. If it says "hydrogenated oil," leave it alone. The best margarine is derived from vegetables, safflower, soy or corn oil. Soft margarine is hydrogenated less, leaving more of the natural oils intact. It is lower in hard fats.

Use vegetables oils. But make sure they are cold- or expeller-pressed (unhydrogenated). They are readily available from health food stores. A hydraulic press is used on the nuts, seeds, grains, olives or vegetables. The oil is extracted without heat. Virgin or crude unrefined oils like olive oil are processed the same way.

Canola oil is derived from the rapeseed plant and like olive oil, it is high in monounsaturated fats and helps prevent heart disease. Canola oil, unlike olive oil, has no distinct flavor, so it is good to use if you do not like the flavor of olive oil.

Keep these four rules in mind when changing your diet from unhealthy fats to healthy fats:

1. Avoid all saturated animal fat.
2. Saturated fats are solid or semisolid at room temperature, i.e.. butter, lard, or fat that is seen in meats.
3. Fish contains unsaturated fats. *Omega-3* fatty acids aid in lowering cholesterol and are found in fish oils, especially cold water fish.
4. Unsaturated fats are liquid or very soft like vegetable oils.

See recipe section for Garlic Oil a valuable cooking and salad oil. The Good Things Salad Dressing (see recipes), is the best you will ever taste and is good for all health problems.

Be aware of any product labeled "saturated fats", coconut, and/or palm kernel oils. If the label doesn't list the source of "vegetable oils" avoid them. **Coconut and palm kernel oils are as high in saturated fat as animal fat, but they are labeled as vegetable oils.**

Salad dressings, butter, choice margarines, shortening, and oils are the most concentrated sources of fat, and red meat is still at the top of the list for fat.

All fried foods should be avoided, they cause premature aging and worse. Isn't this reason enough to avoid the saturated fats or at least cut back on their consumption to once weekly instead of daily?

Begin to improve your health by removing red meat from the diet. Avoid marbled cuts of beef and hamburgers. If you must eat meat trim all fat before cooking. Remove the skin and fat from poultry.

There are several valuable hints to follow when using oils:
1. Purchase cold- or expeller-pressed oils (unrefined)
2. Avoid hardened oils (hydrogenated)
3. Never re-use oil that has been used for frying
4. Refrigerate all oils after opening
5. All oils should be stored in a cool dark cupboard
6. Never consume oil that smells rancid
7. Olive oil maintains a longer shelf life than most oils
8. Don't let oils heat to smoking
9. To saute or stir fry, use 2 tablespoons of water in the oil

BEST OILS	WORST OILS
Olive	Coconut
Canola	Peanut
Walnut	Palm
Safflower	Palm Kernel
Avocado	Cottonseed
Almond	
Rice bran	
Sesame	
Flax seed	

Commercial Products to Reduce or Eliminate

Hot dogs	Fried foods	Egg yolks	Aerosol whipped cream
Shellfish	Cream cheese	Spare rips	Chow mein noodles
Salami	Chocolate	Cream	Packaged potatoes
Shrimp	Pork & Lamb	Smoked meats	Black olives
"Organ" meats	Coconut oil	Poultry skin	Hydrogenated margarine
Coconut	Lunchmeats	Cheese (soft)	Imitation dairy products
Bologna	Gravies	Duck	Non-dairy cream
Ice cream	Palm oil	Peanuts	Toaster pastries
Butter/lard	Most chips	Cocoa	Lobster/crab Sardines
Many desserts	*Cookies	*Cereals	Corned beef Goose
*Refried beans	Sausages	Yellow cheeses	Microwave popcorn
Packaged rice	Liver sausage	Palm kernel oil	Processed granola
Peanut butter	*Ground turkey	*Muffin mixes	*All packaged cakes
Mayonnaise	Whole milk	Corned beef	Creamy dressings
Hamburger	Bacon	*Crackers	

The items listed above with an * may be eaten if they are homemade and the fat content is controlled. Cake and muffin mixes (i.e. Fearn) found in a health food store, have all natural ingredients and you can add the sweetener and a healthy oil.

If you don't purchase these foods you will not be tempted to eat them.

Read Your Labels

It is very important to read and understand labels. The term "light" or "lite" usually refers to texture and does not refer to low-fat or salt content.

High-Fat Terms

Fried - any form	Buttery/buttered	Breaded	Scalloped	Rich
Au gratin/cheese	Creamy/cream sauce	Hollandaise	Cream or creamed	
Pan gravy - in its own sauce				

Low-Fat Terms

Stir-fried	Roasted	Steamed	Poached	Grilled	Broiled

Naringin - a bioflavonoid found in the fruit, rind and flowers of a grapefruit. Aids in preventing cataracts and nerve destruction, especially in diabetics. Naringin inhibits the action of aldose reductase, preventing the conversion of glucose into sorbitol and can slow or even prevent the formation of cataracts, *Varma D Prog Clin Biol Res* 86;213:343.

Quercetin - found in grapefruit, broccoli, shallots, summer squash and especially onions. (It is also found in many red wines.) Quercetin also inhibits the aldose reductase enzyme, although it is much harder for the body to absorb. As an alternative, to avoid the assimilation problem, the pineapple derived digestive enzyme bromelain, can be taken , *European J Clin Pharmaco* 84;33:33.

Catechin - another underutilized bioflavonoid. Has been successfully used in treatment of liver diseases, especially hepatitis. Green and black Indian teas contain as many as four different catechins. Works well for those with food allergies by blocking the formation of histamine in the stomach tissue to reduce or prevent allergic reactions and skin wheals or hives, *Acta Pharm* (Suppl) 80;13:23. Catechin also has strong anti-viral effects, especially against the Lupus Simplex Virus. (*Prong Clin Biol Res* 86;213:521-36.) Teas (green and black varities) contain as many as four different catechins. Researchers in Japan, France, Canada and Russia have reported that these catechins work as powerful antioxidants. They have been using them medicinally to protect against blood vessel damage and to supress cancer, *Mutation Research* 85;150:127-132. Although Catechin can only be ordered by physicians, these green and black teas are found in Oriental markets and health food stores.

Sensible Alternatives

American Diet	Healthy Alternative
Haddock breaded and fried	Haddock broiled
Tuna canned in oil	Tuna canned in water
Fried Potatoes	Baked potatoes, no butter or sour cream - plain yogurt or seasoning and a little sesame or canola oil (melted butter is basically melted oil)
Vegetables with cheese sauce	Vegetables with lemon juice
Potato chips	Plain popcorn
Danish pastry	Whole grain muffins
Ice cream	Frozen fruit or sherbet
Bologna	Baked breast of turkey
Hamburgers	Soy or veggie burgers
Beef	Broiled fish or turkey breast
Canned soups	Homemade soups or health Valley and Hain's brand soups
Canned biscuits	Homemade with plain low-fat yogurt, whole wheat flour, aluminum free baking power and canola
One whole egg	2 Egg whites

Replace High-Fat Foods with these High-Protein Foods

Skinless turkey or chicken breast
Water-packed tuna
Poached or broiled fish
Brown rice with steamed vegetables
Meatless veggie chili
Beans and brown rice
Tofu products

Lentil and bean soups
Vegetable soups
Pasta and vegetables
Spaghetti with soy chunks
In casseroles, stews, and tacos, use beans in place of meat
Top vegetable dishes with sesame seeds or raw nuts

Remove the skin from turkey and chicken, and keep fish on a rack out of the drippings.
Use paper towels to clean anything that comes into contact with raw poultry. Sponges or cloth towels are extremely difficult to sterilize. You'll be tempted to reuse them before you launder them.

Fat Content in Nuts and Seeds

Food	Fat (g)	Saturated Fat (g)	Cholesterol (mg)
Almonds, 1oz.	15	1	0
Cashews, dry roasted, 1 oz.	13	3	0
Chestnuts, roasted, 1 oz.	1	0	0
Hazelnuts, 1 oz.	18	1	0
Macadamia, roasted in oil, 1 oz.	22	2	0
Peanuts, roasted in oil, 1 oz	14	2	0
Peanut Butter, 2 tablespoons	16	3	0
Pecans, 1 oz.	19	2	0
Pistachios, 1 oz.	14	2	0
Sesame seeds, 1 tablespoon	4	1	0
Sunflower seeds, 1 oz.	14	2	0
Walnuts, 1 oz.	16	2	0

All nuts contain high amounts of compounds called *protease inhibitors*, known to block cancer in test animals. *Dr. Walter Troll of New York University* puts nuts high on the list of possible antidotes to cancer. Nuts are also rich in certain *polyphenols*, chemicals shown to thwart cancer in animals. The oil from walnuts, for example, is polyunsaturated and tends to lower blood cholesterol. However, while most nuts are generally healthy, peanuts (especially those used for commercially-prepared peanut butter) are often contaminated by a mold called aflatoxin, which is a carcinogen.

Almonds: The King of nuts. High in potassium, magnesium, phosphorus and protein. Cancer clinics around the world recommend 10 raw almonds per day because of the laetrile content. Laetrile acts as an anti-cancer agent. Both almond oil and almond butter are nutritious.

Cashews: Grown primarily in India. High in potassium, magnesium, vitamin A and fat. Don't consume large amounts as they contain high amounts of bad fat.

Chestnuts: Good raw, boiled or roasted. Lowest in fat content.

Filbert or Hazelnuts: High in potassium, sulphur and calcium. They have a mild flavor and are good cooked with vegetables and grains.

Peanuts: Has the highest fat content of all nuts. Are a complete protein, but are often contaminated with aflatoxin, a known carcinogen. (Peanuts are actually a legume, rather than a nut.)

Pecans: A member of hickory family. High in potassium and vitamin A. Rich in essential fats. Good for baking, candy, etc.

Pine nuts (Pignolia): Used in Middle Eastern and Italian dishes. Chewy and sweet which makes them good for salads or combined with fruits.

Pistachios: A sweet, mild flavor. May see holes in these nuts made by a tiny worm which gives each nut its unique flavor.

Walnuts: The oil is used in cooking, high in potassium, magnesium and vitamin A. Good in all baking, salads and topping on desserts.

Never use roasted nuts or seeds because the oils become rancid when exposed to light and air. Consume only raw seeds and those tightly sealed in bags.

HOW MUCH FAT SHOULD I EAT?

Here is a formula to find the percent of fat in foods. Your goal should be 10% fat, no more than 15% fat. Read labels carefully!

1. Look at the label listed on the product for the grams of fat and the number of calories per serving.

2. Multiply the number of fat grams by 9. This is the number of fat calories.

3. Take the number you calculated and divide this by the number or calories per serving listed on the label. The answer will be less than one.

4. Now to get the percent of calories from the fat, multiply this number by 100.

For example: *Low Salt Ritz Crackers*

1. 1 serving: 4 grams of fat, 70 calories per serving

2. 4 gm x 9 = 36 fat calories per serving

3. 36/70 = .514

4. .514 x 100 = 51.4% of the calories per serving of crackers is from the fat content

NEW SUGGESTIONS FOR REDUCING FAT IN YOUR DIET:

1. Consume broiled fish containing high amounts of omega-3 fatty acids at least 3 times per week.

2. Make your own salad dressings so you can use an oil that is good for you.

Another method of testing the fat in your favorite cracker is by rubbing it on a paper napkin. A grease mark indicates a high fat content. The fat content is usually from an oil that's not good for you, like the hydrogenated oils, or the palm, or coconut oils.

---

3. Use raw apple cider vinegar and oil instead of creamy salad dressings.

4. Add flavor without fat to baked potatoes with plain yogurt and chives. Mash tofu with a little low-fat (egg free) mayonnaise, add herbs for seasonings.

5. You can replace oil in most recipes with plain low-fat yogurt.

6. In saute pan, cook sliced vegetables with mushrooms in their own juices, instead of butter or oil. Mushrooms, onions, and garlic add flavor.

7. Steam cook all vegetables.

8. Steam in canola oil and add a tablespoon of water to prevent the oil from getting too hot.

9. Try poaching in place of frying for firm-fleshed fish. Use 4 parts water and 1 part lemon juice and herbs. For chicken, try a blend of 4 parts water to 1 part tamari sauce and/or pineapple juice for an excellent flavor. Add fresh or granulated garlic to everything, for flavor enhancement and your health.

10. When baking chicken turkey and fish place on a rack to prevent it from cooking in the fat drippings. Cover the pan to keep the food moist instead of basting with its own drippings or using oil. Trim all fat and remove skin before cooking poultry.

11. Defat soups, meat stocks, chili, and stew by refrigerating them for a few hours. Fat is then easily skimmed off the top.

12. For low-fat sauces, puree vegetables or use potato flakes as the thickening base. Arrowroot is also good as a thickener.

13. In sauces that call for cream, substitute nonfat dry milk, or plain low-fat yogurt. You may substitute sour cream with yogurt in all recipes.

14. Substitute mashed tofu for ricotta and cottage cheese recipes.

15. Use tuna packed in water rather than oil.

16. Butter melts and looks like other oils when placed on potatoes or steamed vegetables. Replace butter with sesame or olive oil and top with chopped chives.

17. Use eggless safflower or soy mayonnaise found in health food stores.

18. Consume oil-free breads found in health food stores like macrobiotic bread.

19. Avoid all processed meats, they are very high in saturated fats, like hot dogs, luncheon meats, sausage, bacon, etc.

20. When making muffins, cornbread, biscuits, etc., use low-fat plain yogurt.

21. In place of oil, use liquid lecithin to grease baking pans and casserole dishes.

22. Replace 1 egg with 2 egg whites, or use arrowroot powder or egg replacer.

23. Use walnuts in place of peanuts.

24. Use crackers made without oil.

Essential Fatty Acids

HYDROGENATED is a word to AVOID. Hydrogenation chemically alters oils into saturated fats by adding hydrogen atoms which saturate the unsaturated fats.

Grind your own turkey, use only skinless breast. Store bought ground turkey contains 14 grams of fat in only 4-ounces of meat.

The essential fatty acids (EFA's) are sometimes called vitamin F. The EFAs were discovered in 1930 at the *University of Minnesota by George and Mildred Burr*. Researchers have found that all animals and humans require essential fatty acids in the diet. A partial list of EFA's include *omega-3, alpha-linoleic*, and *omega-6 linoleic acid*. These cannot be synthesized by the human body and therefore are termed "essential". More of these EFAs are required by the body than all other types of fats or nutrients that are "essential". Every single cell, organ, and tissue requires a daily supply of EFA.

Omega-6 is obtained from vegetable oils, but the *omega-3* is often lacking. The vegetable oils that contain the highest amount of *omega-3* include:

Pumpkin seed oil	Flaxseed oil
Canola oil	Soy oil
Walnut oil	

The two most common *omega-3* fatty acids are *eicosapentanoic acid* (EPA) and *decosahexanoic acid* (DHA). The fat content of fish varies. Cold-water fish have a higher fat content and thus contain the largest amounts of EPA and DHA.

All dark green leafy vegetables also contain high amounts of the *omega-3*.

Flaxseed oil has the highest content of omega-3 (52%) and contains twice as much as fish oil. Flaxseed oil is less expensive and more stable. About 2 tablespoons of flax oil daily will add a generous supply of the essential *omega-3* fatty acids. Both flaxseed and flaxseed oil can be found in health food stores. Grind flaxseed just before use, because it becomes rancid quickly. If you purchase ground flaxseed, make certain it is tightly sealed. *Omega-Life, Inc.* has a fortified flaxseed that is very rich in *omega-3*.

COMMERCIALLY FRIED CHICKEN VS. HOME-COOKED

BREAST	FAT (g)	Serving
Extra Crispy	22.3	3.9 oz.
Skinless-home roasted	2.7	2.6 oz.

DRUMSTICK	FAT (g)	Serving
Extra Crispy	13.9	2.4 oz.
Skinless-home roasted	2.7	1.7 oz.

Beware of healthy-sounding cereals and granolas. Although they are advertised to be great for your health, many are loaded with fats, sugars and sodium. Many granolas are saturated with tropical oils, and the nuts are high in fat, neither of which should be in a healthy breakfast.

Breakfast should have a good source of fiber, protein, complex carbohydrates, vitamins from fresh fruit, and a few calories from a little fat. There should be no more than 10% of the calories from fat in your breakfast.

Lunch can also be loaded with unwanted fats. A sandwich with cheese can increase your fat intake by 100 calories per slice. Sixty-six percent of those calories are fat. The processed luncheon meats are full of fat and sodium, too. Even luncheon meat, made from turkey, can have up to 90% of the fat calories.

To cut down on fat in your lunch, try eating skinless turkey breast, tuna that is packed in water instead of oil, and low calorie mayonnaise.

Linseed oil is made from flaxseed. Some chemists do not classify linseed oil as edible, but some nutritionists recommend linseed oil. **We prefer and recommend using flaxseed oil.**

To add these valuable essential fatty acids to your diet, consume canola, walnut, or flaxseed oil daily. It is best to purchase unrefined oils. Do not heat these oils as heating will destroy the nutrients. Use these oils in salad dressings. Also consume at least one serving of dark-green leafy vegetables daily for *omega-3* requirements.

THE CORRECT BALANCED DIET	
FAT (Approximately)	10 - 15%
PROTEIN	15%
CARBOHYDRATES	70 - 75%

Causes of an EFA Deficiency

1. A diet rich in saturated fats
2. Consumption of processed vegetable oils containing trans-fatty acids that prevent the proper formation of linoleic acid
3. Excess alcohol consumption
4. Diabetes
5. Aging
6. Lack of magnesium, zinc, and vitamins E, C, and B-6 (pyridoxine)
7. Viral infections
8. Radiation, chemotherapy, and cancer
9. Smoking tobacco
10. Environmental toxins
11. Using certain drugs

A study, conducted at the *University of Maryland,* found large amounts of trans-fatty acids (TFAs) in margarine, cooking fats, bread, cakes, french fries, pretzels, chips, frostings, puddings, and highly processed foods. Your body needs EFAs, not TFAs.

Udo Erasmus states in his book, Fats and Oils, that over 80% of the United State's population has an *omega-3* deficiency.

Omega-3 has the ability to thin the blood. If taking blood thinners like aspirin, avoid high amounts of *omega-3*. It is better to take the EFA and avoid the aspirin, as aspirin can be toxic. Blood clots can cause heart attacks and stroke, but fish oils prevent blood clotting by reducing the tendency of blood platelets to clump. Avoid high amounts of cod-liver oil since its high content of vitamins A and D can be toxic--take only 1 teaspoon daily, and never drink alcoholic beverages when taking cod-liver oil.

Consume more fish in place of oil supplements. Saltwater fish from cold, deep waters are less likely to be polluted than lake fish. In general, a four-ounce serving of fish will supply about 1,400 mg. of *omega-3*. Three capsules of fish oil, 500 mg. each, supplies 1,500 mg. If you are a vegetarian and do not want to consume fish, add flaxseed oil to your diet.

Be sure to take vitamin E along with fish-oil supplements. This will protect your cells. *Carleson Labs* have an excellent salmon oil capsule that has vitamin E added for protection.

Omega-3 Fatty Acids

*Beneficial for rheumatoid arthritis
*Good for all forms of arthritis
*Helps control viral infections
*Reduces cholesterol and triglycerides
*Lowers risk of stroke or heart attack
*Reduces risk of artereosclerosis
*Improves psoriasis
*Improves immune response
*Lowers harmful effects of prostaglandins aiding in preventing breast cancer
*Reduces severity of migraine headaches
*Improves brain function
*Improves function of the glandular system

84

The Fish Story

Researchers found that Eskimos in Greenland, whose diets consisted of fatty fish, had less arteriosclerosis and fewer deaths from heart disease than in the United States. The Japanese also consume more fish than Americans and have a lower risk of heart disease. From the *University of Leidi in Holland,* researchers studied 852 Dutchmen who ate 7 to 11 ounces of fish weekly. **There was a 50% lower death rate from heart disease among those who ate fish versus those who did not consume any fish weekly.**

A *Consumer Report* team conducted a six-month investigation in urban and suburban New York City, Chicago, and the San Jose-Santa Cruz area of California. They went to grocery stores and specialty stores sampling salmon, flounder, sole, catfish, swordfish, lake whitefish and clams. They found 40 % of the fish were either contaminated or beginning to spoil and 30% were rated poor, due to bacterial contamination, PCBs or mercury. Fish requires storage temperatures between 30-32° F and some store display cases reach 45° F. Many markets defrost frozen fish and sell it for fresh, letting it sit for days in their display cases.

If your fish smells fishy, the fish oils are becoming rancid. Your best buy is frozen fish, because it is frozen within hours of being caught, whereas fresh fish is often transported for days before reaching the market, unless you live in a coastal area.

To avoid the mercury content in fish, broil on a rack so the fish is cooked above the juices that run off.

HIGHEST SOURCES OF *OMEGA-3*

FISH	GRAMS
Norway Sardines	5.1
Mackerel, Atlantic	2.6
Herring, Atlantic	1.7
Tuna, bluefin	1.6
Sablefish	1.5
Salmon, sockeye	1.3
Bluefish	1.2
Mullet	1.1
Bass, striped	0.8
Hake, silver	0.6
Pompano, Florida	0.6
Shark	0.5
Swordfish	0.2

Salt-Water Fish

Fatty fish include canned sardines, mackerel, salmon, smelt, anchovies, mullet, and herring.

Medium fat fish include halibut, ocean perch, red snapper, sole, sea trout, and albacore tuna.

Low-fat salt-water fish include flounder, haddock, swordfish, cod, shellfish, and whiting.

All of the fish listed above are the best to consume, as they contain good fats.

Fresh Water Fish

Fatty fish include lake trout, mullet, smelt, catfish, and rainbow trout.

Medium-fat fish include carp.

Low-fat fish include bass, bream, pike, and lake perch.

SEAFOOD NUTRITION INFORMATION CHART

■ SEAFOOD 3oz, edible, cooked, without skin	Total Calories	Protein	Carbohydrate	Total Fat	Saturated Fatty Acids	Cholesterol	Sodium	Vitamin A	Vitamin C	Calcium	Iron
	kcal	g	g	g	g	mg	mg	\% U.S. RDA			
Blue Crab, steamed	90	19	0	1	0	80	310	*	*	9	4
Catfish, baked	120	19	0	5	1	60	65	*	*	3	5
Clam, steamed, 12 small	130	22	4	2	0	60	95	10	*	8	130
Cod, broiled	90	19	0	1	0	50	60	*	2	*	2
Flounder, baked	100	20	0	1	0	50	85	*	*	2	2
Haddock, baked	90	20	0	1	0	60	70	*	*	4	6
Halibut, broiled	120	22	0	2	0	30	60	3	*	5	5
Lobster, boiled	100	20	1	1	0	100	320	*	*	5	2
Mackerel,											
Atlantic/Pacific & Jack, broiled	190	21	0	12	3	60	95	7	*	*	9
Ocean Perch, baked	100	20	0	2	0	50	80	*	*	10	6
Orange Roughy, broiled	70	16	0	1	0	20	70	*	*	*	*
Oyster, steamed, 12 medium	120	12	7	4	1	90	190	*	*	8	65
Pollock, broiled	100	21	0	1	0	80	90	*	*	*	*
Rainbow Trout, broiled	130	22	0	4	1	60	30	*	5	7	10
Rockfish, baked	100	20	0	2	0	40	65	4	*	*	3
Salmon, Atlantic/Coho, baked	150	22	0	7	1	50	50	*	2	*	4
Scallop, broiled, 6 large or 14 small	150	29	2	1	0	60	275	*	3	2	*
Shrimp, boiled	110	22	0	2	0	160	155	*	3	3	15
Sole, broiled	100	21	0	1	0	60	90	*	*	2	2
Whiting, baked	100	19	0	1	0	70	75	2	*	5	2

* Contains less than 2% of U.S. RDA

(Data Source: FDA)   **Serving Size:** 3 oz. cooked portion-skinless, broiled/grilled, baked, microwaved, boiled or steamed without additional fat, sodium or sauces.

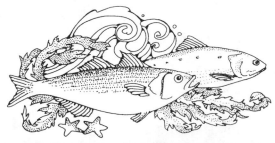

A seafood hot line is available through the American Seafood Institute. For free information on the purchase, preparation and nutritional value of seafood products, call (1-800) 328-3474 between 9 a.m. and 5 p.m. Eastern time on weekdays.

FDA CONSUMER, July-August 1992, pg. 35

Low-Fat Recipes

This pumpkin pie recipe tastes fresh and as good as any ever made, and without the use of eggs, canned cream (fat), salt, and sugar. It contains only 2 grams of fat per serving and 5 grams of protein, and no cholesterol.

Low-Fat No Cholesterol Pumpkin Pie

FILLING:

1 pound drained tofu
2 tablespoons arrowroot powder
2 cups canned pumpkin, nothing added
1/2 cup fructose or honey or use
1 tablespoon barley malt concentrate or
1 cup barley malt syrup or 1 cup rice syrup
2 teaspoons ground cinnamon
1/2 teaspoon ground allspice
1/2 teaspoon ground ginger
1/2 teaspoon ground nutmeg

Preheat oven to 400 degrees. Thoroughly mix all ingredients in a blender or food processor. Pour into a 9" unbaked pie shell and bake for 15 minutes. Reduce temperature to 350 degrees and bake an additional 50-55 minutes. It's done when a toothpick comes out clean after being inserted in the center of the pie. May top with pecans. Let cool and serve.

Low-Fat Whipping Cream

Make before serving, because this cannot be stored, it will separate in about 15-25 minutes, but it is great on desserts and fruit.

Place 1/2 cup skim milk into a stainless steel bowl (stainless steel is best because it retains in the cold).

Place in the freezer for 20 minutes or just until ice crystals begin to form on top.

Use a hand-held electric mixer and beat in 1/4 cup of non-fat dry milk solids slowly until the mixture thickens and soft peaks form. Add 1/2 teaspoon barley malt sweetener or 1 tablespoon of honey. Continue to beat for about 3 minutes.

Low-Fat Salmon Cakes

8 ounce drained salmon
1/4 cup chopped green pepper
1/4 cup whole wheat bread crumbs
1/4 cup plain low-fat yogurt
1/4 teaspoon dried mustard
1/4 cup chopped onion
1/4 teaspoon granulated or
  fresh crushed garlic
1 egg white *(optional)* or
2 teaspoons arrowroot powder

Combine all ingredients and place into four oiled custard cups. Bake at 350 degrees for 20-25 minutes. Serve with sauce listed below.

SAUCE:
1 cup plain low-fat yogurt
1/2 cup cucumber (chopped, seeded, and peeled)
2 tablespoons chopped onion
1/2 teaspoon dried dillweed
1/2 teaspoon fresh lemon juice *(optional)*

Mix all ingredients in saucepan and heat. Pour over salmon cakes. Can also add fresh peas to sauce. Serves four.

Hain's Cheese Soup mix is fast and also good for topping salmon cakes. Use 1 cup plain yogurt and water to add to the soup mix.

Low-Fat Miracle Spread

At low speed with a hand mixer or food processor, blend:

1 tub *Hain's* soft safflower margarine
(found in health food stores)
1/2 cup unrefined canola oil
1/2 cup homemade lowfat yogurt*(optional)*

Spoon into a tub and refrigerate. Use in place of butter or margarine for all recipes and for spreading on top of all vegetables, potatoes, etc.

Low-Fat Sour Cream

1/2 pound tofu
2 tablespoons lemon juice
3 tablespoons canola oil

Place tofu and lemon juice in a blender or food processor. Blend until creamy. While mixing add oil through the feeder tube and continue to process until mixture is thick. If too thick, blend in a little water as needed. Makes a one-cup serving with only 3 grams of fat.

High Tech Foods

Genetic engineering is the genetic manipulation of food, adding genes foreign to produce to increase shelf life and diminish damage during shipping.

Many are concerned that genetic engineering may introduce potential allergens that unsuspecting shoppers will have to deal with. A peanut gene could be introduced into a food and someone with a peanut allergy would not connect the two. The industry has tested tomatoes with founder genes, corn with a fire fly gene and potatoes with chicken genes. Other foods to be tested are potatoes that resist rotting and fruit trees that the cold won't damage.

Currently there is a no-labeling policy that may create dilemmas for vegetarians and some religious groups who would have no idea of the alterations.

Wheat-Free Protein Waffles

These waffles are high in omega-3 and protein.

1 cup ground whole millet
1/4 cup powdered nonfat milk
1/2 cup plain yogurt or use all yogurt in place of powdered milk
1/2 cup canola oil
4 tablespoons ground flaxseed
1/2 cup water

Blend millet and flaxseed in blender or food processor until powdered. Add nonfat dry milk and mix. Pour in canola oil and water and mix well. Preheat waffle iron while mixing ingredients. Have a little extra water on hand. The flax soaks up a lot of moisture and more water may need to be added to mix. Pour mixture in hot waffle iron and cook 3 - 6 minutes. Top with fresh fruit and pure maple syrup.

Since 1930, the increased use of pasteurized dairy products and hydrogenated oils increased in direct proportion to deaths from heart attacks.

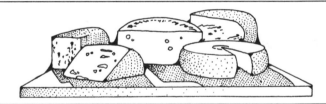

In the recent years, hundreds of cases of hepatitis A, a viral infection that inflames the liver and causes gastroenteritis (a mild flu-like illness), has been linked to consumption of raw clams and oysters. Also, some ocean fish are contaminated with parasites that can cause infection in humans. Cook all fish to at least 140 degrees or freeze below zero to kill these parasites. Unless the fish used to prepare *sushi* has been frozen, it should be considered contaminated and dangerous.

Fast Healthy Food

Eat healthy foods found in health food stores to replace foods with high amounts of salt, sugar, animal fat, and chemical additives.

Just Add Water to Prepare

Cabash Natural Foods
Breakfast Cup
Couscous
Rice Pilaf, Lentil Pilaf
Humus Mix
Tahini Dip and Sauce (mix)
Tabouli
Edward's and Son
Miso Cup and Miso Cup with Seaweed
Fantastic Foods
Humus Mix
Taste Adventure
Instant Black Bean Soup
Instant Split Pea Soup
Chili
Westbrae
Instant Hearty Red Miso Soup

Preparation 5-10 minutes

Arrowhead Mills
Mashed Potato Flakes
Organic Beans
Organic Chick-peas
Lentils (red and green)
Sesame Tahini
Brown Rice
Steel Cut Oats
Raw Wheat Germ
Buckwheat Pancake (mix)
Multi-Grain Pancake (mix)
Multi-Grain Cornbread (mix)

Casadian Farms-frozen
Sorbet
Mixed Vegetables
Broccoli
Carrots
Green Beans
Hash Browns
Strawberries
Peas
Fantastic Foods
Instant Black Beans
Instant Refried Beans
Health Valley-frozen
Turkey or Chicken Wieners
Baby Lima beans, Whole Kernel Corn
Spinach, Broccoli, Green Beans
Light Foods, Inc.
Tofu Browners (knockwurst)
Tofu Light Links
Lightlife Foods
Fakin Bakin
Tofu Pups
Foney Boloney
Lundberg
Short and Sweet Rice
Wild Country Rice
Riz-Cous Dinners
Shelton's
Turkey Chili
Chicken Chili with Black Beans
Dressing (mix)
Soy Deli
Savory Baked Tofu
Tofu Tempeh Burgers
Tofu Burger Teriyaki

That's Some Din Sum
Vegetable Wonton
Vegetable Powza

White Wave
Lemon Broil Tempeh
Healthy Franks
Tempeh Chili
Tempeh Cutlet
Templeh Burgers
Vegetarian Sloppy Joes
Meatless Bologna

Westbrae
Cashew Butter
Almond Butter
Instant Ramen Soups
Whole Wheat Spaghetti

10-15 minutes

Basmati rice
Buckwheat
Grainnaissance Mochi
Harvest Moon Mochi
Quinoa
White texmati rice

Arrowhead Mills
Quick Brown Rice
  Plain
  Spanish Style
  Vegetable Herb
  Wild Rice and Herbs

Deboles
Noodles and Cheese Dinner
Shells and Chedder Dinner
Rotini
Lasagna
Rigatoni
 Corn Spaghetti

Fantastic Foods
Nature's Burger (mix)
Pasta Salads
Tofu Burger (mix)
Tofu Scrambler
Country Potatoes

Love Burger
Mayacama's Soup
Potato Leek Soup
Garden Pea Soup
French Onion Soup
Creamy Mushroom Soup
Creamy Tomato Soup

Health is Wealth-frozen
Vegetarian Egg Rolls
Pizza Tofu Munchies
Spinach Cheese Egg Rolls
Veggie Munchies

Jaclyn's
Breaded Cauliflower
Breaded Mushrooms
Barley and Mushroom Soup
Minestrone Soup
Split Pea Soup
Vegetable Soup

Ken and Robert's
Veggie Pockets
Greek Veggie Pocket
Pizza Veggie Pocket
Tex Mex Veggie Pocket

Northwest Natural-frozen
Medallion Halibut
Salmon Patties

Shelton's
Italian Turkey Sausage
Breakfast Sausage
Chicken Franks
Turkey Hot Dogs
Chicken Pot Pies

20-25 minutes

Vegetarian Health
Vegetarian Beef (tofu)
  Chunks & Bits
Vegetarian Hamburger Bits
  (tofu)
Bulgur Wheat
Red Lentils
Tempeh

Cabash Natural Foods
Falafel Mix
Nutted Pilaf
Rice Pilaf
Spanish Pilaf
Wheat Pilaf

Fantastic Foods
Falafel Mix
Polenta
Potatoes Au Gratin
Potatoes Country Style

Tofu Classics Pasta and Sauce
Shells n' Curry
Mandarin Chow Mein
Creamy Stroganoff

25-30 minutes

Fantastic Foods
Vegetarian Chili
Fearn
Baking Mix
Banana Cake Mix
Spice Cake Mix
Carrot Cake Mix
Sunflower Burger Mix
Sesame Burger Mix

Hain's
3 Grain Herb Side Dish
Rice Almondine Side Dish
Kashi Pilaf

30-45 minutes

Brown Rice
Green Lentils
   Casbah Natural Foods
Lentil Pilaf
Tabouli
   Amy's Kitchen--frozen
Broccoli Pot Pie
Macaroni n' Cheese
Macaroni n' Soy Cheese
Vegetable Pot Pie
Apple Pie
   Au Naturel Cuisine-frozen
French Bread Pizza
Boneless Trout Dinner
Roast Turkey
   Legume (**tofu**)-frozen
Enchilada Tofu
Manicotti Florentine
Stuffed Shells
Lasagna Vegetable/Tofu
   Mud Pie
Vegie Burgers

Healthy Products

Organic Baby Food

Earth's Best
Mixed Grain Cereal
Instant Brown Rice Cereal
Oatmeal and Prunes
Juices-Pear and Apple
Pears
Carrots
Sweet Potatoes
Bananas
Apple-Blueberry
Peas-Brown Rice
Plums-Bananas-Rice
   Simply Pure
Winter Squash
Applesauce
Beets
Diced Carrots and Potatoes
Green Beans
Carrots

Frozen Breads

Garden of Eatin'
Bagels
Bible Bread
Pita Pockets
Tortillas (flour and blue corn)
Chapatis
   Nature's Garden-frozen
Macrobiotic Bread
Rye Bread
Oatbran Diet Muffins

Cereals

Arrowhead Mills
Bran Flakes
Corn Flakes
Puffed Corn
Puffed Brown Rice Cereal
   Barbara's
Crunchy Oat Bran
Breakfast Biscuits
Raisin Bran
   Elam's
Miller's Bran Flakes
Steel Cut Oatmeal
Oat-Bran Granola
   Golden Temple
Lite-n-Crunchy
Blueberry Granola
Muesli-Date and Almond
Muesli-Swiss Style
Coconut/Almond Granola
   Health Valley
Oat Bran Flakes
Fruit & Nut Oat Bran O's
Fiber 7 Flakes
Amaranth with Raisins
   Lundberg
Creamy Rye and Rice
Crown Rice Crunchies
   New Morning
Apple & Cinnamon Oatios
Honey Almond Oatios
Fruit-E-Os

Perky's

Nutty Rice with Raisins
Crispy Brown Rice-Apple/
   Cinnamon
Crispy Brown Rice-Carob
   Roman Meal
Cream of Rye
Old Fashioned Oats
Flax with Bran, Rye, and
   Wheat

Dressings

Hain's
Safflower Mayonnaise
Light Mayonnaise
Eggless Mayonnaise
Light Canola Mayonnaise
No Oil Salad Dressing Mix
Pourable Dressings
Crackers
Chili Seasoning (mix)
Bean Dips
   Nasoya
Mayonnaise (no eggs tofu)
Creamy Dill Veggie Dip
French Onion Dip
Garlic and Herb Dip
   San-J
Wheat Free Tamari
Shoyu
Teriyaki

Drinks

R.W. Knudsen
Frozen Cranberry Juice
Frozen Lemonade
   Pero
Coffee substitute (malted
   barley, chicory, rye)

Entrees

American Prairie
Garbanzo Beans
Great Northern Beans
Kidney Beans
Black Beans

Cedarland Foods
Soypreme French Bread
    Pizza
    (Dr. Balch's favorite)
China Rose
Fresh Organic Tofu
Garden Gourmet-frozen
Vege-Cutlets
Vege-Links
Vege-Patties
Vegetarian Franks and
Beans
    Tofu Enchiladas
Nasoya
Stuffed shells
Ravioli
Manicotti
Tortellini
SoyBoy
Tofu Ravioli
Soypreme-frozen
Cheese Pizza
Garden Pizza
Tofu Stroganoff
Tofu Luau
Stuff n' Spuds
Sunberry Farms-frozen
Apple Fiber muffins
Raisin Muffins
Date and Nut Muffins
Macaroni and Cheese
Pizza-Rolla Sandwich
Worthington Food, Inc.
Beef-Style Pie
Chili
Meatless Salami
Country Stew
Vegetarian Burger
Smoked Turkey Roll

Vegetable Scallops
Super Links
Veja-links
Vegetarian Cutlets

Nutritional Substitutes

Ener G
Egg Replacer
Nut Quik
Soy Quick
Brown Rice Baking Mix
Corn Mix
Oat Mix
Esculent-a Tree of Life
Fructose
Turbinado Sugar
Skim Milk Powder
Lecithin
Arrowroot Powder
Wheat Bran Flakes
Sca Salt
Sucant
Organic Evaporated Cane
  Juice Sweetner

Sauces

Pritikin Foods
Rice Cakes
Mexican Sauce
Spaghetti Sauce
Fruit Spreads
Salad Dressings
Pasta
Canned Soups
Enrico's
Ketchup
BBQ Sauce
Salsa
All Natural Spaghetti Sauce

Tumaro's
Black Bean Enchilada
Empanadas
All-Natural Cereals
Arrowhead Mills
Bran Flakes
Corn Flakes
Puffed Corn
Puffed Brown Rice Cereal
Health Valley
Oat Bran Flakes
Fruit & Fiber Oat Bran O's
Fiber 7 Flakes
Amaranth with Raisins
Perky's
Nutty Rice with Raisins
Crispy Brown Rice-Apple/
    Cinnamon
Crispy Brown Rice-Carob
New Morning
Honey Almond Oatis
Apple & Cinnamon Oatis
Fruit-E-O's
Barbara's
Crunchy Oat Bran
Lundberg
Hot and Creamy Rice Cereal
    -Cinnamon/Raisin
American Prairie
Creamy Rye and Rice
Golden Temple
Lite-n-CrunchyGranola
Muesli Lite
Elam's
Miller's Bran
Steel Cut Oatmeal
Roman Meal
Old Fashioned Oats
Cream of Rye
Cereal with Oats, (wheat,
    rye, bran and flax)

There are many wholesome products in a health food store that can be made quickly for those with a busy schedule. You don't have to feed anyone chemicals, colorings, salt, sugar, white flour, saturated fats, and fiberless meals.

High Fiber Foods

Fiber helps to lower the **blood-cholesterol** and stabilize the **blood-sugar** levels. It also helps to prevent **colon cancer**, **constipation**, **hemorrhoids**, **obesity** and much more. The American diet is lacking in fiber, because refined foods have their natural fiber removed.

There are more than 85,000 colon cancer cases, the most common form of cancer in the United States, diagnosed each year and the number is growing. In contrast, colon cancer is rare in those who eat a diet low in meat and high in fiber-rich foods. Fiber collects carcinogens and binds them so they can be removed from the body.

Apples are high in fiber. There's more truth to the old saying, "An apple a day keeps the doctor away," than we ever realized.

There are two kinds of fiber, soluble and insoluble. Most plants contain a mixture of both types.

Pectins and gums are considered soluble fiber. This type of fiber forms a gel in the gastrointestinal tract by absorbing water and swelling as much as 10 times its weight. It slows down the passage of food and gives us a feeling of being full. That full feeling aids weight loss.

Insoluble fiber does not break down during digestion. This type fiber is also called roughage, and is found in grain cereals and breads as well as fruits and vegetables. Because it is not absorbed into the bloodstream, its calories are not added to the body.

The advantages of the following fibers is that they are known to reduce the risks of **obesity**, cut down on **blood-sugar** swings, reduce **heart disease**, **bowel disorders**, and **cancer**. There are six forms of fiber, each with a function of its own. You should start with small amounts of fiber and gradually increase your intake until stools are the proper consistency.

Pectin

Good for diabetics because it slows down food absorption after meals, removes unwanted metals and toxins. Pectin is valuable during treatment with radiation therapy or **X-rays**, and it helps lower cholesterol, lessens the risk of **heart disease** and **gallstones**. Pectin is found in apples, carrots, beets, bananas, the cabbage family, the citrus family, in dried peas, and okra.

Cellulose

Good for **hemorrhoids**, **varicose veins**, **colitis**, and **diverticulitis**. It is excellent for removal of cancer-causing substances from the **colon** wall, **constipation** and a boost for **weight loss**. Cellulose is found in apples, pears, the cabbage family, carrots, broccoli, lima beans, peas, whole grains, Brazil nuts, green beans and beets.

Hemicellulose

Good for **weight loss**, **constipation** and **colon cancer**. It fights carcinogens in the intestinal tract. Hemicellulose is found in apples, beets, whole grain cereals, cabbage, brussel sprouts, bananas, green beans, corn, peppers, broccoli, mustard greens and pears.

Lignin

Good for lowering **cholesterol** levels, protecting against **colon cancer** and preventing **gall stone** formation. It binds with bile acids to remove them. It's recommended for diabetics. Lignin is found in the cabbage family (cauliflower, etc.), carrots, green beans, peas, whole grains, Brazil nuts, peaches, tomatoes, strawberries and potatoes.

Gums & Mucilages

They regulate blood **glucose levels**, aid in lowering **cholesterol** levels and help in the removal of **toxins**. These are found in oatmeal, oat bran, sesame seeds and dried beans.

> Fiber helps to remove fat from the colon wall and unwanted metals and toxins from our bodies. In today's polluted environment our bodies need help in excreting this overload. Increase your intake of raw foods and supplement your diet with extra fiber!

One of the following should be part of your daily meal planning:

Oat bran to help lower blood cholesterol.

Cooked beans, one cup contains the same amount of soluble fiber as 2/3 cup of oat bran.

"People with low-fiber, high sugar diets are more prone to cancer," *Science News,* November 10, 1990.

Glucomannan picks up fat from the colon wall and moves it out. It is good for **diabetes** and **obesity** because it is a fat mobilizer. It expands to 10 times its own size. You must wash the capsule down with a large glass of water. Because it expands so much, it helps to curb the appetite if you take two or three capsules 30 minutes before meals.

Psyllium seed is a good intestinal cleanser and stool softener, it is one of the most popular fibers.

Fennel seeds help rid the intestinal tract of **mucus.**

Flaxseed is an excellent fiber with the added benefits of the essential fatty acids.

Kelp is good and helps keep your **weight** under control.

For the optimal diet, it is best to alternate the supplemental fibers. There are several to choose from besides the ones previously mentioned. Corn, brown rice, apple bran, apple pectin and agar agar are good for removing certain toxic metals.

The correct foods will add fiber to the diet. Among foods that will add the greatest amount of useful fiber to your diet are whole grain cereals, flours, brown rice, all kinds of bran, apricots, dried prunes, apples, most fruits. However, oranges are too acidic. They are bad for **arthritis** and are highly allergenic. Nuts, seeds, beans, lentils, peas, and vegetables (cabbage, broccoli, beets, cauliflower, carrots, and dark green leafy vegetables) are also good sources of fiber. Be sure to eat several of these foods daily.

Laxatives are habit-forming and irritating to the colon. Periodic internal cleansing is a good idea, along with a liquid diet for one to three days (diabetics or pregnant women should not fast on liquids, but could benefit from a raw food fast). **Hypoglycemics** do very well on a liquid fast using spirulina. It contains vitamins, minerals, chlorophyll, and the needed protein to keep the blood-sugar level up. Hypoglycemics benefit from using spirulina between meals to prevent a drop in blood-sugar and as a replacement for snacks. It helps to **control weight** and adds beneficial nutrients.

A study in the *Drug Store News* revealed the top-selling products across the nation are Fleet enemas, Bayer aspirin, Mylanta, Actifed and Visine. This list says a lot about the American public. First, people are constipated. Second, they are in pain. Next they suffer from heartburn and ulcers, and are miserable with colds, flu and sinus problems. Lastly, they have tired, bloodshot eyes.

Many of these problems are a direct result of a weakened immune system and a life-style that punishes our bodies. Much of the food we eat exerts extra pressure on an already overburdened body. The American diet of fat, sugar and salt strikes fear into the hearts of most of the nation's medical professionals and frustrates the efforts of nutritionists.

The latest Census Bureau statistics show that the average American consumes each year

    13.8 pounds of coffee
    106.2 pounds of beef
    Only 13.6 pounds of fish
    65.5 pounds of pork
    40 gallons of soft drinks
    6.9 gallons of milk

Do you see fresh vegetables or whole grains listed? Raw foods are important in your diet! Raw foods are filling and keep you from overeating, plus, they are full of needed nutrients and enzymes to help you stay healthy. Eating raw foods that are naturally high in fiber does not leave you with a craving for more food the way processed foods can.

> Do not consume fiber the same time as medications or other supplements. They will lose much of their effectiveness and strength because some fibers are so absorbent they pick up the beneficial elements as well as bad.
>
> Replace lost minerals the fiber absorbs with a mineral supplement taken at another time.

Remember, doctor bills, hospital bills and funeral bills are costly. Correcting your diet and changing your life-style, will not only keep you in good health but will add years to your life, and in time will save you a lot of money. Do not short change yourself.

For **weight loss**, fiber and exercise should be part of your program. Find the fiber that works best for you. We have found one-fourth cup of aloe vera juice, added to your morning juice and before bed, works wonders. Also, unsalted, unbuttered popcorn is excellent for added fiber.

Rice bran fiber may provide a source of dietary fiber that is superior to oat bran. When rice bran fiber is properly processed it can contain 27% dietary fiber by weight, 20% insoluble and 7% soluble.

Wheat bran contains 22% fiber, whereas stabilized rice germ and bran contain 34% fiber. These are also rich in linoleic and oleic acid, a monounsaturated acid. These unsaturated fatty acids, help lower cholesterol levels. Stabilized rice bran and germ fiber have a nutty taste. Due to the proportions and amounts of protein, carbohydrate, and unsaturated oils in them. Highly refined sources of fiber tend to be tasteless, or can even have a bitter aftertaste.

The highest fiber vegetable is the baked potato with its skin, and one serving of *Pritikin* Navy Bean Soup has twice the fiber content of a bowl of All Bran cereal.

Both soluble and insoluble natural fibers absorb many times their weight in water in the gastrointestinal tract. Psyllium absorbs 40 times its weight in water, while wheat bran absorbs three times its weight. The water absorption causes the bowel movement to be softer and to have greater bulk. The increased bulk puts pressure against the intestinal walls, this eases and regulates movement through the intestines. Fiber provides the bulk needed to encourage the expulsion of fecal material. During the digestive process, insoluble fiber remains unchanged.

Soluble fibers breaks down to form a gel in the small intestines that retards the absorption of glucose. This makes soluble fibers useful in the management of **diabetes, hypoglycemia, hyperglycemia,** and other conditions that are affected by the quick breakdown of carbohydrates. The body then can convert these carbohydrates into glucose, a form of sugar, slowly.

Soluble fibers increase the frequency of bowel movements and slow down the time it takes food to go through the system. In comparison, water insoluble fibers can also absorb water, increase fecal size, and frequency of bowel movements. The primary differences are that the insoluble fibers speed up the transit time and gastric emptying.

Soluble fibers have a strong effect on reducing serum **cholesterol** and fats by giving the body a full feeling, satisfying the **appetite**, stabilizing the **blood sugar**, reducing bacterial **toxins**, speeding up **bile-acid** excretion, and reducing gas. These fibers are less effective at speeding elimination of waste, absorbing toxins, softening stools, and improving bowel disorders. They do not block mineral absorption. Insoluble fibers are also effective at appeasing the **appetite**, reducing bacterial **toxins**, speeding the **elimination** of waste, absorbing toxins, softening stools, improving **bowel** disorders, and blocking mineral absorption. They are less effective at lowering serum cholesterol, speeding bile acid excretion, and reducing gas. Water insoluble fibers are not effective at giving a full feeling for a longer period or stabilizing blood sugar.

Scientists are learning how the various fibers act in the body. Some bind with bile acids and carry them out of the intestine so they cannot form cholesterol. Soluble pectin fiber in fruits and beta-glucan in oat bran seem to absorb harmful fatty acids. In some cases, the fiber's oily substance interferes with cholesterol synthesis, or perhaps blocks the action of carcinogens.

Psyllium acts like both a soluble fiber, preventing cholesterol absorption, and an insoluble fiber, scrubbing through the intestines and cleaning it of potential carcinogens. **Rice bran** and **oat bran** may both act as cholesterol reducers, but rice bran is not a soluble fiber.

Some scientists have theorized that the bile acids carried out of the intestines by some types of soluble fiber may act as cancer promoters once they reach the colon. A high fiber level then may be a trade off between **cholesterol** lowering and **cancer** risk. Although, an insoluble fiber would supposedly sweep out the colon with regular bowel movements.

The four components of fiber that do not dissolve in water are collectively referred to as insoluble dietary fiber. These include *cellulose, hemicelluloses, lignins, and waxes*. The main structural fiber of the plant cell wall is cellulose, hemicelluloses tie the cellulose fibers together. Within some plants are elements that make the plant cell wall rigid, these are the lignins. Good sources of cellulose are unpeeled apples, pears, canned peas, fresh carrots, and coarse bran. Hemicellulose is found in whole grain breads, beets, bran cereals, eggplant, and radishes. Pears, toasted whole grain breads, and browned potatoes also contain lignin.

Food Combining Guide

Combine Foods For Better Digestion

Correct food combinations are important for proper digestion, utilization and assimilation of the nutrients. If our food is not digested properly, it can pass through the intestinal tract without being completely broken down, getting caught in crevices in the intestinal tract and causing toxic wastes that putrefy. Then toxic particles pass into the bloodstream, where they can cause allergic reactions. Foods that the body cannot utilize waste the body's energy and overwork its organs. Additionally, the undigested food particles become food for unhealthy bacteria to feed upon. Even with a good diet, food must be properly prepared for the body to assimilate its nutrients. This is especially important for those who have hypoglycemia, diabetes, digestive disorders, and food allergies.

All sugars slow down digestion. The secreation of gastric juices needed for the breakdown of protein is almost stopped by sugar.

Sugar breaks down in the intestine and proteins break down in the stomach. Sugar can be held up in the stomach by meat until it ferments and creates problems. The result is foul smelling gas and stools, bloat and even heartburn. The body must work overtime getting rid of the toxins and poisons from wrong food combinations. Whenever our organs are overworked they can not function properly. This imbalance will generally give us a warning signal, however, if we do not act upon it, our whole system may malfunction. Problems such as obesity, high cholesterol, high and low blood sugar, among others, may be result of long-term consukption of the wrong food combinations.

> **Vegetables combine well with protein or starches.**

Let us start now and combine our foods properly to help our body. Food combining should be part of meal planning. Most important, remember not to eat sweet fruits with a protein meal, fruits should always be eaten alone. All melons should be eaten alone. Try not to combine acid fruits with sweet fruits.

Only those few people who have no digestive problems whatsoever, who chew their food extremely well and who eat mostly vegetables and all-natural foods may be able to get by without worrying about the rules of food combining.

Proteins are made up of amino acids. These are complete and incomplete proteins. The incomplete proteins lack one or more of the eight essential amino acids. We must supply them to our body. Proteins are the building blocks for all tissue and cells. Proteins provide energy and are also converted to fat.

Our bodies contain more protein than any other substance besides water. Although we need protein we do not require proteins derived from other animal products. Too much animal protein will lead to many health problems because of the high fat content and toxins. Meats are hard on the digestive system. See Meat & Dairy section.

Excessive protein consumption can damage the kidneys. Too much protein results in a buildup of nitrogen, which is eliminated as urea in the urine. Those with kidney disorders like nephritis and chronic kidney infections must follow a low-protein diet.

The eldery should also reduce protein intake because kidney function decreases with age.

People with liver disease need to limit protein intake. Excess protein also interferes with calcium metabolism, and those with osteoporosis should watch their protein intake.

The athelete needs complex carbohydrates because they are quickly metabolized into blood glucose and used during times of increased energy consumption. They don't need to increase their protein intake.

A pregnant woman needs extra protein to build the baby's tissues, brain and placenta, in addition to her own body's needs. Two to five ounces per day and after the fifth month three to five ounces may be needed. If the baby will be breast fed, the mother may need as much as four to five ounces daily. This protein should come partly from vegetable sources because ther is a chance of pesticide residues that are found in animal fats being passed along to the baby through the placenta, and later via the breast milk.

An optimal diet should consist of at least 50% vegetables. Combining is important for correct digestion and to utilize the nutrients fully.

Combining the following foods make up a complete protein. These foods lack one or more of the amino acids by themselves, but when put together they make a complete protein and are easier to digest than meat.

Combine for complete proteins	
Food	**Combined with**
Beans	Rice, cheese, wheat, sesame seeds, corn, all nuts or seeds
Corn Meal	L-Lysine
Rice	Cheese, sesame seeds, beans, wheat, seeds or nuts
Legumes	Combine any grain (beans, peas or peanuts) all nuts or seeds

By adding any of the above combinations to meals, you do not need animal protein. For instance, veggie chili or beans over brown rice makes a complete protein. Eat bread with nut butters or add nuts or seeds to meals. All soybean products: tofu, cheese, soy milk, or tempeh are complete proteins. The availability of complete proteins is limited without combining foods, even though vegetables contain protein, you would have to eat a large amount to fulfill the body's needs.

Vegetables combined with either grains, seeds, nuts, or dairy products are complete proteins. All vegetables contain protein and two or three of them combined complement each other. Remember, a complete protein consists of the eight essential amino acids the body cannot manufacture. Grains are complete proteins.

Strict vegetarians must be careful to get enough B-12, riboflavin, and vitamin D. Children and infant vegetarians need greater amounts of nutrients than adults, and careful planning is necessary to ensure they get a balanced diet. Children have small stomachs and a veggie dish maybe so high in bulk that it may be difficult for them to eat enough to meet their growth and energy needs.

Vitamin B-12 requirements must be met by eating fermented soybean products like tempeh, alfalfa, sea vegetables, kombu, and wakame, and nutritional yeast fortified with B-12. Adults and children have been deficient in B-12 when on strict vegetarian diets, so be sure to supplement your diet with B-12. Spirulina is a good addition to any diet, providing high amounts of B-12, B complex, beta carotene, gamma-linolenic acid (GLA), all eight essential amino acids plus 10 non-essential nutrients, such as vitamin E, folic acid, digestive enzymes, chlorophyll and iron. Spirulina is available in tablet or powder from a health food store.

Proteins combine poorly with all fruit, especially sweet fruit and other starchy foods. Proteins and sugar or starch neutralize the digestive juices needed by each for digestion. Milk ingested with proteins will neutralize the acid needed to break down the protein. Pasta and meat are also a poor combination.

Some additional examples of poor sugar-protein combinations are: ice cream (sugar, milk, and eggs), yogurt with sugar, baked beans, milk shakes, chocolate milk, and fruit with either eggs, cheese or meat.

All meat-protein meals combine best with vegetables (but not those with high starch content). All sources of protein combine well with green vegetables, especially salads.

Some of the basic rules in food combinations

> **The only time fruit can be successfully combined with another food is when the other food is soured (fermented), such as yogurt and cottage cheese.**

are: vegetables combine well with all starches; acids and sweet fruits are a poor combination; any type of melon should be eaten by itself; acidic fruits can be eaten with nuts or cheese.

Breads, crackers, muffins, all starches, do not combine with sweet fruits. Pancakes are poor with syrups and honey. Starches and proteins should not be combined with any form of sugar.

Remember, fruit contains a high percent of sugar, and because of this it should not be eaten with protein. Sugar and protein do not go together. The standard breakfast has been fruit and protein. The best breakfast one can consume is fruit, because of the cleansing effect. It also provides energy. Sweet fruits should be avoided by hypoglycemic or diabetic individuals.

The tongue recognizes four tastes, sweet, salty, bitter, and sour. The food industry plays on the sweet and the salty taste because they know man prefers sweet or salty to bitter or sour flavors. They camouflage foods that are picked before they are ripe by adding sugar to give it the ripe taste. Foods eaten before the acid has had a chance to turn into a natural sugar can be damaging to your health. Unripe fruits can cause indigestion, colitis, diarrhea, cramps, and many other intestinal disorders.

Foods loaded with salt result in excess water retention and the related problems such as obesity, high blood pressure and many more. The latest studies have shown that sodium may play a part in causing colon cancer. Even when they are not needed salt and sugar are added to nearly every commercial food product to enhance the taste. The food industry has made us sugar and salt addicts; don't buy these loaded foods.

Foods are made up of organic compounds: protein, sugar, carbohydrates, starches, fats, fiber (indigestible substances), minerals, trace minerals, vitamins, organic salts, and water. If that sounds familiar it should, because it is essentially what you are made of. Your body uses food for its basic building materials.

The following foods are broken down into categories to enable you to quickly identify the proper foods to combine

To have a basic understanding of why certain foods work the way they do, toy need to know something about the organic compounds from which foods are made. The following brief explanations cover complex and simple carbohydrates, acid and alkaline foods.

Simple Carbohydrates

Simple carbohydrates are found in all forms and types of sugars, some juices, and in processed and refined grains (not whole grains). Simple carbohydrates should be avoided if at all possible. However, glucose, fructose and galactose (which are also simple carbohydrates) are commonly found in our diets.

Two Simple Sugars

Sucrose (refined white sugar) and lactose (milk sugar) must be broken down, digested, before they can be absorbed into the bloodstream. Sucrose breaks down into glucose and fructose, and lactose breaks down into glucose and galactose. Most of us lack the ability to break lactose down into the simple sugar glucose; this is called **lactose intolerance**. It can cause diarrhea, gas, bloating, and cramps. If the problem is not a true allergy to milk but just the lactose intolerance, cheese or soured products such as yogurt will not cause you problems. Health food stores carry enzymes that will assist in breaking down the lactose.

Glucose (a sugar derived from sucrose sugars) is a major concern. Diabetes, for example is a condition characterized by too much glucose in the blood. Hypoglycemia, in a sense, is the opposite of diabetes. **Hypoglycemia** occurs where there is not enough glucose in the body. The percentage of glucose in the blood is normally regulated by insulin, a hormone secreted by the pancreas. When glucoseamounts rise above a normal level the pancreas releases insulin. When glucose levels drop below normal, then glucose is released by the liver to bring the levels back up to normal. When large amounts of glucose are ingested, they are quickly absorbed in the intestines. That quick shot of glucose triggers the pancreas to release insulin to counteract the glucose levels. When too much insulin is released, the blood glucose level falls below normal. This results in fatigue and a feeling of hunger. That is why, after a sugary snack, you still feel hungry and are even more tired than before. It can be a never-ending cycle that can lead to obesity. The constant hunger and the need to eat is real. The hunger and desire for sugar is equally real.

But, you must recognize the problem in order to resolve it. To replace the craving for sugar, eat a protein snack, this will increase your energy levels rather than leaving you feeling tired and hungry. Spirulina tablets, taken between meals, help keep the blood sugar level up.

Obesity, diabetes and hypoglycemia are possible results of a high-sugar (simple carbohydrate) diet. Sugar and fat lurk behind many health problems, heart disease and cancer lead the list.

Complex Carbohydrates

Complex carbohydrates are found in fresh vegetables, fresh fruits, beans, and natural whole grains. They provide dietary fiber and have only one-third the calories found in fats and simple carbohydrates. Proteins and carbohydrates contain a rich amount of vitamins and minerals. Carbohydrates can be converted into fat and provide the body with energy and warmth. A constant flow of energy is supplied from complex carbohydrates, rather than the short-lived energy bursts of simple carbohydrates or starches.To avoid the high energy and fatigue

cycle of unregulated blood sugar resulting from the ingestion of sugar, eat a diet high in complex carbohydrates that avoids all refined, processed foods and all forms of sugars. This is not just a method to reduce or maintain a normal weight, but a credo to be followed for basic good health for everyone.

Two basic steps to be followed that require only very minor changes in dietary habits:

(1) Eat complex carbohydrates during the day, when hungry.

(2) Do not raid the refrigerator late at night or eat a heavy meal late in the evening.

The more starch you consume, the more vitamins the body needs, especially B-vitamins. For weight reduction, lecithin should be added to your foods or liquids. Take one tablespoon before meals to help dissolve fat. For weight reduction, lecithin has the ability to bind water to fat to form an emulsion, which is why it is used in salad dressings and added to foods. It is a good addition to any program to prevent high blood pressure and arteriosclerosis, and to improve memory. The eldery also benefit from lecithin supplements, because of its high choline and inositol (B-vitamins) content.

The following test can help to asses your personal metabolism. It can provide a clue to excessive use of processed foods and simple carbohydrates.

Acid and Alkaline Test

1) Purchase nitrazine paper, available at any drugstore, and apply saliva or urine to the paper (or check both).

2) Check before eating or at least one hour after eating. The paper will change colors to indicate if your system is overly acidic or alkaline. Water is neutral at pH 7.0. Below pH is acid, above pH 7.0 is alkaline.

3) The ideal pH range for saliva and urine is 6.0-6.8 since our body functions best when it is naturally midly acidic. Therefore, values below pH 6.0 are too acidic, and above pH 6.8 are too alkaline.

4) The following foods should be consumed according to your test. If you were overly acid or alkaline omit the acid or alkaline forming foods from your diet, until your pH test returns to the normal range.

Fruits	
Highly Acid	**Mildly Acid**
Cherries	All Berries
Cranberries	Apricots
Dates	Banana
Dried Fruits	Fig
Grapefruit	Grape
Kumquat	Huckleberry
Lemons	Kiwi Fruit
Limes	Loquat
Oranges	Mango
Persimmon	Mulberry
Pineapples	Nectarine
Pomgrante	Papaya
Raisin	Peach
Sour Apples	Pear
Sour Grapes	Strawberries
Sour Peach	Sweet Apples
Sour Plums	Sweet Fruits
Tangerines	Sweet Grapes
Tomato	Sweet Plum

Starch-Free / Sugar-Free Vegetables	
All Lettuces	Fresh Sprouts
All onions	Garlic
Asparagus	Kale
Bamboo Shoots	Kohlrabi
Beet Greens	Leeks
Bell (green/red)	Okra
Broccoli	Parsley
Brussels Sprouts	Radishes
Cabbage	Rhubarb
Cauliflower	Sauerkraut
Celery	Scallion
Chinese Cabbage	Spinach
Chives	String Beans
Collards	Swiss Chard
Cucumber	Tomatos
Dandelion	Turnips/tops
Eggplant	Watercress
Endive	

PH Adjusting Foods	
Acid-Forming	**Alkaline-Forming**
Chicken	Almonds
Dairy products	Apricots
Eggs	Avocados
Fish	Coconut
Grains	Figs
Ham	Grapes
Lamb	Honey
Pork (all forms)	Lemons (not oranges)
Most nuts and seeds	Maple syrup
Meat--Beef	Milk
Turkey	Molasses
Veal	Raisins
All store bought	Umeboshi plums
processed foods	Vegetables (see fruits chart)
	Watermelon (all melons)
	Yogurt (soured products)

NOTE: most fruits turn alkaline in the body

Carbohydrates are both sugars and starches. Sugars are simple carbohydrates and starches are complex carbohydrates. Complex is good for you and gives a steady flow of energy.

Complex Carbohydrates

All whole grains, brown rice
All vegetables
Artichokes
Avacodos
Banana squash
Corn
Dried peas, beans and lentils
Fresh and dried fruits
Hubbard squash
Pastas
Potatoes, yams, pumpkin
Sweet potatoes
Water chestnuts
See also starch list

Food Enhancers for Health

Herbs and spices can change the most ordinary food into a memorable dish. They must be used with a light touch and soaked for 10-30 minutes in some of the liquid to be used in the recipe to release the flavor. To alter the flavor of any basic dish, prepare it with different combinations of herbs or spices:

> *Italian:* Basil, oregano, rosemary, thyme, marjoram
> *Oriental:* Fennel, anise, ginger, licorice root, cinnamon, clove
> *Continental:* Parsley, thyme, bay leaf, marjoram, tarragon

Combine equal amounts of the above mixtures in small jars and keep on hand for easy use.
Use 2 to 3 times the amount of fresh herbs in place of dried herbs.

Allspice

A berry used whole, ground or pressed with the leaves for their oil. The flavor is a blend of to cinnamon, cloves and nutmeg. Good in meat broths, broiled fish, gravies, desserts, and pickling.

Anise

The volatile oil of anise is helpful for bronchitis and spasmodic asthma. Five drops of anise oil placed in a teaspoon of honey half an hour before meals can help relieve those suffering from **emphysema**.

Anise has a licorice flavor, use in baked goods and oriental dishes, soups and cakes.

Basil, Sweet Basil

Basil is from the mint family, the leaves are cut and dried before the plant flowers. It has an aromatic, warm, and sweet flavor. Used in flavoring sauces tomatoes, fish, savory dishes poultry, and salads. Medicinally used as a disinfectant, an **immune stimulant**, for **intestinal parasites**, for the **stomach, lungs, spleen**, and **large intestines**. This spice can cause problems in large amounts, so use sparingly.

Bay Leaves

Leaves of the plant are picked and dried, the fruits and oils can also be used. It has a spicy and bitter flavor. Used in flavoring meats, fish, poultry, vegetables, and stews. Remove the leaf after cooking. Good for **stress management**, **infection**, also can be used to keep cockroaches away, spread around infested area. Place in grain to deter insects.

Caraway & Caraway Seed

The caraway root is eaten as a vegetable, the leaves as a seasoning, the oil is also used. The flavor tends to be sweet, warm and acrid, but pleasant. The seeds are used in flavoring breads, cakes, cheeses, and cookies. The oil is used in canning, flavoring meats, gargles, and antibacterial soaps. The most popular use is in sauerkraut and dishes with a sour flavor.

Cardamom

A member of the ginger family, the seeds and oil are used. Its flavor is sweet, aromatic, and pungent. The seeds can be ground and used in pastries, buns, and pies and to flavor coffee. It is also a breath freshener. Cardamom is used by the Bedu tribes of the Arabian Peninsula as an **energy booster**.

Cayenne, African Pepper & Chilies

A member of the nightshade family, the fruit of the plant is picked when it has turned red, and then it is left to dry. It flavors hot, spicy dishes, eggs, and

101

beans. Good for **circulation**, **colon disorders** and the **heart**. Also good for chronic pain such as **arthritis** in a cream form. Avoid contact with the eyes.

Celery Seed

A member of the parsley family, the roots and stalks are used.The flavor is lightly bitter and is used to flavor a wide variety of foods. The oil is used in soaps and perfumes.

Chervil

Use this in soups, stews and salads. Use in any dish as you could use parsley

Chia

This tiny black seed is found in the Southwestern part of the United States and Mexico. Indians have used it for years to sustain life and energy on long hunting trips. The seeds are high in protein. They can be sprinkled, in seed form, on foods or ground in a blender. Try them on sandwiches, cottage cheese, or salads.

Chives

A grasslike plant, only the greens or leaves are used. Has a mild, onion-like flavor. Used in broths, eggs, vegetable dishes, and as garnish.

Cinnamon & Cassia Bark

The bark of this plant is peeled and dried. A mildly strong, acidic flavor, that sweetens.Used in cakes, breads, pickling, and flavoring drinks and by some of the people of Eritrea (a province of Northern Ethiopia) as a general flavoring in their food. The bark is also used by them as an activating ingredient for a mildly alcoholic drink made with honey. Good for **back and neck pain**, **chest pain**, and **menopause**.

> Chinese researchers report a number of common spices that are effective in relieving **arthritis** pain. These include: ginger, parsley, basil, oregano, sage, marjoram, clove, thyme, and cinnamon.

Cloves

The petals on the plant are picked and dried. The flavor is sweet, strong, and highly aromatic. Cloves are used in baked goods and desserts, when ground. The spikes are used to flavor meats, pickles, fruits, and syrups. A good **anesthetic** for **toothaches**, **a digestive aid**, **kills intestinal parasites**, for **hernia**, **hiccupping**, **upset stomach**, and **abdominal pain**.

Coriander

A member of the parsley family, the seed and the leaf of the plant are used. Has a mild, sweet, and pungent flavor. Similar to lemon and sage. Used in curry powder, to flavor meats, candy, and also used to disguise the nauseating qualities in some medicines. It **kills bacteria**, **fungi and is good on cuts and wounds** to kill micro-organisms.

Cumin

A member of the parsley family, the plant is dried and threshed when it withers. Has a strong smell, and is bitterly hot. Used in stews, soups, sauces, also as a flavoring for cheeses, breads and chutney. Use seeds sparingly.

Dill

Of the parsley family, the primary part of the plant used is the seeds. Has a taste similar to caraway. May be used ground up or whole to flavor breads, salads, and seafood, but it is mostly used as a condiment. Good for **poor appetite**, **circulation**, **kidneys**, **spleen**, and **lowers the blood pressure**.

Fennel

Of the parsley family, the leaves, stalks, roots, and seeds are used. Has a flavor like licorice, a smell stronger than dill, but tastes milder. Used to flavor fish, soups, teas, and salads. The seeds are used in breads and pickles. Good for **stomachaches**, **lumbago**, also aids in function of the **kidneys**, **bladder**, and **stomach**. It has a gentle **laxative** effect and is good as a tea for nursing mothers to **increase** their **milk** or for **infant colic**.

Fenugreek

Of the bean family, the plant is dried and threshed. A bittersweet burnt taste, the oil smells similar to celery. Used in breads, chutneys, curry powders, and as a condiment.

Reduces mucus in sinus and **asthmatic conditions**. Latest research found that it **lowers cholesterol**. This seed makes an excellent tea for **intestinal irritation** or as a gargle for **sore throats**. It can also be ground as a poultice for **wounds** or **inflamed areas**.

Flax

Linseed oil is made from flaxseeds. These good tasting seeds are high in unsaturated fatty acids. They can be used as a tea or ground to sprinkle on cereal, yogurt, salads, and so on. They are good for **brittle hair, constipation, bronchial conditions** and for all health problems.

Garlic

Perhaps the most significant effect of garlic is on the lipid profile of the blood and tissues. It lowers cholesterol, triglycerides, and LDL cholesterol levels, while increasing the beneficial cholesterol HDL. Onions have the same effect.

The bulb of the plant is a relative of onions and chives. The flavor is very strong and powerful. When garlic is whole, it is essentially odorless. When crushed, an enzyme, alliinase, combines with a main sulfur component, alliin, to produce allicin, which has the strong odor. Use chopped, minced, and powdered to season many dishes. Very good for lowering blood pressure, strengthening the heart, and as a natural deterrent to insects. A potent immune enhancer. It is good for the **heart, stomach, spleen**, and **lungs**.

Researchers at *Loma Linda University* have found that compounds in garlic activate enzymes in the liver that **destroy aflatoxin**, a potent carcinogen produced by mold that can grow on peanuts and grains. Aflatoxins are a leading cause of liver cancer. Garlic may also **protect against cancer causing agents** found in cigarette smoke, charbroiled meat, and polluted air. See the Garlic section for more information.

Ginger

Ginger is a favorite ingredient used medicinally and in Chinese cooking. The rhizomes or underground stalks of the plant are used. The flavor is strong, spicy, and sweet. It is used in breads, pickles, soft drinks, puddings, cookies, and oriental dishes. A good digestive aid, it **thins the blood, lowers blood cholesterol**, and **reduces fever**. Also good as a **tonic**, for **colds, cough, asthma**, and **relieves vomiting**. Good for the **lungs, stomach**, and **spleen**. Ginger contains a substance called ginerol, which may prevent so called "little strokes."

Marjoram

Of the mint family, the leaves and tops of the plant are harvested and dried. Has a sweet and delicate flavor. Used ground or whole to flavor cheeses, meats, and vegetables dishes. Good for **fever, colds, flu, jaundice**, and **vomiting**.

Horseradish

Of the mustard family, the root of the plant is used. The flavor is sharp, hot and pungent. The root is grated and used with meats and seafood sauces. Is good for all **bronchial** and **lung disorders, loosens** and **removes mucus for bronchitis** and **asthma**.

Mint

Use in herb teas, sauces, on new potatoes, salads and fruit salads. Good for **digestion**.

Mustard Seed

Has a hot, spicy, and strong flavor. The oil of the seed is used as a condiment.

Nutmeg

The inside of a nut of a specific evergreen. Has a aromatic, bitter, strong, and warm flavor. Used ground up to flavor beverages, and baked goods. The oil is used medicinally. Aids in **relieving pain, abdominal swelling, indigestion**, and **diarrhea**.

Onion

The bulb of the plant has a strong pungent flavor, not as overwhelming as garlic. Used widely in cooking. The skins are used to make paper. Has been used by *Dr. Victor Gurewich, Professor of Medicine at Tufts University* to increase HDL levels by about 30% while decreasing LDL (unhealthy cholesterol) levels. During his research *Dr. Gurewich* found that as little as one-half a medium sized, raw onion per day was sufficient to produce these positive, healthful results. Additional research at *Tufts University* indicates that onions, cooked or raw, greatly **reduce platelet clumping** by reducing the levels of fibrinogen, the basic clot-forming substance. By lowering the blood's ability to clot, some of the dangerous effects of high blood pressure are reduced. Even though cholesterol levels and blood-clotting are two different matters. Chemically, *Dr. Gurewich* has identified some 150 compounds in onions some or all of which are involved in these beneficial effects.

Oregano, Wild Marjoram & Wintersweet

Of the mint family, the leaves are dried and and have a spicy, aromatic flavor. Used in omelets, tomato dishes, salads, stews, and vegetables.

Paprika, Hungarian Pepper & Sweet Pepper

A member of the nightshade family, the pods are dried, the flavor is pungent and savory. Used on meats, salads, relishes, eggs, and vinegar.

Parsley

Leaves and seeds of the plant are used. Has a mild, agreeable flavor. Used in soups, stews, salads, as a garnish and is good for freshening breath. The oil

of the seed is used in medicines. Good for **indigestion, measles, lungs**, and **spleen**.

Poppy Seed

The seeds can be black or white but black seeds have been found to be higher in quality. Has a nutty flavor. Used as a condiment on rolls and pastries, is crushed for sweet fillings and used to flavor fish, vegetables, rice, and noodles.

Psyllium

This seed is used primarily as fiber and as a lubricant. It is effective for combating **constipation**. It can be added to cereals or blended to drinks. Use 2 to 3 full tablespoons (or 4-5 capsules) daily for **colon problems**.

Pumpkin

This seed is rich in zinc, calcium and B vitamins. Some doctors use the oil and seeds to treat the **prostate gland**. It has been used to **destroy parasites** (worms) in the intestinal tract. It is also available in capsule form.

Rosemary

From the mint family, the fragrant leaves are used to flavor stews, potatoes, soups, vegetables, and lamb dishes. Mix with food which spoils easily. It helps to **prevent food poisoning**, **fight infection** and ward off **headaches**.

Saffron

The stigmas of the flower of the plant are used. Pleasantly spicy, bitter taste, has an odd odor. Used to spice rice dishes, cakes, breads, and dressings. Also used in medicines for **congestion of the chest, abdominal pain after childbirth**, to **improve circulation, affects the heart, liver** and **promotes energy**.

Sage

Seeds or cuttings can be used from this plant. Has a warm, bitter flavor. Leaves used to flavor salads, pickles and cheeses. Good for **canker sores, bleeding gums, sore throat, lungs, diabetes, wounds**, preservative for meats that spoil, and as an **antioxidant**. Sage contains a volatile oil, tannin, resin, and is bitter. The oil is composed of pinene, camphor, salveve, and cineol. *Ursolic acid* was also found in sage leaves. The oil contains bactericidal properties. Medical herbalists use the sage for **tonsillitis, ulceration of the mouth** and **throat**, as a tea and a gargle.

Savory

A popular spice used for stuffings, soups and bean dishes. Good for **flatulence (gas)** when added to beans, **coughs, colds, stomachaches** and **diarrhea**.

Sesame

This seed is very tiny, but rich in calcium, potassium, iron, phosphorus and protein. It is also a good source of unsaturated oil. Sesame is also made into butter, which is good when used in sauces or over vegetables to make a complete protein meal. Seeds easily become rancid, if not properly packaged and refrigerated. They should be light in color.

Star Anise

The flavor is similar to licorice and is used in seasoning dishes and sweets. The seeds can be chewed as a **breath freshener**.

Tarragon

The leaves of the plant are dried. The flavor is bittersweet. Used in salads, vinegars, and general seasonings.

Sunflower

These wonderful seeds are full of the B vitamins, phosphorus, potassium, and much more. Make sure the seeds have not been overcooked in "bad" oils or that they are not rancid. They should not be too dark in color, nor should there be several colors. Look for fresh, medium gray seeds that are sealed, or kept under refrigeration.

Thyme

The flowering tops are cut and dried. Has a warm, pleasant flavor. Used to flavor meats, cheeses, and vegetables. Good for **acute bronchitis, laryngitis**, and **whooping cough**. A *Scottish researcher, Biochemist Stan Deans, Ph. D., of the Scottish Agricultural College in Auchincruive* concludes that thyme may provide **protection from free radicals**, marauding molecules, that can undermine cells throughout the body, thus **protecting the brain, liver, kidneys, heart** and **retinas** in lab rats.

Turmeric

Is a root from the ginger family. The rhizomes are used. Has a ginger-pepper pungent flavor. Used to flavor curry powder, prepared mustard, dressings cheeses, and butter.

Vanilla

Pods of the plant are picked and dried. A spicy, delicate flavor. Used to flavor desserts and in perfumes.

Vanilla beans are derived from a tropical climbing plant that belongs to the orchid family. The pods are aged for about six months until they start to ferment. Pure vanilla extract is made by macerating the pods in a 35 to 40% solution of food grade alcohol. You should take care to buy the pure extract rather than an extract made from vanillin, a synthetic product made in a laboratory; if it is pure it will state this on the bottle.

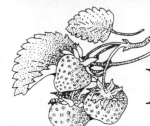
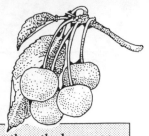

Fruits & Healing

Most fruits ripen faster when left in a plastic or paper bag, since the bag traps the ethylene gas that is produced by the fruit and acts as a ripening agent. Apples give off large amounts of gas, so you can help speed the ripening of other fruits by placing an apple (or apple slices) in the bag with them, *University of California at Berkeley Wellness Letter,* Vol. 8, Issue 9. You can also place sliced apples in fructose or granulated sugar that has hardened and it will soften overnight.

Apples

Chronic enteritis
Bladder cleanser
Intestinal infections
Inflammation of the colon
Diarrhea
Arthritis
Herpes and viruses
Acid stomach
Excellent fiber
Aid in detoxifying metals
Protect against danger from x-rays,
   radiation therapy
Lower blood cholesterol
Lower blood pressure
Stabilize blood sugar

They contain 84% pure water, carbohydrates, protein, minerals, vitamins A, B, and C. Also high in iron, potassium and many nutrients.

Apricots

Constipation
Cancer
Muscle and nerve tissue
All bowel disorders
Skin
Excellent fiber

The seeds are used in cancer treatment in some clinics. They contain *laetrile* which is believed to be beneficial in controlling cancer. Apricots contain good amounts of carotene, potassium, and iron.

Avocado

Fatigue
Hypoglycemia
Urinary infections
Convalescence after surgery
Nerves

Avocados contain high amounts of the good fats, making them important for the hypoglycemic. However, they should be consumed in moderation by diabetics.

Bananas

Nerves
Alcoholism
Hypertension
Hemorrhoids
Heart disorders
Ulcers
Diarrhea
Potassium deficiency
High blood pressure
Edema
Intestinal disturbances
Muscular system
Feed the good bacteria in colon

Excellent for children and infants. Low in fat, good for reducing diets. Good for convalescents because bananas are soft and high in needed nutrients, especially potassium and vitamin C.

All dried fruits should be soaked in boiling water a few minutes to kill bacteria that forms during drying.

Aldicarb, a toxic insecticide used on bananas, was suspended after levels above permitted tolerances were found in bananas grown in five trial sites in Central and South America. The manufacturer, Rhone-Poulenc, has suspended its use on bananas pending a study by the firm and the EPA. The study is also probing the safety of aldicarb use on pecans, soybeans, oranges, grapefruit, potatoes, and sweet potatoes.

Blueberry

Hypoglycemia
Tinnitus (ringing in the ears)
Rejuvenates pancreas

High in manganese and vitamin A, also contains potassium, silicon, and iron, an excellent source of fiber. The high amounts of manganese make this very good for many disorders. The blue pigment may be a powerful liver protector, also found in bilberry (herb).

Blackberry

Leucorrhea
Enteritis
Chronic appendicitis
Constipation
Diarrhea
Blood builder
Anemia

All berries are high in fiber. The leaves are used to make medicinal herbal teas in herbal medicines.

Cherries

Excellent for gout
Lumbago
Rheumatism
Paralysis
Arthritis
Stunted growth
Obesity

Black cherry juice prevents tooth decay by stopping plaque formation. Good for the glandular system, removes toxic waste from tissues. Aids in gall bladder and liver function.

Grapefruit seed extract is a natural antibiotic, it fights bacteria, including candida, as well as viruses and parasites. Works fast and is safe. Some side effects experienced are mild stomach irritation and flatulence. The extract comes from ground grapefruit seeds. A good natural alternative to pharmaceutical antibiotics. It should never be taken in straight liquid form as it could burn the mouth, throat and stomach. Either mix it with juices or take in capsule form.

Cranberry

Kidneys and bladder
Asthma
Skin
Intestinal antiseptic
High in Vitamin C

A glass of quality cranberry juice in the morning and afternoon will control many female bladder infections.

Figs

Kill bacteria
Destroy roundworms
Hemorrhoids
Anti-cancer agent
A restorative for the ill
Aid digestion

Fig juice is good for destroying intestinal parasites. Contain high amounts of fiber.

Grapes

Combat toxins
Stimulate the liver
Increase energy
Skin
Fever
Constipation
Cancer
Edema
Palpitations of the heart
Cleansing effect on all
   tissues and glands

Grapefruit

Cardiovascular system
Chest congestion
Protect the arteries
Lower risk of cancer
Lower blood cholesterol

The whole fruit, pectin, pulp, and fibrous content are important. Good for a healthy heart. High in potassium and vitamin C, with no fat. The seeds are available in pill form because experiments show they aid in healing candida and other infections, due to their antibiotic action.

Lemons & Pineapple

Cleanses the bloodstream and liver
Inflammation
Colds, influenza, and sore throat
Bronchitis
Asthma
Digestion
Heartburn
Diabetes
Scurvy
Fevers
Rheumatism

Lemons are a wonderful liver stimulant and a solvent for uric acid and other toxins.

Fresh pineapple contains manganese which is an essential part of certain enzymes needed to metabolize protein and carbohydrates.

Melons

Cantaloupe and honeydew are the most available melons year round. One half cantaloupe provides more vitamin A (beta-carotene) and vitamin C than most other types of fruit. It is also high in potassium and only 95 calories per serving.

Choose cantaloupes with thick close netting, avoid those with smooth areas or soft mushy spots. When ready to eat, the ends should yield slightly to the pressure of your finger. If it is too hard it will never ripen properly or become sweet enough.

Honeydew melon is slightly larger, yellowish-white (cream) colored on the outside and a light green on the inside. Test for ripeness, the same as for cantaloupes. Honeydews have a smooth surface. If you cannot find one ripe enough, let one stand at room temperature until ripe, then store it in the refrigerator.

Warning: Scrub the rind with a mild detergent and thoroughly rinse it before cutting to prevent spreading the bacteria into the flesh of the melons. This is good for all fresh produce which may be contaminated. The *Food and Drug Administration* reported that over 200 cases of salmonella, food-born illness, were caused by cantaloupe harvested in Texas. Most of the victims ate contaminated melons at salad bars in the Midwest and Eastern parts of the U.S. Consumers purchasing melon to eat at home are in less risk as they normally eat the melon immediately after slicing it.

Smoldering orange and grapefruit peels are highly effective mosquito fumigants, according to recent research. The peels were dried for 3 days, crushed, then .2 pounds were ignited in a mosquito infested room. After 1 hour 60% of the insects were dead. To avoid respiratory irritation do not enter the room for 3 hours. *HerbalGram,* No.25, 1991.

Oranges

Oranges are mainly used for juice in our country. They contain high amounts of vitamins C and A. Because of the over-consumption of oranges, many people have an allergic reaction to oranges. They often do not connect their symptoms to the juice they consume each morning. Choose oranges that do not look like they are a wax imitation. They have been picked green before the acid can turn to fructose, this is why most people cannot tolerate them. They are sprayed orange to look appealing. Choose those that do not look perfect. **If you have joint pains, or bladder trouble, omit oranges from your diet.**

Oranges are beneficial for reasons other than their high vitamin content. Studies have shown that the oil in the peel has been found to lower the incidence of chemically-induced cancers. *Terpenes* in orange oil, in addition to *d-limonenes*, contain anti-cancer qualities. *D-limonene* has been found to reverse tumors. In addition, d-limonene is a natural cholesterol-lowering substance and can dissolve gallstones. Researchers at the *University of Wisconsin* have found that tumors, in 90% of a group of mice being studied, completely disappeared after being fed *d-limonene*.

Oranges, if picked green, may cause "joint-like" arthritic pains and make those who suffer with arthritis worse. The citric acid in these green oranges has not had time to be converted to fructose sugar and they have very little vitamin C content. Also, some oranges are colored orange with a red dye to appear ripe and then waxed to prolong storage life. They are also sprayed with a fungicide to retard rotting. Be sure oranges are organic if you must have them. Some of those beautiful oranges may not be so beautiful for your body.

Ellagic acid found in strawberries and cherries counteracts both human and naturally occurring cancer-causing agents. *American Health Foundation* research reported in *Natural Health*, March/April 1992.

Papaya

Acidosis
Colon disorders
Enzymes
Chronic illness
Digestion of protein
Ulcers

Breaks down unwanted substances, including uric and toxic acids in the body. Good to add to infant formula to help digestion.

Peaches

Peaches contain beta-carotene (vitamin A), potassium, and fiber, in addition to being low in calories. They are good for those suffering from cancer, heart disease or any type of illness. They are soft and easy to digest. The elderly should include this fruit in their diet. Do not buy peaches that are rock hard or have a green tint. Choose ones that have a creamy yellow and red color, and a peachy smell. Store ripe fruit in the refrigerator.

Pears

Natural laxative
Chronic gall bladder disorders
Arthritis
Gout
Lungs and stomach
Pears have a very high insoluble fiber content.

Pomegranate

The fruit is red, and it is the size of an orange. It is eaten and the juice is used to make refreshing drinks in the Middle East.

Used to treat diarrhea, excessive perspiration, a gargle for sore throats, for fevers, leucorrhea, and tapeworm infestation (using the root bark).

The peel contains about 30 percent tannin, which is an active astringent substance.

Prunes

Lower blood cholesterol
Constipation
Parasites
The *benzoic acid* present in plums is used for liver disease, blood poisoning, and kidney disorders. High fiber content is found in the prune, not the juice. Remember, a prune is a dried plum.

Raspberry

Liver tonic
Diarrhea remedy
Frequent urination
Impotence
The dried leaves, used as an herb are made into tea for all female disorders.

Strawberries

Protect against viruses and cancer
Protect against DNA damage
Protect against herpes simplex
virus, skin disorders, and acne
Strawberries contain high amounts of vitamin C and have more fiber than a slice of whole grain bread. High in potassium and certain *polythenols*, good antioxidants. Strawberries can block the transformation of nitrosamine, a powerful cancer causing substance. The viruses that strawberries can destroy in the body are retro-viruses and herpes viruses.

Do not remove the strawberry caps until they are ready to eat, to keep the vitamin C in tact. Avoid moldy berries because the mold will spread very rapidly. Do not wash until they are ready to eat.

Berries are high in fiber, potassium, and vitamin C. They come in many varieties including blackberries, blueberries, boysenberries, currants, dewberries, elderberries, gooseberries, huckleberries, loganberries, raspberries, and strawberries.

Watermelon

Natural diuretic
Blood purifier
Cleanses tissues
Canker sores in mouth

Dr. Linus Pauling believes vitamin C works to strengthen the immune system, keeps tumors from spreading and migrates through the body to find and destroy stray cancer cells. Vitamin C has "remarkable general detoxifying powers for toxic substances that enter the human body, including carcinogens." Ten grams a day is a conservative dose of vitamin C for those diagnosed with cancer. Dr. Pauling recommends much more as part of a comprehensive nutrition program for those with cancer. From Dr. Pauling's studies, and additional research, it appears that cancer is neither inevitable nor out of our control, *Let's Live*, September 1991.

109

PRODUCE NUTRITION INFORMATION CHART

■ FRUITS (RAW)	Total Calories	Protein	Carbohydrate	Total Fat	Dietary Fiber	Sodium	Vitamin A	Vitamin C	Calcium	Iron
	kcal	g	g	g	g	mg	\% U.S. RDA			
Apple, 1 medium (5.5oz/154g)	80	0	18	1	5	0	*	6	*	*
Avocado, ⅓ medium (2oz/55g)	120	1	3	12	2	5	*	5	*	*
Banana, 1 medium (4.5oz/126g)	120	1	28	1	3	0	*	15	*	2
Cantaloupe, ¼ medium (5oz/134g)	50	1	11	0	0	35	80	90	2	2
Cherry, Sweet, 21 cherries, 1cup (5oz/140g)	90	1	19	1	3	0	*	10	2	*
Grape, 1½ cups (5oz/138g)	85	1	24	0	2	3	3	9	2	2
Grapefruit, ½ medium (5.5oz/154g)	50	1	14	0	6	0	6	90	4	*
Honeydew, 1/10 medium (5oz/134g)	50	1	12	0	1	50	*	40	*	2
Kiwifruit, 2 medium (5.5oz/148g)	90	1	18	1	4	0	2	230	4	4
Lemon, 1 medium (2oz/58g)	18	0	4	0	0	10	*	35	2	*
Lime, 1 medium (2.5oz/67g)	20	0	7	0	3	1	*	35	2	2
Nectarine, 1 medium (5oz/140g)	70	1	16	1	3	0	20	10	*	*
Orange, 1 medium (5.5oz/154g)	50	1	13	0	6	0	*	120	4	*
Peach, 2 medium (6oz/174g)	70	1	19	0	1	0	20	20	*	*
Pear, 1 medium (6oz/166g)	100	1	25	1	4	1	*	10	2	2
Pineapple, 2 slices (3″ diameter, ¾″ thick), (4oz/112g)	90	1	21	1	2	10	*	35	*	*
Plum, 2 medium (4.5oz/132g)	70	1	17	1	1	0	9	20	*	*
Strawberry, 8 medium (5.5oz/147g)	50	1	13	0	3	0	*	140	2	2
Tangerine, 2 medium (2⅜″ diameter) (6oz/168g)	70	1	19	0	2	2	30	85	2	*
Watermelon, 1/18 medium (2cups diced), (10oz/280g)	80	1	19	0	1	10	8	25	*	2

(Data source: FDA)

* Contains less than 2% of U.S. RDA

The waxes that are commonly applied to various fruits and vegetables are made of shellac, paraffin, palm oil or synthetic resins, and they are recognized as safe by the U.S. Food and Drug Administration. The fruit and vegetable industry uses waxes to make products look shiny and fresh as well as to seal in moisture and prevent wilting and shriveling.

However, fungicides are often mixed with waxes to prevent mold and rot. Animal studies suggest that some of these fungicides may increase the risk of cancer and other disorders. Because waxes are insoluble, rinsing waxed produce with water won't remove them. The only way to avoid ingestion is to peel the food--especially for produce commonly eaten with the peel, such as apples, tomatoes, cucumbers, peppers and potatoes.

Lifetime Health Letter, June 1992, pg.8

The *Food and Nutrition Board of the National Academy of Sciences* recommends that you eat five servings of fruits and vegetables daily. The reason: Fruits and vegetables can help you control your weight and reduce your risk of coronary heart disease and cancer.

Fruits and vegetables contain virtually no fat and most have fiber. They also are rich in a variety of vitamins, minerals and other chemicals that scientists suspect may be related to disease prevention, particulary cancer prevention.

Mayo Clinic Health Letter, July 1992, pg. 1

Pectin Zaps Tumors

The citrus pectin in fruits may inhibit tumor cell growth. In the *Journal of the National Cancer Institute*, researchers reported that once their studies are confirmed, injections of pectin could be given to patients before and after surgery.

HOW TO BUY FRUIT

	Best Buy	Avoid
Apples	Firm, well-colored fruit. Immature apples lack color and may look shriveled after being stored.	Fruit which yields to slight pressure on the skin and which has soft, mealy flesh, and fruit with bruised areas.
Apricots	Plump fruit with uniform golden-orange color. Ripe apricots will yield to gentle pressure on the skin.	Dull-looking, soft, or mushy fruit and very firm, pale yellow or greenish yellow fruit.
Bananas	Fruit which is free from bruises or injury. Best eating quality when skin is solid yellow and newly speckled with brown spots.	Bruised fruit, discolored skins, or a dull, grayish appearance. At times, the skin may be entirely brown and the flesh still in prime condition.
Blueberries	A dark blue color with silvery bloom, plump, firm, uniform size, dry and free from stems or leaves.	Moldy, bruised or green berries.
Cantaloupes (muskmelons)	Thick, coarse, corky surface with veins standing out on surface. No stem. Yellowish rind. Will yield slightly to thumb pressure on non-stem end. Ripens at room temperature. Small bruises OK.	Pronounced yellow rind color, softening over entire rind, or mold growth, particularly in stem scar.
Cherries	A very deep maroon or mahogany red to black. Bright, glossy, plump-looking surfaces, and fresh looking stems.	Shriveled fruit, dried stems, soft, leaking flesh, brown discoloration, mold growth and a dull appearance.
Grapefruit	Smooth, firm, well-shaped fruits, heavy for their size. Skin defects such as scars and discolorations do not affect the quality.	Rough, ridged, or wrinkled skin, soft discolored areas on the peel at the stem end and a soft and tender peel that breaks with pressure.
Grapes	Well-colored, plump grapes that are firmly attached to the stem	Soft or wrinkled grapes and grapes with lighter areas around the stem end.
Honeydew Melons	A soft, velvety feel, a slight softening at the blossom end and a yellowish white to creamy rind color.	Fruit with flat white or greenish-white color and hard, smooth feel; large bruised areas; surface cuts. Small sunken spots ok for quick use.
Lemons	Firm and heavy fruit with rich yellow color and smooth texture with a slight gloss. Pale or greenish color means more acidity.	Fruit with darker yellow or dull color, hardening or shriveling of the skin, or soft spots or moldy surface.

111

HOW TO BUY FRUIT

	Best Buy	Avoid
Limes	Glossy skin and heavy weight for the size. Dark green without yellowing.	Dull, dry skin, soft spots, or mold. Purplish or brownish mottling does not indicate damage in early stages.
Nectarines	Rich color, plump and soft along the seam. Orange-yellow in color, but some varieties are greenish.	Hard, dull fruit, slightly shriveled fruit, soft fruit, or fruit with a cracking skin.
Oranges	Firm and heavy oranges with fresh, bright-looking skin which is reasonably smooth for the variety.	Lightweight, rough skin texture, dull, dry skin, spongy texture, spots on the surface, discolorations, dyed and perfect appearing.
Peaches	Firm or becoming a bit soft. The skin color between the red areas should be yellow or creamy.	Hard or very firm fruit with green color. Also, very soft fruit with large bruises or any sign of decay.
Pears	Firm fruit. Bartletts-pale to rich yellow; Anjou or Comice-light green to yellowish green.	Wilted or shriveled fruit with a dull appearing skin and weakening of the flesh toward the stem. Avoid spots.
Pineapples	Bright color, fragrant pineapple odor, usually dark green, firm, plump and heavy when mature.	Fruit with sunken, slightly pointed, dark, or watery eyes; dull yellowish-green color; dried apperance, soft spots.
Plums	Fruit that is fairly firm to slightly soft.	Overly hard or soft fruit. Fruit with skin breaks or brownish discolorations.
Raspberries & Boysenberries	Uniform good color. Plump and tender but not mushy. No attached stem caps.	Leaky and moldy berries and wet or stained spots on the container.
Strawberries	Clean and dry berries with full red color and a bright luster, firm flesh, and a cap stem still attached.	Large colorless or seedy areas, a dull shrunken appearance, softness, or mold.
Tangerines	Deep yellow or orange color and a bright luster.	Very pale yellow or greenish fruits, small green areas on deeply-colored fruit is ok. Fruit with cuts or punctured areas.
Watermelons	Firm, juicy flesh with a good red color, free from white streaks; dark brown or black seeds. Smooth, dull surface, hollow sounding when thumped. Cream-colored belly.	Pale colored, dry, mealy, watery, or stringy flesh with white streaks and whitish seeds.

U.S. Department of Agriculture

Garlic

A Miracle Healer bridging medicine and herbs

Garlic has been known since ancient Biblical times (Numbers 11:5), as a staple food that provided remarkable preventative and healing properties. World-wide research presented at the *First World Conference on Garlic*, Washington, D.C., July 1990, reinforced this knowledge, bringing to our attention the marvelous potential of garlic as a vital resource to our "Healing Power Within." A wide range of health benefits were identified. These scientific revelations included how garlic lowers serum **cholesterol**, especially the LDL component called "bad cholesterol," how it significantly and safely lowered blood pressure, how garlic improved circulation by reducing the "stickiness of the blood", how garlic helped arthritis, and probably most important, how garlic potentiates the human **immune system**. *Kyolic,* the odorless, aged garlic extract known as "sociable garlic," was discovered to be even more potent because of the enhanced therapeutic activity.

Paavo Airola, considerd a leading authority on biological medicine, described garlic as, "A much neglected wonder food, with amazing nutritional and medical properties, and The King of the vegetable kingdom." His research of the world's scientific literature confirms these facts: Garlic was proven effective in treating **allergies, arthritis, arteriosclerosis, cancer, diabetes** and **hypoglycemia, fungus disease (candidiasis), gastrointestinal disorders (colitis),** and **pulmonary disease (asthma, bronchitis, and pneumonia)**. It may seem impossible to believe, but these are the facts, and physicians have known about this miracle food for centuries.

We have always been intrigued with garlic because of its potential to enhance the immune system. Recent research indicates the trace minerals, germanium and selenium, both rich in garlic, are extremely important in normal immune function. The unusual form of sulfur found in garlic, *sulfhydryl amino acid,* is also known to enhance immunity.

Kyolic garlic is grown in volcanic soils that are saturated with these important substances and that is one reason for its effectiveness in many immune-deficient disorders. The aging process further increases its potential, at the same time making Kyolic garlic odor-free.

Kyolic and *SGP* (Special Garlic Preparation) are the only aged garlic extracts available in the U.S. Nutrients formed during the aging and cold-extraction process are precursors of *sulfhydryl* compounds. These are very potent antioxidants that work against cell-damaging free radicals. SGP recently was the recipient of the *Science and Technology Award from the Ministry of Science and Technology of Japan,* 1991.

Aged garlic extract has recieved patents or has patents pending for use as an **anti-oxidant, anti-tumor agent, immune enhancer, liver protective agent, anti-stress agent, acidophilus growth stimulant, and an anti-fungal agent**. Kyolic is available in tablet form, capsules, and liquid.

Kyolic is the world's most researched and scientifically-documented garlic. *Kyolic* undergoes a special 20-month aging process that enhances the therapeutic properties beyond those of raw garlic. The aging process transforms the oxidizing action of raw garlic into potent antioxidants. Kyolic is one of nature's most potent immune boosters. Clinical studies of *Kyolic* in leading universities have been focused on its effect on **heavy metals, melanoma, breast cancer, tumors, viruses, radiation, cardiovascular disease, candida, benzopyrene (an air pollutant), aflatoxin, high cholesterol, and cancer**. *Kyolic* does not cure or kill, but activates healthy cells to defend and protect the body. *Kyolic* is standardized by *s-allyl cysteine*. Recently, the *National Cancer Institute* developed a $20.5 million-dollar program to study the effect of medicinal plants including garlic, *Nutrition & the M.D.,* Vol. 17, No. 5, May 1991. At long last, medical science is showing some humility toward the virtues of garlic.

Kyolic Garlic

This liquid garlic by *Wakunaga* is odorless and nearly tasteless. It is good added to juices such as *R.W. Knudesen's* Very Veggie Chili Cocktail. *Kyolic* comes in tablet, pill and liquid forms.

> ## GARLIC-THE PROTECTOR
>
> **Research at *Loma Linda University, California,* found that a compound in garlic can protect against the most powerfully know natural carcinogen, aflatoxin B1. Aflatoxins are most often found in nuts, mainly peanuts and peanut butter. Traces are found in corn, wheat and other grains.**

Liquid Garlic, It's Healing Uses

Eye Problems

Conjunctivitis, sties, pink eye, irritations, etc.

Place liquid garlic in an eye dropper with an equal amount of steam distilled water and place two drops in each eye every four hours as needed.

Ear Infections

Add two to four drops of liquid garlic warm (not hot) in each ear--do not use the same dropper for each ear for it may spread the infection. Place only in the ear infected if that is the case. Especially helpful for children.

Mouth Sores

Place one teaspoon in the mouth and swish around and hold for a few minutes. Mix one capsule of golden seal with the garlic for added healing.

Hemorrhoids

Insert with a cotton swab or can insert a Kyolic capsule in the rectum.

Vaginal Yeast Infections

Douche with one tablespoon liquid garlic.

Finger or Toe Fungus

Place in a cotton ball that is saturated with liquid garlic on infected areas, use a bandaid to hold in place--you can wear cotton sox to hold it in place. Change the saturated cotton daily.

Cholesterol

Four to six capsules daily for two months, then four daily thereafter.

For Pets

If you have animals, especially cats, place a couple of drops in the ears to avoid ear mites. Also, place 1/4 to 1/2 teaspoon on their food daily, this will aid in getting rid of ticks and fleas, and enhance immune function. A big plus--garlic is good for them. Liquid Kylolic has been used by veterinarians for many animal ailments, including infections, and Parvo virus. We also mix garlic capsules in brewer's yeast. This is very nutritious and no flea, tick or mite will make their home on your pet.

Mosquito Repellent

Take four liquid capsules with vitamin B-1 and B-12 one hour before going outside. Marvelous results.

> **To remove the skin of garlic before using, press the side of a knife or bottle on the clove. The skin will split and can easily be taken off.**

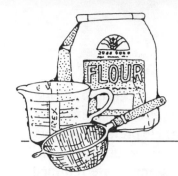

Grains & Flours

Grains have particular attributes which make them unique. Rice is non-allergenic and gluten-free, except for sweet glutinous rice. While oats are relatively high in fat for a grain, they contain an antioxidant which delays rancidity. Wheat contains gluten and is the only grain suitable for baking leavened breads without the addition of any other grains. Quinoa is the only grain to contain a complete protein source.

Whole grains are high fiber, complex carbohydrate foods, they are rich in both fat and sodium. They are a good source of minerals and the B vitamins. Grains have been a staple food throughout the world's history. Grains are a complex carbohydrate that promotes energy, which is vital to the body. All whole grains, except wheat, help reduce fat in the body. Grains are an excellent source of complex carbohydrates needed by body builders to ensure a steady blood sugar level. Grains are good for all blood sugar disorders.

A whole grain is made up of these basic parts: the bran, the germ, and the endosperm and exosperm. When grains are refined they are stripped of the bran, and sometimes the germ. The bran is the outermost part of the grain, and a good source of roughage, as well as B vitamins, proteins, fats, and minerals. Each part of a whole grain has nutritional value. The exosperm is rich in bran, the endosperm is principally starch, the husk is primarily fiber; and the germ, is rich in protein, polyunsaturated fatty acids, vitamins, and minerals.

Whole grains, like corn, oats, rice, and wheat account for some of the most sought-after foods found in a natural-foods outlet.

Whole grains provide complete nourishment when complemented with legumes, beans, or vegetables. These foods eaten together will form a complete protein.

Labels

It is important to know what a label means when you read it. The ingredients are listed in the order of whatever is in the largest quantity first and so on. When wheat flour is listed first in the ingredients, you may be getting mostly white flour, since white and wheat flour are used synonymously.

When a label reads "white bread" or "just bread", the loaf of bread is made of refined flour. A loaf of bread is truly whole wheat bread when the ingredients read whole wheat flour. When a manufacturer or bakery uses the term "whole wheat" the loaf must be made from 100% whole wheat flour containing everything in the same proportion as in the original wheat kernel.

There are several terms used on labels when describing grain products, some of the terms are significant, others inconsequential. The federal Food and Drug Administration (FDA) does not have any regulations for the use of "natural," although most manufacturers use it to mean that preservatives were not used in the product. When a product is labeled enriched, it must meet government specifications for certain B vitamins and iron, and the bread is required to contain a certain amount of thiamine, riboflavin, niacin, and iron per pound. Unbleached means that the flour or grain was not treated with chlorine, benzoyl peroxide, or any other bleach to give it a white appearance. It is ironic that bleached flours are supposedly more appetizing. The FDA has not set any standards for dietary fiber, so when a product touts its high-fiber content, it means nothing. When a bread is termed reduced calorie, by law it must contain one-third fewer calories than an equivalent non-diet slice. When a product contains malted barley flour, this means the barley flour has been partially germinated, dried and powdered or made into syrup. It is used to feed the yeast, which helps the bread to rise.

One slice of whole wheat, multi-grain, rye, or pumpernickel provides almost as much fiber as two slices of wheat or three of white bread. Not only do you obtain a more significant amount of fiber, but the levels of protein and minerals are higher. The body burns carbohydrates most efficiently when all B vitamins are consumed at the same time, whole grains contain both B vitamins and carbohydrates.

When you read calcium propionate, although it sounds questionable it prevents mold and adds calcium.

Michael Jacobson, Executive Director, Center for Science in the Public Interest, believes that "enriched" is a deceptive term. He prefers the phrase "partially restored," since when the grain is processed not all the nutrients that are stripped are returned. Processing normally removes many of the beneficial trace elements, such as potassium, magnesium, and zinc.

Types of Grains and Flours

Amaranth Flour

This is the ancient grain of the Aztecs. It is higher in nutrients than most other grains, and second only to quinoa for its high protein content. The protein content of amaranth is twice that of corn and rice. Use it as you would wheat, though it is not technically a grain. It has a distinct taste, so start out by substituting a small amount at first: use 1/3 cup amaranth flour to 1 cup of whole wheat. You can make a highly nutritious breakfast using 1/3 cup of the flour in 1 cup boiling water, and cook for a few minutes. It is primarily used in making crackers and flatbreads.

Grain salads are a great way to add protein to your diet. Your cooking method will make the difference in how your salad turns out. Add grain to boiling liquid, cover, and cook a few minutes less than the recipe calls for, this will give your grain a nice crunch. After removing from the heat, immediately rinse with cold water, to prevent further cooking which will cause softness and swelling. Add chopped raw veggies and, your choice of dressing.

Barley

Mugi, a barley miso, is made from a specific type of barley shown to reduce tumors and fat in the body.

This grain is rich in potassium, sulfur and phosphorus acids. The outer hull can not be easily digested so the hull is removed and the remaining grain is called pearled barley. For gluten-free diets, barley flour can be used because it contains very little gluten. This grain is good for soups, and the broth is excellent for the ill and convalescing as well as those with heart problems. Barley stimulates the liver and lymphatic system, enhancing the discharge of toxic waste from the body. Add to vegetable soups and stews. Whole barley (with hulls) is a dark grain and larger in size than most other grains, except corn. It is higher in calcium, iron, protein and potassium than pearled barley.

Barley contains *tocotrienol* which aids the suppression of cholesterol production in the liver. *Beta-glucans* in barley work with other soluble fibers to aid in preventing dietary fats and cholesterol from being absorbed in the intestines, *Nutrition & Dietary Consultant,* April 1990.

Buckwheat

Not part of the wheat family, buckwheat is known for its use in pancakes and as a form of honey. Kasha or buckwheat groats are popular. It is high in potassium, rutin, phosphorus, especially vitamin E, calcium, and the B vitamins. Its high rutin content makes this grain good for arteriosclerosis, for strengthening the capillaries and for lowering the likelihood of hemorrhages. (Rutin also can be purchased in pill form. It is a citrus-free bioflavonoid.) Buckwheat is a good blood builder and neutralizes acidic wastes. It is beneficial for the kidneys, also.

Kasha (or buckwheat groats) is a staple grain in the Russian and Eurasian diet. To cook, boil 2 cups of water and add 1 cup of kasha. Cover and simmer for 10 minutes. To make buckwheat, roast 1 cup over high heat, stirring constantly, for 3-5 minutes. The longer it is roasted the deeper the flavor and color. Then cook it the same as the kasha. Both taste good with fish, chicken, or vegetables.

Bulgur Wheat

This is used in cereals, stews, soups, pilafs, baked goods, salads, and even desserts. You can soak the cracked grain for 30 minutes and use it in salads, such as a taco salad and sandwich fillings. The form usually found in health food stores has been parboiled, dried and then cracked. There is a new process called "whirling" which removes the bran but retains all the choline, niacin and minerals.

Corn

The grain is ground and used primarily for cornbread. It can be used as breading on fish, chicken etc. before baking. Some varieties have added lysine, with this added nutrient it becomes a complete protein source. This is an excellent grain and was used as a staple by the Indians.

Corn Germ

Corn germ is high in nutrients, higher in some than wheat germ. It contains ten times more zinc than wheat germ. Corn germ makes a great breading for chicken or fish. It is also good added to cereals and toppings. Corn germ has a longer shelf life than wheat germ. A product by *Fearn* carries corn germ in tightly sealed packs and can be found in health food stores.

Corn Grits or Hominy

Good as a cereal or side dish. There are several grains in grit form: barley, buckwheat, brown rice, soy and wheat. They all are excellent for hot cereals, adding to breads and for breading on fish and chicken.

Durham Wheat Flour

This is used in cereals, stews, soups, pilafs, baked goods, salads, and even desserts. A diabetic can eat more of this flour because it contains only about one fourth the carbohydrates of other gluten flours, such as wheat. It makes sprouted breads lighter.

Gluten Flour

This flour is extracted from wheat and the starch removed. Gluten is what helps breads and other baked goods to rise. Wheat has the highest gluten content. Combined with other flours, it helps give breads a lighter texture and is high in protein. If you desire to increase the protein content in your baked goods, add some of this flour. Gluten is not recommended for the ill.

Graham Flour

The kernel is ground to the consistency of white flour. The outside bran is left course and flaky. Graham flour is good for all baked goods. It is derived from the whole wheat known as "winter wheat." If you have a recipe calling for this flour, you can substitute whole wheat flour, using the same amount. This flour was named after a physician, Sylvester Graham. He rebelled against white bread, which he called, "even less than useless." Graham crackers were named after him.

Jerusalem Artichoke Flour

This popular flour is used to make pasta. Use 1/10 of this flour to whatever other flour you are using. The pasta will have better flavor and texture without sticking together. This flour (used in the ratio above) is good to use for all baking. It is especially good for diabetics because it is a non-digestible flour carbohydrate, and will not affect blood sugar levels

117

Kamut

This grain is a relative of durum wheat, tolerated by many people with wheat allergies. Nutritionally better than wheat, kamut is high in minerals and protein, magnesium and zinc. The flavor is rich and buttery, it makes an excellent pasta.

Millet

This grain has the most complete protein of any grain, except for quinoa and amaranth. It is a primary food of the Hunza people. Millet was an important staple food in Biblical times, and is considered a sacred food by the Chinese. Millet also has significant amounts of iron, lecithin, and choline, which help keep cholesterol in check and stop the formation of certain types of gall stones. It is the only grain that because it is alkaline, it is good for the spleen, pancreas, and stomach. Millet can also benefit those who suffer from acidosis, which is a common ailment with those who are ill. It is also good for colitis, ulcers, and urinary disorders.

The whole grain makes a good tasting cereal and should be included in your diet. It can be added to breads and homemade granola. It can be ground into a flour or meal if desired. Millet is the oldest grain known and is used in our country primarily as bird seed.

Yale University experiments have shown millet's protein, vitamins, minerals, and unsaturated fat content to be higher than any other grain.

Oats

Oats and oat flour have the ability to normalize blood glucose in diabetes. They are good for a slow working thyroid. Oats contain the highest amount of fat of all grains creating warmth and stamina in the body.

There are steel-cut oats, rolled oats, oat groats, flakes and instant oats. Oats retain more of their food value through processing than wheat. Use oat flour in part or all of your baking as it adds exceptional flavor to any bread recipes. The best form for the most value is rolled or flaked (crushed) oats; these do take a little longer cooking time, around 20-30 minutes. Steel-cut oats are sliced and untampered

with, and have the highest amount of nutrients left in the grain. Oats can be used as a very good thickener in stews, soups, stuffings, pancakes, granola. Cook one cup steel-cut oats in two cups of water for thirty minutes. All whole-grain cereals can be made in a thermos jug. Use boiling water and grain, let sit overnight and the next morning it will be hot, delicious and nutritious.

The protein content in oats is easily assimilated and helps neutralize excess cholesterol. It contains high amounts of calcium, iodine, phosphorus, iron, vitamin E, thiamine, riboflavin, niacin, and the whole B-complex. Oats are the most acidic of cereals and have a high gluten content.

Potato Flour

This is good added to soups as a thickener and adds flavor. It can also be added to gravies, sauces, stews, muffins and breads. One pound of this flour equals five pounds of whole potatoes. It also comes in flake form, which can be used for instant mashed potatoes and in soups as a thickener.

Quinoa

Pronounced kee-no'-ah, it is known for building strength and endurance with its high source of protein, B vitamins, iron and fiber, calcium and phosphorus. It can be made into a finely ground whole flour that lends a nutty taste to baked goods, cookies, and pie crusts. Like amaranth and buckwheat, it can usually be tolerated by those who are allergic to various cereal grains. Each grain of quinoa is wrapped with *saponins*, a naturally occurring compound that repels harmful insects and birds.

A basic recipe for quinoa is to mix 1 cup, with 2 cups of water or stock, and a pinch of salt. Rinse the quinoa, bring the water and salt to a boil, add the quinoa and return to a boil, simmer covered on medium heat for 15 minutes. Remove from heat and let stand, covered, for 10 minutes before serving.

Rice

Research recently conducted at the U.S. Department of Agriculture indicates that a low-fat diet including 10% dietary fiber from rice bran can reduce blood cholesterol levels by 15%.

There are four forms of rice: brown rice, parboiled, regular milled and pre-cooked. It comes in short, medium, and long grained varieties. *Phytic acid* found in the germ aids in expelling poisons from the body. Because of its high B-complex vitamins, it is soothing to the nervous system and the brain.

Brown rice is high in all the B vitamins, calcium, phosphorus, iron and protein. Combine rice with beans or vegetables and you have a complete protein. Brown rice keeps the blood sugar stablilized so you do not feel hungry for longer periods and, therefore, you eat less often. Serve broiled fish, chicken and steamed vegetables over brown rice. Many people make a gallon at one time (it keeps well if refrigerated). Later the desired amount can be added to soups, on top of salads or used in rice salad (see recipe section of this book). There are "Rice Cream" breakfast cereals, also. Wild rice is very high in nutrients, but more expensive. We sometimes mix half brown and half wild rice before cooking. **Basmati rice** is a long-grain, cream-colored rice with a nutty flavor, originally from India and Pakistan. Brown rice is the easiest grain to digest, making it good for those with food allergies.

Parboiled rice has been steamed and dried before milling, to ensure the grains remain separated after cooking.

Pre-cooked rice has been milled, cooked and dehydrated, which makes it convenient with a short cooking time.

White rice has been milled, which removes the brown bran coating. Do not use white rice, which has been processed and the nutrients destroyed. It is very mucus-forming.

Rye

This grain has been cultivated for more than 2,000 years. It has a stronger flavor than most grains. There are very few allergenic reactions to this grain. Rye has the highest amount of lysine of all grains. (*There is now a new cornmeal available which is also high in lysine.*) Rye is low in gluten and needs to be used with flours that have more gluten, such as wheat. The whole grain can be cooked as a cereal or there is "Cream of Rye," which is an excellent change of pace.

Rye aids in developing a superior glandular system. Good for weight loss because it does not rise as much, due to the lack of gluten, and therefore fills you up faster.

Soy Flour

This is made from the soy bean, making it a high protein flour. It adds lecithin and B vitamins to foods. It also contains vitamin E. It is good used in baking, adding 1/4 part soy flour to the primary flour called for. It can be added to hot cereals, soups, stews, loaves, pancakes, cookies--almost anything. Be sure to add this valuable flour to your foods. Soy comes in many different forms.

Spelt

Better tolerated than any other grain. High in carbohydrates, spelt contains more crude fiber and more protein than wheat, including all eight essential amino acids, that are needed in the daily diet to insure proper cell maintenance. The fiber in spelt helps lower cholesterol and plays a role in helping blood to clot. High in the B vitamins. It's the only grain containing *mucopolysaccharides*. Occasionally referred to as "The Rice of Europe."

Over 5000 years old, spelt is once again resuming a place of prominence among preferred grains. Particularly attractive to the wheat sensitive, spelt is easily substituted for wheat in recipes and offers a subtle, nutty flavor that is welcomed by all.

Spelt can be obtained from Purity Foods, Inc., 2871 W. Jolly Road, Okemos, MI 48864.

More on Spelt

Spelt has a high nutritional value and is better tolerated by the body than any other grain.

The immune-stimulating properties of spelt are in its *cyanogenic glucosides* or *nitrilosides*, called the "anti-neoplastic vitamin B17." They support the body's cancer fighting system, *W. Weuffen et al., Nah-Z.f. Ernaehrungswiss*, 18, 1979, pp. 16-22. Spelt also contains special carbohydrates called *mucopolysaccharides* which play a decisive role in blood clotting and stimulate the body's immune system, *H Wagner et al., Economic and Medicinal Plant Research*, Vol. 1, 1985, Academic Press, London, 113.

Sunflower Seed Flour

This seed can add lots of nutrients to baked goods. Use it to replace a portion of the flour called for. It is good in cookies. Make sure the sunflower seeds are fresh, although fresh raw seeds are difficult to find. If the package contains many colored seeds or a large proportion of dark seeds, pass them by. For best results, grind your own just before use because the seeds may become rancid once they have been exposed to air.

Tapioca Flour

This can be used the same as cornstarch or arrowroot for thickness. It is recommended for use in fruit pies, gravies, or stir fries.

Triticale

This is the first man-made grain. It is a combination of wheat (triticum) and rye (secale). This flour has a higher content of protein than either wheat or rye. Use part triticale flour in your baking to add proteins, especially cystine, methionine and lysine.

Nutrients per 1/2 cup of Brown Rice	
Calories	354
Protein	7.7
Carbohydrate	77.5
Fat	2.19
Sodium	4mg
Thiamine	0.29mg
Riboflavin	0.05mg
Niacin	4.53mg
Calcium	33mg
Iron	1.6mg
Phosphorus	231mg
Fiber	1.0mg

Wheat

Wheat has a high gluten content, which is what makes bread rise. Gluten is a tough, sticky, nitrogenous substance that forms mucus and coats the villi of the intestines. If the villi get too heavily coated, nutrients cannot be absorbed, resulting in malabsorption. This also affects on the myelin sheath of nerves.

The American diet includes a lot of wheat daily and this is connected to many ailments. Wheat will clog up the digestive system and cause nervous problems. Wheat products should be consumed in moderation or not at all if you suffer from intestinal disorders. Barley and oats also contain gluten, but in lesser amount. Alternate your flours.

There are two varieties of flour, used primarily for baking. **Soft wheat** is higher in carbohydrates and is good for pastries. **Hard wheat** is higher in protein and good for breads because it has a higher gluten content. Cracked grains are good for hot cereals and can be sprouted. There is also **rolled wheat** which is similar to rolled oats and can be used in granola and cookies. Use unbleached types if you prefer a healthier flour.

Wheat Flours

All-Purpose

A combination of hard or hard and soft wheat combined, without the bran.

Bread

Similar in composition to all-purpose, but with added gluten.

Cake

This flour is milled from soft wheat and is very low in gluten.

Cooking Guide For Grains

There are a few rules to follow when cooking grains: (1) bring liquid to a boil; (2) add grain and boil five minutes; (3) turn heat to very low and simmer with a tight-fitting lid -- do not lift the lid until time recommended in the following guide.

Grain	Amount	Water, Milk or broth	Time (minutes)	Yield (Approximate)
Barley, flaked	1 cup	3 cups	15	3 cups
Barley, pearled	2 cups	2 cups	30-40	2-1/2 cups
Buckwheat Groats	1 cup	2 cups	20	3 cups
Bulgur	1 cup	2 cups	15	2-1/2 cups
Millet	1 cup	3 cups	30	4 cups
Oat Groats	1 cup	3 cups	40-50	2-1/2 cups
Rolled Oats	1 cup	2-3 cups	15-20	4 cups
Quick Oats	1 cup	2 cups	1	2 cups
Brown Rice	1 cup	2 cups	35-40	2-1/2 cups
Wheat Groats	1 cup	2-1/2 cups	35	3 cups
Rye Berries	1 cup	3 cups	35	3 cups
Rye Flakes	1 cup	3 cups	20	3 cups
Cornmeal	1 cup	3-1/2 cups	30	3 cups

What we are trying to do is steam the grain. Heating longer than the time listed will not hurt, as long as the heat is sufficiently low. You can also turn the heat off without lifting the lid so the steam will not escape, and let the grain sit for awhile

An easy way to make whole grain cereal in the morning is to place grain and boiling water in a thermos, the night before, and the cereal will be ready to eat in the morning, with all the nutrients intact.

Stoneground grains are best. All the nutrients have been left intact, without the use of heat. Purchase only flours which meet this criteria. Purchase from a store that keeps grains refrigerated or in a freezer. Keep all whole grain flours under refrigeration.

Farina

Coarsely ground hard wheat, commonly used in inexpensive pastas and cereals.

Gluten

Mostly used with low-protein flours. Wheat is high in gluten.

Pastry

Very similar to cake flour, but with less starch.

121

Self-rising

An all-purpose flour containing salt and leavening.

Semolina

This flour is coarsely ground from durum wheat, and used primarily in pasta and couscous.

Spelt Tacos or Tortilla Shells

2 cups spelt flour or 1-1/2 cup flour and 1/2 cup cornmeal
1 teaspoon sea salt
1/4 cup butter or vegetable oil
1/2 cup lukewarm water

Combine flour and salt. Add butter, cutting it in until crumbly. When particles are fine, add water. Knead thoroughly until smooth and flecked with air bubbles. Divide dough into 10-12 balls and roll as thin as possible on lightly floured board. Fry on a hot ungreased heavy skillet for 30-60 seconds until light brown. Turn over and bake on other side. Serve hot, or cool and freeze for later use. Warm up in the oven in a tightly covered dish

Quinoa Veggie Pie

Chill a pie plate and press cooked quinoa into the bottom (see the Basic Recipe on page 124). Bake quinoa crust for 10 minutes at 400°. Steam your favorite veggies and place into the baked crust. Sprinkle grated soy cheese (or your choice) over the top of the veggies and bake for 15 minutes. Season lightly with Spike or sea salt and cayenne pepper and serve hot.

Whole Wheat

This flour uses the complete wheat kernel, it is also called graham flour.

Wheat Germ

Fresh wheat germ is almost impossible to find. It becomes rancid within a few hours of being separated from the grain. **Unless it is vacuum sealed, it can do more harm than good.**

Spelt Bread

No fat, eggs, or dairy
2 packages dry yeast or 1 cake compressed yeast
1 tablespoon sweetener of your choice
7 cups flour, fine and coarse (at least 3 cups fine flour are necessary)
2 cups water
1 tablespoon sea salt

Boil water and then let it cool to a lukewarm temperature. Stir yeast and sugar, gradually adding lukewarm water. Add about half the flour and the salt and beat well. Add the remainder of the flour gradually to acquire a stiff dough. It may require more or less than the 7 cups given in the recipe. Knead 5 to 10 minutes until smooth and elastic. Put dough into a buttered bowl and turn once to butter surface. Cover with a towel and let rise until doubled, keeping it between 80 and 90 ° F. during the entire rising time. It will take about 2 hours for the bread to rise. Preheat the oven to 350°. Grease two 9x5 inch loaf pans. Punch down with your fist and divide into two. Knead and shape into 2 loaves and place into loaf pans. Cover again and allow dough to rise to top of pans. Bake for 50 minutes. Variations: add spoonfuls of flaxseed, fennel, caraway and/or thyme for spicy bread.

Tuft's University Diet & Nutrition Letter, Vol. 9, No. 7, September 1991. "That a bread is brown doesn't mean it's whole grain. It may simply mean molasses or caramel coloring was added to darken the loaf. Thus, typically dark breads like pumpernickel and rye are <u>not whole grain unless the ingredients list says so.</u>"

Spelt Muffins

2-1/4 cup of spelt flour, fine or coarse
1/4 cup honey
1 tablespoon baking powder (Rumford's aluminum-free)
1/2 teaspoon sea salt
1-1/4 cups soy or Rice Dream milk
3 eggs, beaten or egg substitute
1 tablespoon expeller-pressed oil

Preheat oven to 425°. Oil and flour 12 muffin cups. Combine all dry ingredients. Add milk, eggs and oil and mix until moistened. Fill muffin cups 2/3 full with batter and bake for 17 minutes or until brown. Variations: add 1/2 cup chopped almonds or 1/2 cup chopped dates or raisins or 1/4 cup of each to batter before baking.

There will soon be a quick spelt muffin mix on the market.

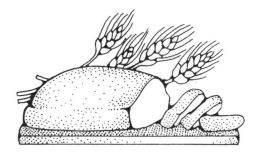

Buttermilk Biscuits

2 cups finely ground spelt flour
1 tablespoon Rumford's aluminum-free baking powder
1/4 teaspoon sea salt
1 cup buttermilk

Preheat oven 425°. Oil baking sheet. Combine all dry ingredients and add buttermilk until just blended. Drop batter by heaping spoonfuls onto baking sheet. Bake for 12 to 15 minutes or until lightly browned.

Handy Biscuit Mix

4 tablespoons aluminum free baking powder
8 cups sifted whole wheat or unbleached flour-*I like half and half*
1 tablespoon sea salt
1-1/4 cups cold-pressed canola oil

Sift flour, salt and baking powder togher. Cut butter or oil into flour mixture thoroughly. Store in glass jar with tight lid in refrigerator until ready to use. Add 3/4 cup buttermilk or yogurt to 2-1/2 cups mix. Knead a few times and roll out to desired thickness and cut out biscuits. Bake 450° for 12-15 minutes.

Commercial bread and flour manufacturers and distributors use a number of terms that, although they appear helpful, actually only serve to obscure the ingredients and processes they subject grains to before they reach a grocer's shelves.

Here are a few of their words to watch out for:

Wheat - used for bleached white bread flour also

Enriched - thiamin, riboflavin, niacin, and iron have been added to the flour (after refining)

Oat bran or oatmeal bread - the manufacturer has added some oat bran or oatmeal to wheat bread. There are no guidelines on just how much oats are needed before wheat bread becomes oatmeal bread

In addition, here are a few words you're likely to see that mean whatever the manufacturer wants: Stone ground, natural, whole-grain goodness, and high fiber.

Green & Leafy

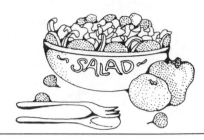

Green is a powerful healing color. God created more green on our planet than all other colors combined. Looking at a landscape or forest can calm us and release stress. Green has the same peaceful effect when used inside our bodies.

Use all these magnificient raw greens in your power juice. Because of the high content of *chlorophyll, carotenoids,* calcium and high mineral content, these greens are essential in the healing process.

Green and leafy vegetables should become a part of your daily diet. We often forget these high nutrient, valuable greens that add vitamins, minerals, usable calcium and the beta-carotene needed for the **immune system**. They also ward off diseases such as **cancer**. Leafy greens are excellent for the **gall bladder, spleen, heart and blood**, and are a good **brain food**.

Greens can be cooked in many ways to make them appetizing, used as fresh juices and added in salads. To clean them: soak in the sink for a few minutes and swirl around, then drain the water. Pat dry. Tear the leaves into small pieces, trim the ends of the stems, then chop. All greens are good when miso is added as a seasoner in soups, stews, casseroles, and cooked in defatted turkey broth with a little chopped onion, carrots, and celery. They are also good just steamed and seasoned before serving. Keep in mind all leafy greens contain chlorophyll, iron, magnesium calcium, manganese, vitamin C, potassium, vitamin A, and a bonus of the essential fatty acids and **no cholesterol**. The vegetables with the darkest, most intense colors, tend to contain the highest levels of nutrients.

To make a broth: cook a finely chopped onion, a couple of cloves of minced garlic, 1 finely chopped carrot, with 1/2 cup reduced-sodium chicken or turkey broth (miso is good for vegetarians) in a large covered skillet until the onion is completely wilted - about 10 to 15 minutes. Because greens contain sodium, you need not add additional salt when preparing. The sodium, content varies from 22 mg. (milligrams) per cup in cooked mustard greens to 316 mg. in a cup of swiss chard. Keep in mind this is a natural form of sodium needed by the body for a correct potassium balance.

Know Your Leafy Greens

Arugula

From the mustard family, this green is peppery and tart, it mixes well with other greens, is also known as roquette. It adds pizazz to any raw salad, and is high in vitamins A, C, and niacin; and iron and phosphorus. Good for normalizing body acid with its high alkalinity.

Beet greens

Best used in juices, they are very high in nutrients, especially iron and calcium. These greens can be used in cooking also. A must in juices for enemas, blood disorders, liver function and the flow of bile.

Belgian Endive

Good in a salad with a raspberry vinaigrette dressing, can also be cooked in liquid. Has pale yellow or white leaves, a root of the chicory plant. Kin to chicory with similar healing qualities and nutrient content.

Butterhead

Also known as Boston Bibb, this is a very tender leaf, with an almost buttery taste. Makes a good salad when used with spinach, endive, or watercress. Lettuce is said to calm the nerves.

Chicory

A bitter green, with curly leaves, the young leaves are best in salads. High in vitamins C and A, and calcium and iron. Aids in liver function and blood disorders.

Try radiccho, often called red-leaf chicory, good in salads.

Collards

A member of the cabbage family. Use only the leaves, they tend to be tough, cook for 8 to 10 minutes on medium heat. Can be used in salads as a substitute for cabbage and is great for juicing. No leafy green is more valuable in the body for disorders of the colon, respiratory system, lymphatic system and skeletal system.

Crisphead

This crisp and mild leaf is best known as iceberg lettuce. It holds up well over time, and mixes well with other leaves.

Dandelion greens

The young leaves have a tangy taste. Are good for gall bladder disorders, rheumatism, gout, eczema, and skin disorders. Dandelion is also an excellent liver rejuvenator. Cooks the same as any leafy green. Rich in calcium, potassium, vitamins A and C. This is a must to add to juices. It is also available in tea and capsule form.

Escarole & Endive

From the chicory family, the leaves are very dark green, with a slightly bitter taste. Makes a good salad with a warm citrus-flavored dressing.

Cook as any leafy green. Very rich in vitamin A, calcium, minerals, B-vitamins, iron and potassium. Good for most infections, for liver function, and internal cleansing.

Kale

The King of Calcium. Use only the leaves of this plant, the taste is like cabbage. Its juice is good added to carrot juice. High in usable calcium. Excellent for osteoporosis.

Loose-leaf Lettuce

The leaves are green, red, or curly. The plant does not grow in a head, and the flavor is mild and slightly sweet. Lettuce is good for the nervous system.

Mache

This lettuce has a nutty taste, and it is good when tossed with crunchier, tarter greens. Very perishable.

Mustard & Turnip greens

These greens have a nippy taste with flavors varying from mild to hot. They are good sauteed with a little garlic and oil or steamed. Also, suitable for juicing. High in calcium and vitamin C. Good for infections, colon disorders, colds, flu and elimination of kidney stones due to excess uric acid.

Parsley

All types of this plant are rich in vitamin A, B-complex, C, minerals, potassium, manganese. It contains mucilage, starch, *opinol* and volatile oil. It is very crisp and tangy. This green has an "odor eating" quality, that restores fresh breath after a meal with garlic or onion.

Add to fresh juices to provide needed daily nutrients. Good for digestive disorders, also an excellent diuretic.

Try cilantro, a Chinese and Mexican parsley. Essential in many Chinese, Spanish, Mexican, and Thai dishes. Try it in salsa, tacos, and chicken salad.

Romaine

A very crunchy green. Highest in nutrients of all types of lettuce. Good in salads. Not good for cooking.

Sorrel

A green with a pleasantly sour and slightly lemon flavor. It is perishable and best bought fresh. Try sorrel in salads, or as a seasoning in soups, casseroles, and omelettes. Sorrel is a powerful antioxidant with the same healing properties as kale.

Spinach

Its tender bright green leaves are most beneficial when eaten raw. Because of the oxalic acid content, the calcium becomes unavailable to the body. Contains many valuable nutrients and high in iron.

Swiss Chard

From the beet family, this green has a mild taste, and is good with walnuts or pine nuts added. Has the highest content of sodium of all greens.

Eat in moderation if on a low-sodium diet.

Watercress

Has young, tender leaves which should be picked before the plant flowers. The spicy-flavored green goes well with iceberg lettuce. Highest in nutrient content of most greens. Excellent for vitamin deficiencies and illnesses of all types. Good added to fresh juices.

Green Cooking

Those of western cultures, especially Americans, do not eat enough vegetables, particularly greens which are essential for healing and good health.

The following recipes are a quick and easy way to make your greens tasty and nutritious. They should be included in all diets, especially in those afflicted with varied diseases, particularly colon disorders, heart disorders, and high blood pressure.

Use only the leaves of collards, kale, mustard, and turnip greens. When preparing bok choy and broccoli de rabe, the whole vegetable is edible, although the ends should be trimmed off.

Braised Greens

This is good for the heart, colon, and all those who need extra nourishment.

1 chopped onion
1/2 cup miso broth or veggie stock
Optional: 2 cloves minced garlic
1 teaspoon grated ginger
1 tablespoon apple cider vinegar
1 finely chopped or shredded carrot
1 pound of greens (can use any type of greens)

Cook onion with the broth or stock in a large covered skillet until the onion is clear. For additional flavor, add garlic, ginger or carrots. Add greens, cut or torn into small pieces. If the greens don't all fit in the pan, cook half, when those have wilted down the others will fit. Cook covered until completely tender, 10 to 50 minutes depending on the toughness of the leaf. Stir in 1/3 cup plain, nonfat yogurt and 1 teaspoon prepared mustard for a creamier texture. Season with Spike or sea salt, nutmeg, allspice, or curry powder, to taste. Makes 4 servings.

Robust Red Cabbage

1 medium cabbage
1/2 teaspoon sea salt or Spike
1 bay leaf
1 minced small onion
2 apples, cut in 8 wedges
1/2 teaspoon ground cloves
2 cups water
1-1/2 tablespoon Sucanat (powdered whole cane sugar juice)
1 tablespoon wine vinegar
3 tablespoons safflower oil
1 tablespoon lemon juice

Shred cabbage. Mix vinegar, lemon juice, sea salt, and Sucanat. Over medium heat, saute onions in oil. Add cabbage to vinegar and mix. Saute 5 minutes. Add water, bay leaf, cloves, and apples. Boil, then simmer for 25 minutes. Remove bay leaf and serve. Goes well with potatoes and your favorite dish.

Quick & Easy Collards

1 bunch shredded collard leaves
2 cloves minced garlic
1 tablespoon olive oil
Dash of Spike seasoning *(optional)* or sea salt
2 teaspoons fresh lemon juice or apple cider
   vinegar

Saute collard leaves with minced garlic in the olive oil, over medium high heat. Stir constantly until the leaves are wilted, approximately 10 minutes. Mix in lemon juice, and season to taste.

Curried Lentils & Mustard Greens

1 pound lentils
1 tablespoon curry powder
1 teaspoon ground cumin
2 tablespoons olive oil or your choice
2 cloves minced garlic
1 chopped carrot
1 large minced onion
1 stalk of chopped celery
3 cups of water or miso broth
1 large bunch of mustard or turnip greens

Saute onion, curry powder, cumin, garlic, carrot, and celery with the olive oil in a large saucepan for 5 minutes. Stir in 1 cup of water or stock. Simmer, covered for 20 minutes. Add lentils, mustard or turnip leaves and an additional 2 cups of water or stock, heat to a boil. Reduce the heat and simmer in a covered pan for about 45 minutes, until the liquid is absorbed. Stir occasionally. Top with plain yogurt and chopped chives if desired.

Cabbage Soup

1 large shredded carrot
1 large chopped onion
1 tablespoon canola oil
1 small head of green cabbage, chopped fine
6 cups of vegetable stock or miso and water
parsley for garnish

Saute onion in oil until soft. Simmer stock, add cabbage and onion, simmer 15 minutes. Season to taste, garnish and serve.

Baked Barley and Kale

One of the best calcium builders and heart tonic recipes.

1 cup pearl barley
2 tablespoons expeller-pressed canola or
   olive oil
3 cups miso or vegetable stock
1 minced onion
1 stalk celery chopped
3 sliced carrots
1/2 pound of sliced mushrooms
1 large bunch of kale leaves

Saute onion, celery, carrots, and mushrooms in the oil, stirring often for about 5 minutes, do not brown. Add the stock, barley, and the torn kale leaves. Bring to a boil.

Cover and place in preheated, 350 degree oven for 90 minutes. Makes 6 servings.

Low-fat Spinach Salad

1 pound fresh spinach
8 to 10 Shiitike or plain mushrooms
1-1/2 tablespoons olive oil
1 teaspoon tamari
1 shallot or green onion, minced
1 clove garlic, minced
1/2 teaspoon Dijon mustard or your choice
1/4 cup balsamic (rice) vinegar
Dash of Spike seasoning or sea salt

Remove the tough stems from the spinach. Rinse the leaves, changing the water, until the leaves are clean. Pat dry, tear into bite-size pieces. Place in a salad bowl. Remove stems from mushrooms and slice caps into thin strips. Heat two teaspoons of oil in a skillet over medium heat. Add mushrooms, garlic, green onion, tamari and saute, stirring constantly. Cook until tender but not brown, scatter over the spinach. Add remaining oil to the pan, stir in mustard, vinegar, and cook, stirring constantly for a few seconds until the dressing is bubbling hot. Pour over spinach and toss. Top with sunflower seeds, sesame seeds, and raisins or toasted croutons.

Juices for Speed Healing

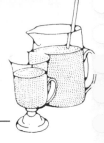

Nothing is as powerful for healing as fresh raw juices! Always dilute juices with distilled water or blend with half herb tea. See Healthy Drinks section for nutritional drinks without using a juicer, Fruits and Healing, Green and Leafy sections and Wellness Charts.

Apple

This juice is good for the **gall bladder** and is known for its cleansing and healing effects on internal **inflammation**. It contains **pectin** and **malic acid**. Be sure to include the skins when juicing. Apples are loaded with nutrients and one large apple has only 129 calories. Apples can lower blood **cholesterol**, aid **liver** function, rid the body of toxins and lessen the effects of X-rays. Five apples make one glass.

Beet

This is one of the most valuable juices for the **liver**, **gall bladder**, **red corpuscles**, **anemia**, cancer, blood cleansing and stimulation of the **lymph glands**. It is rich in iron, potassium, calcium and chlorine, plus many other nutrients. Juice the tops, too. Be sure to dilute the juice with distilled water. One pound of beets makes one glass.

Cabbage

This is used by *Hans Nieper, M.D. of Germany,* a cancer expert, in the treatment of **colon cancer**. The juice heals inflammation of the colon and **stomach**, **ulcers**, **heartburn**, etc. Prepare it fresh and drink immediately, as the vitamin U is destroyed very rapidly by air and cooking. This vegetable should be in your diet! It is high in calcium, vitamin C, sulfur, vitamin A and much more. The raw juice does wonders for all colon disorders and acts quickly. Use shredded in salads. Cabbage has also helped **eczema**, **seborrhea** and infection. It stabilizes chemical reactions in the body, and the leaves make a good poultice for leg ulcers.

Carrot

This is used in the treatment of all forms of **cancer**. It is a good source of beta-carotene. Beta-carotene is converted to vitamin A in the body. Best for liver problems because a pill form of vitamin A should be used sparingly and, in some cases, not at all. A good source of minerals, vitamins A, C and B vitamins. In a recent study by *J. L. Freudenheim, Ph.D., State University of Buffalo, New York,* found carotenoid-rich vegetables contain powerful **antioxidants** and may protect against laryngeal cancer. Carrots and their juice are excellent for **diarrhea** (even for infants), intestinal infection and intestinal disorders. Among other conditions, it aids in the treatment or prevention of **stunted growth**, **rickets**, **colitis**, **gout** and **constipation**, all forms **arthritis** and skin disorders. One pound of carrots yields 1 glass, dilute with 1/3 water.

Celery

Celery is an excellent source of magnesium, iron, vitamins A, B, C and E, calcium and potassium. It has a natural **diuretic** effect and aids in the elimination of **carbon dioxide** from the body. It can also have a relaxing effect. Add a couple of stalks to other juices. It is good for **arthritis**, appetite, **adrenal** function and **weight loss**. Six stalks yield one glass of juice. The sodium content will neutralize acid in the body. Celery is a good **brain** tonic, enhances memory, is good for **dizziness**, **headache**, and **arthritis**.

According to the *Composition of Foods Handbook No. 8* from the *U.S. Department of Agriculture,* a half-pound of carrots, juiced, produces one glass of juice that contains 2 g. of protein, 18 g. of carbohydrate, 69 mg. of calcium, 1.3 mg. of iron, 635 mg. of potassium, 20,460 units of vitamin A (beta-carotene), 15 mg. of vitamin C and small amounts of the B vitamins.

Cranberry

Cranberry juice is good for **bladder infections**. Use brands from health food stores that are made without sugar. It is useful for low blood sugar problems, as it raises the blood sugar level without a jolt to the system.

Cucumber

Promotes urination, good for the **spleen**, **stomach** and **large intestine**. Also good for **acne** and as a **blood cleanser**. Try cutting it open and applying it to burns for relief from pain.

Dandelion

This is known as a weed, but it's rich in many minerals like calcium, magnesium, potassium, phosphorus, sulphur, silicon, iron and chlorophyll. The juice is good for liver disorders and helps cleanse the blood. Calcium, magnesium, and silicon are easily assimilated. Pick leaves before flowers appear to get tender leaves that are not bitter. Carrots are also a good source of vitamins A, C and B complex. Both promote the flow of bile in the **liver**, remove wastes from the bloodstream and liver and have a healing effect on the **kidneys** and all **infections**. Grandma knew what she was doing when she prepared dandelion salads. Somehow, dandelions have disappeared from our tables. These are powerhouse greens for healing, giving strength and acting as an excellent tonic.

Grape

Grape juice is highly recommended for healing and cleansing. The list of good grape varieties is very long. Grape juice assists in all bodily functions and is a good source of minerals, vitamins, sugar and protein. Good for **edema**, **cancer**, and combats **toxins**. Three cups of fruit make one glass.

FRUIT & VEGETABLE CLEANSER

Unless you use organic fruits and vegetables, treat your produce with a special bath to destroy all types of sprays, fungus, metallics, and germs.

Use 1 teaspoon of Clorox bleach to 1 gallon of water. Soak 10-20 minutes. Rinse thoroughly.

Kale

Rich in vitamins A and K, chlorophyll, iron, calcium, sulphur, potassium and high in vitamin C. Kale is a must for your diet! You can add small amounts to all of your juices. A deficiency of vitamin K is linked to **intestinal disorders** and is needed for **blood clotting**.

All Leafy Greens

See Leafy and Green section. Each day use different greens in your juices.

Lemon

Lemon juice is excellent as a **blood purifier**. Upon rising in the morning, drink the juice of one lemon in a cup of warm, steam-distilled water. It is excellent for use in **cleansing enemas**, as it balances the pH in the colon. It helps detoxify the system. Mix with distilled water. No drink can compare with the valuable properties, internally or externally. As a cleanser it neutralizes and promotes healing.

If you have **ulcers**, avoid lemons and other citrus fruits.

Papaya

Chymopapain contained in papaya softens tight muscles and is the reason it is the main ingredient in meat tenderizers. Papaya is also good for **inflammation**, **heartburn**, **ulcers**, **back pain** and any disorder involving the **digestive system**. Chew a couple of the seeds to aid in healing. Papaya juice was studied at *California's Oakland Naval Hospital*, researchers injected *chymopapain* into 50 patients who had undergone **surgery** and 80% found **pain** relief. A new study at the *French Academy* headed by *Dr. Gilles Tangrieve* used fresh papaya juice with excellent results.

Parsley

Parsley is a rich source of all vitamins. It helps maintain the **thyroid** and **adrenal** functions. It is very powerful, so use only small amounts because parsley is very concentrated. Add to other juices. Parsley is also a natural **diuretic** and aids in **digestion**, so do not leave that decorative sprig of parsley on your dinner plate, eat it!

Spinach

This juice is rich in all minerals and organic substances and good as a cleansing blood tonic, healing the **intestinal tract**, **hemorrhoids**, **anemia** and **vitamin deficiencies**. **Those who have known liver disease, kidney stones or arthritis should not use the juice and should eat spinach sparingly.** There is controversy over using spinach for anemia, we believe some of the iron content is available to the body. The oxalic acid content may prohibit the absorption of the calcium found in spinach.

Turnips

This juice has twice the amount of vitamin C as oranges or tomatoes. If you have arthritis, you need to omit oranges and tomatoes from your diet, so use turnips to provide yourself with a source rich in the vitamin C you need. Use the tops, too. This vegetable is often overlooked, although it is rich in all vitamins and sulfur. Turnips are also good for the elimination of uric acid and kidney stones derived from uric acid. This is good for the overweight person and for **gout** sufferers. It is excellent mixed with cabbage or carrot juice.

Brain and Immune Boosting Drink

8 drops siberian ginseng extract
8 drops echinacea and/or astragalus extract
8 drops Ginko biloba extract
1 bunch seedless grapes
1 apple
1/2 banana

Mix in blender.

Watercress

Rich in potassium, calcium, sulphur, sodium, chlorine, magnesium, phosphorus, iron, and iodine. It also contains vitamins A, B complex, C and E. As much as one-third of the mineral content may be sulphur. This is an acid-forming vegetable and should not be used alone but in combination with highly alkaline vegetables such as carrots or celery.

Watercress is a powerful **intestinal cleanser**, **blood cleanser** and builder. Rich in all nutrients. Combine watercress, green pepper, carrot, dandelion and cucumber for hair, nails, skin, bones, collagen formation, muscle, and vitamin deficiencies.

Wheatgrass

This is the king of juices! It is very high in chlorophyll and will stop the development of unfriendly bacteria. It is actually akin to human red blood cells and is the best **blood purifier** we have. Red blood cell counts have been known to return to normal using this juice. This juice is so potent it can have a nauseating effect in the beginning. Start with a couple cups of weak juice through the day, then work up to more. Wheatgrass is good for **energy** and **body building**. It is the best for expelling elevated metals in the body. Healing uses include effectiveness as a douche and a gargle for **sore throats**. It is beneficial for the blood sugar and is the best for healing of the colon and lungs. Wheatgrass has great healing powers! Have you noticed how animals eat grass when they are ill or have worms? They also turn down food. We can learn much from watching the instinctive actions of animals and all of nature.

See the section on Seeds and Sprouts to find out how easy it is to grow this wondrous food. It is definitely worthwhile to rejuvenate your body by adding this to your juices.

You can purchase wheatgrass in powdered, liquid, and tablet forms from a health food store.

If you do not own a juicer, get one. It could be the best present you ever buy yourself. The Champion or the Omega juicers are heavy duty ones that do not destroy all the live enzymes in the juice. The Omega is ultra-quiet and runs smoothly, has a stainless steel construction, is easy to clean, and has a 10-year guarantee. In the long run, live juices can save you hundreds of dollars in medical bills and, best of all, fresh juices will help keep you healthy.

Good Food Sources of Antioxidants

Vitamin C
Fruits and vegetables

Vitamin E
Wheat germ, sunflower seeds, leafy green vegetables, salmon, lobster, peanuts and peanut butter

Beta-carotene
Dark green and deep yellow or orange fresh vegetables and fruits, including carrots, spinach, kale, peaches, papayas and cantaloupe

Selenium
Garlic and onions are the best sources

Preparing Juice Combinations for Speed Healing
And Continued Good Health

1) Purchase organic herbs, fruits and vegetables when possible, or grow your own. Or be sure to peel and wash produce very thoroughly. Use very small amounts of fresh herbs in your juices, since they are so potent.

2) Strong-flavored vegetables like turnips, rutabaga, broccoli, parsley, onions and celery should be juiced in small amounts, for example, 1/4 turnip would be sufficient per glass. Foods that have a high-water content should be your base, like carrots, cabbage, apples and grapes.

3) Alternate your foods and herbs from the charts on pages 38-49 everyday to recieve all the healing and prevention benefits. Gradually work through the entire list as each has a specific role to play in restoring and balancing your metabolism. Do not mix sweet fruit juices with vegetable juices; only a juiced apple may be added to vegetable juice. (Don't use rhubarb greens or carrot tops as they are toxic when juiced.)

4) It is best to make your juice right before consuming it. You can store it for 24 hours, if it is kept at almost freezing, about 30°, but not frozen. Put pre-chilled (set it in your freezer for 15 minutes) into a pre-chilled glass thermos and place it in the refrigerator to retain more of the enzymes and nutrients.

5) If you are using herbs in capsules, mix 1/2 glass distilled water with 1/2 glass juice and stir the capsule contents into your drink or use the extract form which is more potent. This works especially well when giving herbs that are in capsule foem to children, and many herbs on the list can be found in combination with other herbs in capsules. **Consult your healthcare practitioner, if you are pregnant or nursing, have liver or heart disorders or high blood pressure, before using any herbs unless they are specifically recommended for these disorders.**

6) Green drinks are very powerful and so may cause nausea and headaches at first. Green foods are nature's most protective medicine. They detoxify the organs, reduce tumors and act to overcome all toxic substances in the body. Dilute vegetable drinks with distilled water and sip slowly. Drink your fruit juices in the morning and dilute them with half distilled water or herb tea. Diabetics and hypoglycemics should avoid sweet fruit juices, but may use apple and cranberry and any other low-sugar fruit juices to add to herbal juices. Bok choy, a Chinese cabbage may be used in place of cabbage and beet greens, spinich, garlic, and parsley are rich in magnesium, making them good for endurance and stamina for those who exercise. See Leafy & Green section to add powerful healing greens to your juices.

7) You may drink as many live juices as you wish. It is wise to drink at least 4 glasses per day for speed healing and 2 glasses for health maintenance. Nothing else on our planet supplies the body with so many needed substances like live vegetables, fruits and herbs to enhance speed healing.

8) Fast 3 days per month or one day per week (unless you are diabetic, pregnant, nursing, have advanced heart disease, or kidney disfunction) to keep the body clean, and so it can heal and repair properly.

9) Keep in mind that nothing in the universe stays at peak performance at all times. That includes your body. Everything and everyone has cycles--we experience highs and lows. We must constantly work up to reach higher to avoid feeling low. By following this wellness program, you can acomplish that "up" feeling more often and for longer periods. The "lows" will be shorter in duration and farther apart.

Here's to your health! Phyllis Balch

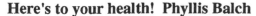

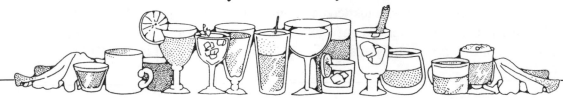

Cleansing for Wellness

Do you desire improved health, increased energy & better absorption?

The primary goal in this cleansing and wellness program is to rid the body of toxins and excess waste. These body-cleansing techniques have been used for centuries to heal the sick. The following program should be repeated at least once every two months.

Most health-oriented people believe that the accumulation of toxins in the system is the main cause of illness and disease. Toxic overload is a primary cause of liver damage.

Fasting

You can add years to your life by fasting periodically. Fasting helps the body to heal faster and gives the organs a much-needed rest. By cleansing the liver, kidneys and blood stream, the body is better able to flush built-up toxins out of the colon. When the colon is toxic, it contains harmful bacteria and maybe parasites. It can be the reason behind malabsorption of nutrients, skin eruptions, bad breath, body odor, mental confusion, liver spots, stiffness of the joints and headaches.

Hypoglycemics should not fast without a quality protein supplement. Spirulina is a good choice and it supplies chlorophyll, too. Fiber and spirulina should not be taken at the same time or with other supplements. Spirulina will also get rid of hunger pangs and is good even when you're not fasting.

Diabetics should not fast on juices or water only. Add fresh vegetables without seasonings or dressings and non-sweet fruits. Plain vegetable broth and herb teas may be used on liquid days.

If you are bothered with **colon problems**, add fresh or powdered wheat grass to your juices; it's loaded with nutrients. Green drinks (made from any green leafy vegetables) are an excellent detoxifier. Chlorophyll, in the form of liquid alfalfa or wheatgrass, found in health food stores, helps decrease body odor. Toxins can also cause mental confusion, liver spots, stiffness of the joints and headaches.

Kyogreen by *Kyolic* gives you the best of land and sea, chlorella, barley grass, wheat grass, kelp and brown rice. It comes in powdered form and is good added to any vegetable juice or water for those who don't own a juicer.

Supplies

Here are a few things you will need for this program:
- steam-distilled water
- fresh sugar-free juices
- fresh lemons, pears, apples
- powdered buffered vitamin C
- fresh beets and tops, leafy greens
- pure, unprocessed virgin olive oil,
- coffee (not instant or decaffeinated)
- fiber (psyllium powder, glucomannan or oat bran)
- 3 herb teas: choose Rose hip, Golden seal, Dandelion, Pau D'Arco, Alfalfa, Echinacea
- spirulina and/or liquid chlorophyll (*optional*)
(see the Wellness Charts and Herb section to choose the herbs that fit your specific disorder)

Enemas

Gentle infusions of warm water or lemon enemas are better than laxatives or drugs. They should become part of your monthly wellness program. Many clinics in the world use this procedure and recommend its use for all disorders and to rejuvenate the body.

There are two types of enemas: retention and cleansing. The cleansing enemas are not retained. They are used to flush out the colon. Retention enemas are designed to aid the absorption of necessary nutrients and substances (i.e. coffee and chlorophyll) through the colon wall. Chlorophyll (wheatgrass) is a standard treatment in many clinics.

Cleansing Enemas

While on this program, the cleansing enema to use daily is as follows: mix the juice of two lemons with two quarts of lukewarm water. The best position for inserting the fluid is head down, bottom up. After the fluid is inserted, lay on your right side, then rotate to your back, then to the left side, simultaneously massaging the colon and helping to loosen fecal matter. If you have trouble with constipation, use the lemon enema alternately with a coffee enema twice weekly until the bowels are moving on their own and the colon is clean and not foul-smelling.

Retention Enemas

For effective detoxification, coffee retention enemas are used during fasting portions of the program. They are used in the treatment of degenerative diseases to stimulate the liver to excrete toxins and to help loosen waste on the colon walls. In some cases fecal matter may have been on the colon walls for months or even years. Add 1-2 ounces liquid chlorophyll, alfalfa or wheatgrass to your coffee enema or use alone for speed healing. This green enema is especially good for those with chronic illness as it provides numerous nutrients that are absorbed by the colon.

Coffee Retention Enemas

Put six heaping tablespoons of ground coffee (not instant or decaffeinated) into two quarts steam distilled water in a saucepan. Boil for 15 minutes, cool and strain. Use only one pint at a time, save the rest and store in the refrigerator. Use this once or twice a day, it's best in the morning, while detoxifying to relieve headaches caused by toxin buildup. When not detoxifying, use only occasionally as needed. If you have trouble retaining the enema, expell and start over. Lie on your right side and hold it for 15 minutes. A good book helps the time pass quickly.

Fiber

At least one of these forms of fiber is recommended every day: rice bran, oat bran, apple pectin, agar, psyllium seed or glucomannan. Avoid wheat bran, as it may irritate the colon wall. For weight loss, take fiber 30 minutes before meals to decrease your appetite. Be sure to drink a large glass of water with fiber capsules because they expand. Aerobic Bulk Cleanser (ABC) is an excellent fiber.

Spirulina tablets or powder should be taken daily, five tablets three times a day or one teaspoon three times a day in juice. Spirulina is a perfect food, high in protein with all the vitamins and minerals the body needs, plus chlorophyll for cleansing. Make sure the spirulina is high-quality. Use Earthrise--a wise choice.

Drink only steam distilled water and plenty of it. You may dilute juices with it, but use only unsweetened juices with no additives. Do not use tomato or orange juice because of their high acidity content.

Skin Brushing

A dry brush massage is important in ridding the body of old dead cells so new ones can form. Dead skin cells prevent your skin from breathing. The massage increases circulation, bringing the blood closer to the surface of the skin. Just before your morning shower, brush with a natural bristle brush in long strokes toward your heart. Your skin will glow and begin to look years younger.

Patients with severe circulatory problems, even those who have difficulty standing for prolonged periods, will improve circulation with dry brush massage.

Exercise

Some form of exercise is important during a fast, like walking or stretching. Continue your normal daily duties.

Take enemas after a bowel movement when possible, and do not overuse them. Prolonged use may develop a dependency on enemas for normal bowel movements.

Six-Day Cleansing and Wellness Diet

Follow once a month to balance your metabolism and stabilize your weight.

Day 1

Breakfast: Drink a glass of steam-distilled water to flush the kidneys. Eat any fresh fruit except oranges. Drink a glass of juice but not orange juice. Diabetics or hypoglycemics should not eat sweet fruits like grapes, pears, papaya, melon, or grapefruit. Add 1,000 mg. of vitamin-C powder to the juice, as well as one tablespoon of a fiber supplement, oat bran, glucommannan or psyllium seed. Take the fiber supplement three times a day, every day.

Lunch: Eat a fresh vegetable salad. Make a dressing of the juice of one lemon, one cup virgin olive oil, a dash of garlic powder or fresh garlic juice, a pinch of dried parsley and 1/4 teaspoon of barley malt or rice malt sweetener or blackstrap molasses. See The Raw Foods Story for a variety of salads for speed healing

Dinner: Steam or boil any vegetable or have a raw salad. This first day is to prepare your body for a cleansing. You may not have any salt, sugar or seasonings except the salad dressing above. To flavor the vegetables, use cold-pressed sesame seed or pure virgin olive oil, chopped chives and a little pure garlic powder. A small amount of kelp is good for minerals and weight loss

You may eat fresh fruit between meals and drink herb teas. Combine herb teas and one-third cup unsweetened fruit or vegetable juice for speed healing. Drink at least six glasses of liquids during the day.

Before retiring, use the lemon cleansing enema(page 133). If you are taking calcium supplements, continue taking them. You can also include vitamin E, but omit other vitamins while cleansing.

Day 2

Upon arising, drink a glass of steam-distilled water. Use a coffee enema(page 133). Drink a glass of fruit juice with 1,000 mg. vitamin C and your fiber supplement. Those with sugar disorders may drink a green drink for speed healing.

Make the following drink, which you can have as often as you like during the day: add the juice of four lemons to one gallon of distilled water. Sweeten with two tablespoons blackstrap molasses or barley malt sweetener. You may also have herb teas mixed with 1/3 fresh juice throughout the day.

You can also use apple juice with the skins and seeds. Drink fruit juices alone and remember to avoid them if you are diabetic or hypoglycemic. You can also make your own applesauce, leave the skins on and place the apples in a food processor or blender. Add a small amount of lemon juice to the applesauce mixture so it will store better. Do not add any sweeteners or use canned applesauce.

Consume only fresh apples on this day for solid food. Eat them alone, not with the broth or the juice.

Before retiring, use the lemon cleansing enema.

If you are using wheat grass or some form of chlorophyll, add it to your juice. If you are including spirulina, take three tablets or one teaspoon of the powered form three times a day.

Day 3

A liquid day.

Drink a glass of distilled water upon arising, then administer the coffee enema. Drink a glass of grapefruit juice or fresh lemon and water, to which you have added two tablespoons pure cold-processed olive oil. (This aids the healing and cleansing of the gallbladder.) You may also add the oil to the juice of 1/2 lemon, if you wish. Repeat the oil and lemon juice drink just after rising in the morning and just before retiring at night for the next three days.

Drink a glass of juice with the vitamin C and fiber supplements. You may drink all the herb teas, lemon juice with distilled water, vegetable broth, and juices you desire. Be sure to dilute all juices with water. Make the fresh vegetable broth or juice to sip on throughout the day. No applesauce on this day, only liquids.

Before going to bed, drink the lemon juice-olive oil combination. If you feel you need a cleansing enema, use it. It is especially good and needed if this is your first fast. You may prefer a laxative, *Nature's Way* Natural Laxative #2 works well.

At this point, you may continue with the six day plan or stay on Day #3 for two more days. Staying on liquids only for three consecutive days will aid in faster **weight loss** and **promote speed healing**. If you have very specific dietary needs (diabetic, etc.) and you decide to continue Day #3 for the extra time, consult your doctor first.

Day 4

Repeat Day #3 but add unsweetened cranberry juice found in health food stores, good for the **urinary tract** and **bladder**.

Lunch: Shred two beets and add one tablespoon olive oil and the juice of one lemon. Drink pear juice on this day, mixed with 1/2 distilled water. If you have sugar problems try diluted apple juice. Drink as much pear juice as you want, but not with the beets. You may also drink beet juice, which is made by putting the beets and the tops into a juicer or blender with distilled water. If you do not have a juicer or beets are not available, beet juice can be found in a health food store.

Day 5

Start the day with the glass of distilled water and juice with the fiber supplements and the olive oil-lemon juice drink.

Follow the instructions for Day #1.

Lunch or Dinner: Add the following: 1/4 head of cabbage, shredded, 1/4 raw onion, one carrot, one turnip and a raw beet. Toss with the olive oil dressing.

You may repeat the last five days at this point for more dramatic results or continue the program if you are already satisfied with your weight and healing results.

Day 6

Breakfast: Drink a glass of distilled water and a glass of juice with the vitamin C and fiber. Have a bowl of fresh fruit or prunes or a bowl of whole grain cereal. Do not eat the cereal and the fresh fruit at the same time. Wait at least half an hour between them.

Lunch: Eat a fresh raw vegetable salad topped with raisins and sunflower seeds. **Be sure to chew food until it is almost liquid.** You can now use the House Dressing in the Salad Dressings section and add raw avocado. Shred the vegetables if you like. Drink the herb tea (remember, do not drink liquids with meals, only before or after).

Dinner: Eat steamed cauliflower, broccoli and carrots over brown rice. Add onions and other vegetables, if desired. Season with lemon juice and a small amount of garlic. Do not eat any processed foods or breads; only freshly prepared foods. Continue with the liquids you have been consuming throughout the program, making sure your body gets at least eight glasses of fluids each day.

You must not return to heavy protein meals at this point! If you do, you will reverse the results you have worked to achieve.

Make these last six days a part of your routine once each month to help stabilize your weight and keep your system clean.

If this is your first cleansing program, it would be wise for you to make either a vegetable drink or broth. If you do not have a juicer, simmer the following vegetables:

2 carrots	2 stalks celery	2 beets and tops
2 turnips	1 clove garlic	1/2 onion
1/2 head cabbage	1/4 bunch parsley	1 gallon quality water

Strain and sip the broth, storing the remaining vegetables for later. Don't eat the vegetables at this time. Even the smallest amount of food will ruin the fast. During the fast there is a total change in the body's metabolism. To suppress the feeling of hunger, drink a large glass of vegetable juice or broth. Use the same amounts for juicing raw, consuming half immediately and the rest an hour later. When making raw juice, make only what you will consume that day.

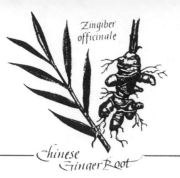

Zingiber officinale

Chinese Ginger Root

Herb Teas
Nature's Potent Healers

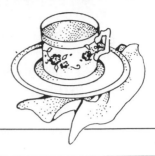

Most herbs are good for aromatherapy (scent therapy) and as essential oils to enhance health. The oils are pleasant added to bath water. **Lavender** has a calming effect, **jasmine** relieves anxiety, **geranium** is uplifting, **eucalyptus** balances energy and is an expectorant, **rosemary** is for acne and is uplifting, **cedar wood** is for stress, **patchouli** regulates the female reproductive system, and **lemon oil** is good for oily skin, uplifting, and soothes anxiety.

Do not use aluminum pots when preparing teas. Do not boil tea. **If pregnant or nursing do not use herbs in high amounts. Use caution with children under 6 years of age.**

The following is a list of terms used in making teas:

Decoction

Made by boiling the bark, root, seed or berry part of a plant.

Herb Vinegars

Use raw apple cider, rice or malt vinegar. Add your favorite fresh or dried herbs. Cap and let stand for two months to let the flavor develop.

Infusion

The leaf, flower or part of the plant is steeped for 3-5 minutes in hot water to make a tea, so you do not destroy the benefits of the herbs. Because these parts are more delicate, do not boil.

Tincture / Extract

Tinctures are the most potent and many contain about 50 percent alcohol. They keep for a long time.

Extracts are potent, and may be created with alcohol or be alcohol free.

Herb teas and their benefits are listed below. For specific illnesses, check the list and choose the ones you need. We have included the top 10 herbs of the 90's (marked with an *) and other important healing herbs.

Alfalfa

Affects colon disorders, blood clotting, arthritis, fungal infections, fluid retention, bad breath, heart disease and stroke, regulate blood cholesterol, cancer, inflammatory diseases, and systematic lupus. Blood purification, calcium deficiency, kidney disorders, rheumatism, ulcers and it's good for weight loss. One of the few plant foods that contains B-12, making alfalfa good for vegetarians and those with colon or blood disorders.

*Astragalus

Contains *saponins* and *gamma-aminobutyric* acid. Stimulates immunity, an antibacterial, anti-fatigue, aids in healing cancer, colds, flus, fevers, arthritis, hepatitis, diabetes, hypertension, AIDS, heart disease, Epstein-Barr virus, adrenal and spleen disorders, kidney, liver, and diuretic disorders and vaginitis. A major tonic, anti-inflammatory agent and an adaptogenic herb. strengthened the focus of

---

Grow your own herbs to juice right along with your vegetables. Chamomile, the mint family, catnip, calendula, borage, echinacea, garlic, and parsley are all easy to grow. Use just a small amount of fresh herbs in your juice because they are very powerful. Remember that dried herbs made into tea can be included in your diet on a daily basis.

astragalus membranaceous as an important immune system herb. Astragalus is often combined with ginseng in Chinese medicine.

Burdock Root

The finest blood purifier. Contains volatile oils, *glucinsides*, inulin, mucilage, tannic acid, vitamin C, iron, niacin plus most minerals. The Japanese boil the root in a small amount of water or eat it with a sauce or drink the water as a tea. Good for sties, cancer and all degenerative diseases (even AIDS) because of its strong cleansing effect on the body.

Black Walnut

Anti-fungal, aids asthmatics, expels parasites.

Buchu

For acute and chronic bladder and kidney disorders. Good for pain when urinating. A good diuretic. Helps the pancreas, diabetes, prostate, liver, spleen, hypoglycemics, as a urinary antiseptic, bloating from PMS, and high blood pressure.

Butcher's Broom

Contains *ruscogenin, neo-ruscogenin* and flavonoids. Good for circulation problems, anti-inflammatory, varicose veins, edema of the legs and hemorrhoids.

Cascara Sagrada, Ginger Root & Licorice Root

All of the above aid those suffering from colitis and diverticulitis. Cascara sagrada is a colon cleanser, for parasites, good for constipation, and disorders of the stomach, liver, gall bladder and pancreas.

Catnip, Lobelia & Echinacea

All of the above are used for fevers and colic. Catnip enemas will reduce a fever quickly for adults and children, quiets the nervous system, and eliminates excess mucus from the body.

Cayenne

Applied directly, it stops the bleeding of wounds. Good for ulcers, as a stimulant, in colds, for circulation, heart disorders, digestive disorders, shingles, chronic pain, cluster headaches, and for the heart, circulation, stomach and kidneys.

Chamomile

Good for inflammation, fever, digestive upsets, anxiety, colon disorders, and ulcers. Also for stomach, kidney, spleen and liver disorders. Relaxes muscles in the digestive tract, and helps menstrual cramps. May be given to children for colic.

Chaparral

Aids in treatment of cancer, arthritis, intestinal parasites, viral illnesses, bruises, venereal diseases, and a potent antioxidant.

Chasteberry

Good for PMS and menstrual disorders. Stimulates the release of leutenizing hormone and inhibits the release of follicle stimulating hormone. Helps to reduce and eliminate some PMS symptoms like anxiety and mood swings.

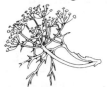

Stop the bleeding following a tooth extraction by chewing softly on a wet black tea bag. Tea contains tannic acid, a natural coagulant.

Cornsilk

Helps prevent bedwetting. Relieves painful urination, water retention, and prostate ailments.

Crampbark

Relieves cramps in painful menstruation. Good for the heart.

Dandelion, Black Radish & Cascara Sagrada

Aids all liver disorders, skin disorders, jaundice, cirrhosis, and hepatitis, a liver cleanser. High in usable calcium and good for osteoporosis. Dandelion is good for blood sugar disorders.

Dandelion, Nettle & Alfalfa

Aids in anemia, arthritis, colon disorders, the glandular functions, liver, and calcium deficiencies.

Dandelion

Good for PMS, high blood pressure, liver disorders, weight loss, cancer, a poultice for breast cancer, a digestive aid, for calcium deficiencies, yeast infections, and bacterial infections. Good for the liver, gall bladder, stomach, pancreas, intestines and blood.

*Dong Quai

For female hormone imbalances, helps hot flashes, menopausal symptoms, stimulates uterine muscle, relieves menstrual cramps, and calms nerves. An immune system stimulant, can overcome vitamin E deficiency symptoms.

For best results, take with herb tea or water, not with fruit juices.

*Echinacea & Golden Seal

Good for inflammation, infections, colds, and flu. Improves lymphatic function, and reduces glandular swelling. Helps to protect the immune system. Is an anti-tumor, anti-fungal, anti-viral, and anti-bacterial agent. Helps urinary tract infections, strep throat, bronchitis, rheumatoid arthritis, and eczema.

Experiments have shown the *polysaccharides*, fatty acids, and *glyosides* in echinacea enhance the function of the immune system making it important in all disorders and illnesses. Also expels toxins and poisons from the body.

False Unicorn

Good for infertility, normalizing ovarian functions and helping menstrual irregularities.

Fennel

Good for obesity, curbs the appetite. Helps an acid stomach and gout. Effective as an eyewash.

Fenugreek

Helps gallbladder troubles, muscle aches, bronchitis, digestive disorders. As a poultice for wounds, boils, and rashes. Good for coughs, sore throats. Lowers cholesterol.

Feverfew

Good for high blood pressure, as a digestive aid, for pain, and stress-related illnesses. A study at the *London Medical Clinic* found this herb reduced headache pain and the frequency of migraines. Avoid alcohol because it destroys feverfew's benefits.

*Garlic

Lowers cholesterol, and blood pressure, improves circulation, stimulates the immune system, good for arthritis, arteriosclerosis, blood-sugar disorders, allergies, bronchitis, asthma, and yeast infections (candida albicans). May help prevent breast cancer, heart disease and stroke, diabetes, lead poisoning, AIDS, herpes, and other viral infections. If you have a problem because of the odor, try odorless *Kyolic Garlic*, an aged garlic extract.

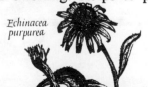

Echinacea purpurea

138

Ginger

Helps nausea, motion sickness and vomiting. Ginger is good for the stomach, indigestion, intestines, joints, muscles, circulation, coughs, asthma,and reduces blood platelet clumping, sore throat discomfort, and cleanses the kidneys and bowels.

*Ginkgo Biloba

Good for memory and brain function, circulation, heart disorders, cholesterol problems, impotence, ringing in the ears, retinal and macular (eye) degeneration, dizziness (vertigo), asthma, Alzheimer's disease, senile dementia, and allergies. The extract, EGb from the plant leaves, is being hailed around the world as the supplement of choice in the fight against problems associated with the aging process. The major active constituents of EGb consist of flavonoid glycosides, *kaempferol, quercitin,* and *isorhamnetine.*

Ginseng & Sarsaparilla

Good for impotence, energy, endurance, stamina, and diabetes.

*Ginseng

Reduces the effects of physical and emotional stress, improves memory, effective against depression and nervous conditions, improves energy, stamina, and resistance to disease, lowers cholesterol, helps diabetes, protects cells from radiation, aids the adrenal glands, a potent immune stimulant, and good for impotence.

There are three primary types of ginseng: red, white, and Siberian. Each has its own unique qualities. **Red ginseng** is stimulating for physical activities, can be used as a sexual tonic. **Women should not use**

GREEN TEA, popular in Japan and other countries in the Far East, though it contains caffeine it significantly inhibits the development of skin, lung, liver and other cancers in mice. An anti-cancer component called EGCG, reduced the number of lung tumors by 38% from nitrosamines in tobacco, *National Cancer Center Research Institute, Tokyo. Call Uncle Lee's Organic Green Tea for information 818/350-3309.*

---

this consistently over long periods, it promotes testosterone production. **White ginseng** is a good for the digestive system, aids recovery of illness, can be used over long periods, and with other tonics for building strength. **American ginseng** is an unprocessed white variety. **Wild American** is the most potent. Grown in the woods, it is a better value and effective. It promotes healing after illness and surgery, and is a powerful adaptogen. **Siberian ginseng** supports the adrenal function, reduces stress, and regulates the blood sugar.

*Golden Seal

Contains *berberine, hydrastine,* and *canadine.* These natural alkaloids support the immune function, the spleen, and lymphatic system. Acts as an antibiotic, good for the stomach, intestines, liver and all mucus membranes. Also good for allergies, asthma, bronchitis, canker sores, diabetes, chicken pox, eczema, bleeding gums, infections, hemorrhoids, herpes, alcoholism, and inflammations. A great healer.

Gotu Kola

An immune stimulant. Good for varicose veins, leprosy, and psoriasis. Accelerates the healing of burns. Also good for the brain's function, nerves, kidneys, heart and circulation, and helps impotence.

Do not confuse with kola nut, the caffeine-containing nut used in soft drinks.

Hawthorne

An excellent heart medicine for long term use. Good for all heart disorders, palpitations, angina pectoris, and high blood pressure. May prevent kidney stones.

Horsetail

Rich in all minerals, especially *silica.* The silica and calcium content is good for the bones, hair, skin, nails, bone formation and connective tissues. Good for the eyes, ears, nose, throat, and glandular functions. Helps rheumatoid arthritis, and ulcers. Highly alkaline to the body, thus good for all diseases. A diuretic that stimulates the kidney function, heart, and lungs. Good for urinary tract infections and to control bedwetting in children.

139

Silica is indispensable for the elasticity of the lung tissue and its function. It helps skin disorders, injuries, bone disease, diseases of the intestinal tract, urinary disorders, bleeding gums, ear, nose, throat disease, and osteoarthritic conditions. Silica is one mineral that has a direct relationship with the absorption of all minerals. Foods with a high content of silica are millet, barley, corn, rye, red beets, potatoes, and onions. Most people are short in this mineral unless their diet is high in fresh vegetables and whole grains. **Best to take for two weeks, then stay off for one week.**

Pregnant woman or children under six should not use horsetail because of the high selenium.

Kelp, Dulse, Irish Moss & Parsley

Good for goiter and thyroid conditions. Relieves water retention, vitamin and mineral deficiencies, preventing obesity. Kelp protects against heart disease and radiation, removes toxic metals (chelator).

Licorice

Contains *glycrrhizic* acid. Good for female disorders. A cough remedy, prevents ulcers, an anti-inflammatory, has anti-viral activities (herpes), enhances immune function, an anti-depressant. Protects the liver, a laxative, helps asthma and arthritis. Good for the throat and injured throat muscles.

American candy is made from synthetic flavorings, not real licorice.

*Pau D'Arco

Has an antibiotic effect, good for yeast infections, an anti-parasite, anti-cancer herb and strengthens immunity. Use an extract form or drink as a tea, after boiling for 10 minutes.

Peppermint

Aids digestion, eases vomiting and nausea, stimulates metabolism and the nervous system. Soothes fever and relieves muscular pain. Can be used as a skin cleanser. Relieves mental strain, depression, and headaches.

Red Clover & Yellow Dock

Good as a blood purifier for skin disorders, and boils.

Red Clover & Dandelion

Good for blood, as a liver cleanser, and for lung congestion. Dandelion is high in calcium.

Red Raspberry

Reduces nausea associated with pregnancy. Helps to strengthen the uterus. Good for female disorders, good combined with Dong Quai.

Red Raspberry Leaves & Black Cohosh

Good for morning sickness, hot flashes, menstrual cramps, fevers, and mouth sores.

Red or Pure Purple Lapacho

According to ancient tradition (and modern practice) it is an excellent source of energy that provides powerful nutrition to the cells. Also helps to protect against the effects of stress, serves as a colon cleanser and helps reduce the impact of many allergies.

Available from *Wisdom of the Ancients*, 640 Perry Lane, Suite 2, Tempe, AZ 85281, in a ready to mix, heat and drink preparation. Many types are available. Most are naturally sweet.

Pumpkin Seeds or Oil & Saw Palmetto Berries

Good for prostate ailments, zinc deficiency, and impotence. Saw Palmetto is good for bronchitis, sterility, enlarged prostate, reproductive organs and kidneys.

Rose Hips

High in vitamin C, helps against infection, also bladder difficulties, flu, mouth sores, PMS, and the common cold.

*Silymarin (Milk Thistle)

In folk history it was widely used to produce milk in nursing mothers. In Germany and Europe it is used for all liver disorders. Milk Thistle increases the liver's *glylathione* content to boost detoxification.

Silymarin compounds help to stimulate protein synthesis, in return the liver produces and maintains healthy new cells. Those exposed to chemicals and alcohol should take two caps, three times per day for detoxification. Silymarin is the best known rejuvenator for the liver.

Slippery Elm

Generally affects the whole body. Good for colitis, diverticulitis, gas, hemorrhoids, lung congestion, stomach disorders, flu, eczema, cystitis and coughs.

Spearmint

Soothes depression and mental fatigue, a digestive aid and breath freshener.

Squaw Vine

For yeast infections, vaginal infections, bladder and colon disorders, urinary irritation and leukorrhea, used to treat water retention.

Strengthens uterus for childbirth.

*St. John's Wort

Fights viruses, such as HIV and EBV, also good for nerves, a sedative, diuretic, for disorders of the lung, stomach, bladder and liver. A blood purifier. Avoid exposure to sunlight while using or a rash may develop.

Do not take if pregnant or nursing or give to children unless under supervision.

Suma (Brazilian Ginseng)

Suma grows up to 8 feet in length in the Amazon Rainforest. Pharmacologists have found natural substances in Suma believed to reduce tumors and regulate blood sugar levels. 152 chemical substances have been identified including plant steroid, *beta-ecdysone*, which facilitates cellular oxygenation, *sitosterol* and *stigmasterol*, plant hormones which encourage estrogen production and reduce high cholesterol levels.

Tea Tree Oil (Not used as tea)

For poison ivy, itchiness, skin irritations, dandruff, and acne. It soothes diaper rash, insect bites, herpes sores, fungal infections, cuts and sprains, vaginitis, and ringworm. Promotes healing of infected wounds and urinary infections and an antiseptic for the respiratory system. *The Medical Journal of Australia* reported that tea tree oil successfully treated diabetic gangrene. Good for vaginal douches of 1% oil in one quart of water for vaginitis (yeast infections). Also helps athletes foot, fungal infections under toe nails, corns, and calluses. For an itchy scalp apply a few drops in your shampoo or apply directly. Massage into joints to ease arthritic pain.

Uva Ursi, Cornsilk & Juniper Berries

Diuretics, good for urinary-tract infections and kidney stones.

*Valerian Root and Skullcap

Good for nerves, stress, insomnia, anxiety, and tension. A relaxant, for convulsions, colic, general pain, and stomach pains. Valerian root is good for viral infections and excellent for insomnia. **Never boil Valerian root.**

White Oak Bark

Tannin, the active principle in white oak bark is used in medicine as an astringent, in the gastro-intestinal tract, on skin abrasions, and burns, for infected and bleeding mouth sores, on hemorrhoids and as a douche for vaginal and cervical discharges. *Tannin* should not be taken internally for long periods of time because in India and South Africa, where many chew a nut high in *tannin*, the users show increased rates of cancer of the esophagus and cheek cavity.

White Willow

Contains *salicin* and is derived from the same bark as aspirin. White Willow is also good for headaches, pain, fever reduction, as a tonic and diuretic. Helps the prostate, urinary tract infections, mouth sores, inflammation and allergies. Reported to work better than aspirin, it is safer and stronger. Aspirin, now being used to prevent heart attacks, has *cyclooxygenase* inhibitors that prevent platelet clumping and blood clots. Mentioned in Egyptian papyri, Hippocrates used it for pain and fever.

Immortal Mushrooms

The Reishi (Ganoderma) and Shiitake Mushrooms

Try power mushrooms, shiitake or reishi, in place of the common button mushroom.

For more than 2,000 years the emperors of Japan and China have used reishi or Ling Zhi mushrooms, known also as Ganoderma lucidum, believing they provided immortality. Shiitake mushrooms are produced primarily in Japan. The extract of *lentinan* from the shiitake is used in treatments. The **reishi** (pronounced ray-she) mushroom is listed in China's pharmacopoeia and is classified as a superior herb. It is a powerful antioxidant, and the *ganoderic acid* it contains is a free-radical scavenger. The *Myasthenia Gravis Association of Japan* encourages the use of reishi for people with debilitating muscle disease. Both mushrooms are used for healing in these countries. Because of their growing popularity they are now commercially cultivated in North America.

In the U.S. herbalists, naturopaths, and ortho-molecular therapists, and even health-oriented doctors, are using them. Canadian herbalist, *Terry Willard, PH.D.* says, "The reishi mushrooms increase disease-resistance and normalize body functions. The reishi mushroom affected positive reports in the treatment of the chronic fatigue syndrome. Japanese pharmacologists have also demonstrated positive results in the treatment of environmental and stress-induced illness. In this country these are two illnesses that are considered "incurable." At the *Wild Rose Health Center* in Vancouver and Alberta, Canada, *Dr. Williard* uses reishi mushrooms to treat cancer, AIDS, CFS and allergic asthma. Further, the Japanese have found the reishi mushroom increases the blood flow and oxygen to the brain which is diminished in Alzheimer's patients.

Reishi inhibits histamine release, which is why it is good against asthma. Also it is used in treatment of chronic bronchitis and heart disease. It contains an anti-tumor polysaccharide know as *B-D glucan,* similar to that found in shiitake.

Reishi contains two major groups of organic compounds, *ganodermic acids,* similar to steroid hormones, and *polysaccharides* which are long chains of naturally occurring sugar molecules, that assist the immune system in preventing tumors by attacking malignant cells and stimulating the body's defenses. Additionally, these components help the immune system recognize and attack harmful yeasts, bacteria and viruses. *Polysaccharides* increase RNA and DNA in the bone marrow where immune cells, like lymphocytes, are made. The long branched chains of sugar, seem to be the main immune modulators in reishi mushrooms. The *triterpenoids* are responsible for the mushroom's bitter taste and for normalizing the circulatory and immune systems, protecting against environmental and physical stress. These compounds are what makes this mushroom a powerful healing herb.

Shiitake mushrooms contain an antiviral substance know as *lentinan* which stimulates the immune system to produce more *interferon,* a natural compound that is known to fight cancer and viruses. Additional studies demonstrate that shiitake extract promotes the activation of macrophages and the proliferation of bone marrow cells, thereby possessing an immunostimulating activity and anti-HIV effect. Shiitake mushrooms also contain an important source of vitamin D, needed for calcium absorption, which is not found in many foods. Shiitake mushrooms contain *lentysine* and *eritadenine,* two ingredients that help lower the level of fat in the blood, which aids in lowering the blood pressure and reducing fatigue. This is also used in the Orient for sexual dysfunction, aging, gallstones, ulcers and diabetes, to name a few. Shiitake are free of the natural carcinogens found in the common white cultivated mushroom (button mushroom). The shiitake does not lose its nutrient value when cooked at high temperatures.

Shiitake's powerful antitumor action reverses the T-cell suppression caused by tumors, making it valuable against cancer, leukemia, lymphosarcoma and Hodgkin's Disease. It further inhibits cell division of viruses, thus impeding their affects. These antiviral actions are due to mycoviral substances present in the spores and mycelia of the fungus. The flu and other viruses are thus hindered by taking shiitake.

Delicious! May/June 1992, pg.39

Vitamin C increases the absorption of the reishi *polysaccharides* improving treatment of cancer and other diseases. Studies have found the following healing properties:

- cholesterol & fat levels lowered
- lowers frequency and severity of migraines
- reduced side effects from radiation & chemotherapy
- improved circulation
- increased stamina
- inhanced immune system
- lowered blood pressure
- alleviated allergic symptoms & auto-immune disease
- regenerated liver
- calmed nervous system
- reduced inflammation in joints
- reduced shoulder & neck pain
- benefits myasthenia gravis, candida, asthma Epstein Barr virus, chronic fatigue syndrome, anxiety, depression, bronchitis, hypoglycemia, & allergic rhinitis

Free-radicals decreased by 50% using reishi, and it protects against **cobalt**, **x-ray**, **radiation**, and has **anti-inflammatory** potential.

Other mushrooms widely used including **poria, polyporus,** and **tremilla** also have powerful healing properties. These mushrooms including reishi and shiitake are used in clinics both in the U.S. and clinics in Europe. Long-term treatment of cancer with reishi has been successful. Reishi is officially listed as a substance for treating **cancer** by the Japanese government.

Recently, *William Stavinoko, Pharmacologist at the University of Texas Health Science Center* in San Antonio, concluded a three-year research study on reishi's **anti-inflammatory** activity. The results were reported at the *Third Academic/Industry Joint Conference* in Sapporo, Japan, August 1990, *Texas Monthly Magazine,* October 1991.

The reishi improved 82% of the heart patients in nine Chinese hospitals. It lowered **triglycerides** in 71% of the patients at risk for **heart disease** improving **blood pressure** and **bad cholesterol,** *Terry Willard, Ph.D.,* Reishi Mushrooms.

Other anti-allergy agents in reishi are **oleic acid, sulphur,** and **protein**. Evidence suggests reishi's ability to alleviate food sensitivities and the ability to inhibit Type I, II, III, and IV **allergic sensitivity** reactions, by limiting **histamine** release.

What is a mushroom? It is a plant that lacks chlorophyll. Most plants get their color from the sun's energy. A mushroom get its nutrients from organic matter, like dead leaves, wood, and waste. They are termed parasites because they also feed off of live organisms like trees. "They are natures decomposers, organisms that recycle all the dead animals and plants that accumulate during the course of a normal life and death cycle. Without mushrooms, and other fungi, the earth would be awash in plant and animal debris. Our soils would not be replenished with fresh humus and our forests would be piled high with leaves, branches and fallen logs," from Reishi Mushrooms by Terry Willard.

Maitake mushroom is found to be a most potent adaptogen by leading mycologists in Japan, Reaserchers claim that Maitake's unique polysaccharide compound, 3-branched Beta 1.6 glucan, makes it another superior mushroom.

Ways to Use Reishi & Shiitake Mushrooms

1) Boil in a small amount of liquid for a few minutes and drink as a tea. This tea is good for food poisoning, stomach/cervical cancer and all colon disorders. Drink 4 times a day for the illnesses listed above.

2) Chop and use in all cooking recipes calling for mushrooms. (Use little salt or soy sauce as the mushroom will absorb these quickly and it will spoil their flavor.)

3) For coughs, use a small amount of the tea. Add 1 teaspoon honey and let it run down your throat.

For those who do not care for the taste of mushrooms, reishi comes in tablet form from Organotech, 7960 Cagnon Road, San Antonio, TX 78252-2202.

Another similar product is from Scandinavian Naturals, Scandinavian Natural Health & Beauty Products, Inc., 13 North Seventh Street, Perkasie, PA 18944.

Maitake can be obtained through Maitake Products, Inc., P.O. Box 1354, Paramus, NJ 07653.

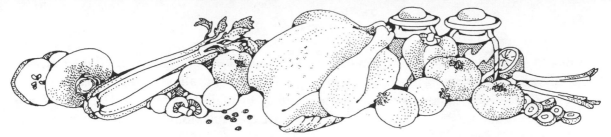

Meat & Dairy Products

Red meat and whole-fat dairy products have in common a high fat content and the possibility of bacterial and chemical contamination. It is common knowledge in the '90s that including little red meat in the diet and using skim or no milk products are healthy practices. Here are some reasons why...

Forty percent of all the antibiotics produced in our country are fed to animals, to increase their growth and prevent bacterial disease. The continued use of antibiotics increases the risk of breeding super drug-resistant bacteria which may be transmitted from the animal to you. Antibiotics given to cattle, hogs, chickens and sheep can produce serious problems in people. These secondary antibiotics contribute to **candidiasis** and all forms of yeast infections. Over a period of time, antibiotics will destroy the "friendly" bacteria, which are sorely needed by the body for protection.

People can build up a tolerance to antibiotics, finally reaching a point where they are ineffective. The *Humane Farming Association* reports that, "veal and hogs are infected with mutant bacteria, requiring lots of antibiotics." The FDA has proposed a ban on the use of penicillin and tetracycline, widely used in animal feed. This has been discussed for several years and most likely the discussions will continue.

Female hormones fed to cattle for growth are possible culprits behind the increases in female disorders like severe **hot flashes, painful menses, breast lumps** and even cancer of the uterus and breast. Because of these hormones, premature development in young girls can lead to precocious sexuality and its associated problems. The hormones can also cause **premature aging** and **impotence** in men, and the chemicals and pesticides found in the foods from the meat of these animals may also be problematic.

Fat is connected to both **cancer** and **heart disease**. Fat in meat is marbled all through the meat and cannot be thoroughly removed. Our populace consumes very large amounts of red meat. Is this why heart disease and cancer are the leading cause of death in the USA?

Carnivorous animals (meat eaters) have many unique characteristics like a relatively short digestive system, approximately three times the length of their body. This is because the flesh they eat decays very quickly, and the products produced by the decay, could rapidly poison the bloodstream if the flesh remains in the body too long.

Other animals live on herbs, grasses, and plants, which are coarse, fibrous, and bulky. This kind of food is first digested in the mouth by ptyalin, an enzyme found in saliva.

To be broken down, grasses and plants must be chewed well and thoroughly mixed with ptyalin. These animals have 24 molar teeth which they use to grind their food with a side to side motion. Carnivorous animals chew up and down, to chop their food. Grass eating animals do not have claws or sharp teeth. They drink by sucking water up compared to the lapping done by carnivores. As they do not eat rapidly-decaying food like carnivores, their food takes longer to pass through their digestive system that is ten times the length of their body.

WHAT ABOUT RED MEAT?

Pork is also red meat, as is veal, even though they are actually pink when raw. Game meats such as venison and rabbit may be lean, but they are still red meat.

Virtually all meats contain about the same amount of cholesterol, what varies is their fat content. As we've often noted, some cuts of beef, pork, and lamb can be leaner than some poultry like a chicken wing, a thigh, or duck. The fact that these are red meat shouldn't scare you, the real red flag is the quantity of fat marbled through the meat and the clumps of fat around it.

Wellness Letter, June 1992, pg.8

Studies have shown that a meat diet is very harmful to the grass- and plant-eating animals. Carnivorous animals however, have an "almost unlimited capacity to handle saturated fats and cholesterol," says *Dr. William Collins of the New York Maimonedes Medical Center.* If a rabbit is fed half a pound of meat daily, in two months the blood vessels become caked with fat and atherosclerosis develops. Like the rabbit, the human digestive system is not designed to digest meat.

Human and anthropoid ape digestive organs are very similar. These apes eat primarily fruits and nuts. They have molars to grind and chew their food, and their saliva contains ptyalin for grass and plant digestion. The intestines in these apes are twelve times the length of their body, for the slow digestion of fruits and vegetables, and their skin has many pores for sweating.

Humans have characteristics like those of the fruit eaters. They are quite similar to those of the grass and plant eaters and are very different from those of the carnivores. The human digestive system, the tooth and jaw structure, and the bodily functions are completely different than carnivorous animals. Just like the ape, the human digestive system is twelve times the length of the body. Physiologically, humans are not carnivores. The anatomy, the digestive system, and instincts of humans are suited to a diet of fruits, nuts, grains, and vegetables.

"And God said, 'Behold, I have given you every herb-bearing seed, which is upon the face of the earth, and every tree, in which are fruits; for you it shall be as meat,'"Genesis 1:29. One of Jesus' disciples, Saint Paul, wrote in a letter to the Romans, "It is good not to eat flesh..." Romans 14:21. Historians have recently found ancient texts similar to the New Testament . "And the flesh of slain beasts in a person's body will become his own tomb. For I tell you truly, he who kills, kills himself, and whosoever eats the flesh of slain beasts eats the body of death," The Essene Gospel of Peace.

Besides other contaminants in meat, animals going to slaughter experience radical biochemical changes. The hormone levels, particularly adrenalin, found in the blood increase drastically when they see animals dying around them and others struggling to stay alive. These high amounts of hormones remain in the tissues of the meat and are later eaten by meat consumers. The *Nutrition Institute of America* reports, "the flesh of an animal carcass is loaded with toxic blood and other waste byproducts."

Animals raised for meat are often infected with diseases which either go undetected or ignored by the meat processors or inspectors. If an animal has cancer or a tumor, that part of the animal will be cut away, leaving the rest of the body to be sold as meat even though the disease may have circulated throughout the animal. Worse yet, the diseased area may be incorporated into mixed meats such as hot dogs or luncheon meats and labeled as parts.

All types of cancers occur at significantly lower rates for Seventh Day Adventists, as compared to another group matched by sex and age. The reason being, that Seventh Day Adventists are vegetarians. They also have a tendency to live longer. A group of Mormons in California has recently been studied. Characteristically, Mormons eat little meat. This group had 50% less cancer than that of the normal population.

The *New England Journal of Medicine* reported that the diets of more than 88,000 women were analyzed over a six-year period. Those who ate the most animal fat were nearly twice as likely to develop colon cancer as those who ate the least. Women who ate red meat as a main course every day were two and half times more likely to develop the disease than those who ate little or none.

People who eat meat have a higher risk of getting cancer because of the carcinogenic preservatives added to meat like nitrites, nitrates, and other preservatives added to mask the green discoloration that occurs as the meat ages. These preservatives are injected into the animal so that they will circulate throughout it's body, often causing death before being slaughtered.

VEGETARIANISM?

We are not advocating strict vegetarianism. Unfortunately, the meat which we would receive with thanksgiving on our tables has been adversely affected by improper handling and processing. If you desire red meat, consume only organic, range-fed beef, farm poultry, and eggs. Some markets are now offering beef, free of these harmful substances.

Urea and uric acid, both nitrogen compounds, are the most prominent wastes collected in the body from a meat diet. Beefsteak contains approximately 15 grams of uric acid per pound. The kidneys have three times the work to eliminate toxic nitrogen compounds from a meat diet, than that of a vegetarian diet. When the body is younger it can handle the extra work of a meat diet without any outward signs of harm, but as the body ages the kidneys become worn out early and cannot work as efficiently. Kidney disease is a frequent result. In 1906 and 1907 *Dr. Irving Fisher of Yale University* conducted endurance tests between vegetarians and meat eaters, and found that vegetarians had nearly twice the stamina of the meat eaters.In summary, the human digestive system was not designed to digest meat. Compare the time it takes the digestive system to pass vegetarian food with that of meat. Vegetarian food will pass out of the system in one and a half days, whereas, meat will pass out of the body in about five days.

Raw meat is in a state of continual decay. It will contaminate everything it comes into contact with, including the cook's hands. The bacteria found in raw meat is frequently not destroyed if the meat is undercooked, barbecued, or roasted, and becomes a source of infection to the unwary consumer.

Did you also know that in two pounds of charcoal-broiled steak there is as much benzopyrene (a cancer causing agent) as in 600 cigarettes? When mice were fed benzopyrene they developed stomach tumors and leukemia. Benzopyrene is an agent that stimulates cancer. But you may say,"I don't eat my steaks charcoal broiled." Did you know when you cook the fat in meat at high temperatures, as is most frequently done to sear it and seal in the juices, methycholantrene is formed, another cancer-stimulating substance. **We know cancer is the second major killer next to heart disease in our country**.

The human body needs protein that consists of the eight essential amino acids. Meat is **not** the only complete protein containing all eight amino acids. Soybeans and milk are complete proteins. They provide all the amino acids humans need. Rice and legumes together also make complete proteins.

Pasteurized and homogenized **milk**, has a high fat content and a conversely low calcium content. The fat content retains toxins that are concentrated in the fat. No other animal on this earth drinks milk as a natural element of their diet after being weaned.

A high-fat diet burdens the body and generates health problems. Do you also know that mice who have breast tumors, pass on their tumors to their newborns who drink their milk? What about the milk of cattle that may have cancers, and we consume their milk? We have no proof that cancer can be transmitted to humans this way but the evidence is pointing in that direction.

> **"Of far greater potential danger to the consumer's health are the hidden contaminants and bacteria like salmonella and residues from the use of pesticides, nitrates, nitrites, hormones, antibiotics, and other chemicals,"** *New York Times*, July 18, 1971.

Lactase is an enzyme found in the small intestines of young children. It is deficient in adults and is necessary for the digestion of milk sugar (lactose) that is in all milk products. Most adults and some children are unable to digest the lactose (**lactose intolerance**) found in milk. According to the April 1991 *Nutrition Action* Health letter, almost 70% of the world's population can't tolerate lactose, the form of sugar in milk.Cheese and soured products are sometimes tolerated in small amounts, because cheese has only about two percent lactose and soured products like yogurt, are already partly "predigested."

The following is a list of common **complaints that can be directly linked to the consumption of meat and dairy products: hives, sinusitis, heart disorders, seborrhea, impaired digestion, obesity, dermatitis, diarrhea, edema, acne, gas and bloating, body odor, dry scaly skin, constipation, allergies, bedwetting, hyperactivity, colitis attacks, headaches, fatigue, colic, anger, depression, congestion** and a runny nose, irritability, excess mucus, hemorrhoids, impotence, malabsorption, hormone imbalance, and hot flashes.

A congressional report concludes that a hormone given to cows to increase **milk** production poses no health hazard to humans. The hormone, technically known as bovine somatotropin, has been the center of a growing debate. There has been a concern that cows treated with the hormone were affected by inflammation of the udder and reproductive problems. If this is true, the result could be that cows would require greater quantities of antibiotics, that would make their way into humans through their digestive systems.

Milk cows were quarantined and milk products recalled in eight states in 1986 after the products were found to contain dangerous amounts of heptachlor, a substance that has been banned from use in the U.S. for years, but still manufactured here.

Chickens often retain estrogen pellets ingested to promote growth and plumpness. Most retailers fail to remove these pellets because they add weight. An antibiotic, tetracycline, added to the chicken's feed, has been linked to severe **food poisoning** by Minnesota health officials. The chickens harbored a highly resistant strain of salmonella bacteria that was passed on to the people who consumed the meat. Several victims had to be hospitalized. This has led many health professionals to petition the FDA to ban the use of antibiotics in chicken and cattle feed. But lobbyists representing the poultry, beef, and pharmaceutical industries, have been successful in protesting the ban, so far.

The *Physician's Committee for Responsible Medicine in Washington, D.C.* is attempting to

remove meat and dairy products from the four basic food groups, long billed as a healthy diet. The group wants to eliminate meat and dairy products, because they are high in cholesterol and saturated fat. They want to add low-fat, fiber-rich legumes, retain whole grain cereals and breads, and split fruits and vegetables into separate groups. Under the proposed new diet, **daily foods would include five or more servings of whole grains, three or more servings of vegetables, two or three servings of legumes, and three or more servings of fruit** (a typical serving is half a cup). This diet has been linked with low rates of cancer and heart disease and revitalized health. Unfortunately, it may take decades before the American public is ready to embrace a meatless diet.

It is apparent that a reduction of meat and dairy products in the diet will lead to a longer and healthier life. *The Journal of the American Medical Association* reported in 1961 that a vegetarian diet can prevent 90-97% of **heart diseases.**

James E. Gern and *Hugh A. Sampson, Research Physicians, Johns Hopkins University School of Medicine in Baltimore,* recently charged that meat processors were incorporating sodium caseinate, a milk derivative, in frankfurters and bologna. But they failed to identify that ingredient for individuals whose allergic reactions to dairy substances could be serious. Many products labeled as "nondairy" contain sodium caseinate, misleading consumers who are sensitive to "milk-contaminated" products. Among the vulnerable are those who have been diagnosed as lactose-intolerant and lack the enzymes to digest dairy products.

Naturally Good Nutrients

The following are products you should incorporate into your cooking in place of things we believe are not healthy. For instance, use arrowroot powder or kuzu to replace cornstarch to thicken sauces, gravies, and fruits--it's great in pies and cobblers. Unlike cornstarch, you do not boil the liquid to thicken it, so arrowroot is ideal for Oriental stir-fry dishes and heat-sensitive fruits.

Agar-Agar

Also called kanten, it grows abundantly in Japan's coastal waters and is high in minerals. One teaspoon of powdered agar-agar can be sprinkled over stewed prunes to aid regular bowel movements.

Arrowroot Powder

The arrowroot plant is a starchy tropical herb. The roots (rhizomes) are used to make a powder. It is easily digested, even for infants and thickens soups, gravies, fruit desserts, fruit pies, and any recipe you would use cornstarch in. Since it thickens before it boils, do not overcook it. As the food cools to room temperature, it will thicken even more, so be careful not to use too much.

Baking Powder

Made of starch and acid, it reacts immediately upon contact with a liquid. The best baking powder to use is cream of tartar, which is made up of sediment deposited in wine casks as a result of fermentation. Cream of tartar is composed of yeast and compounds of grapes. It acts quickly so should be used immediately after being mixed into a batter. Phosphate baking soda, another baking powder, is made of calcium and sodium phosphates. This type of baking powder poses a health problem because of its sodium content (see the note about sodium at end of chapter). Do not use double-acting baking powders, they contain sodium aluminum sulfate. Aluminum is thought to cause neurological disorders, as it collects in the brain stem. We recommend the use of aluminum-free baking powders found in health food stores. *Rumford* Baking Powder is aluminum-free and found in health food stores.

Baking Soda

Not healthy for consumption due to high sodium content. But it is an excellent non-toxic cleanser in the kitchen and a good deodorizer, especially for the refrigerator. Use on bathroom fixtures, countertops and sinks, be sure to rinse well. Great for use by those with extreme sensitivity and chemical allergies.

Barley Malt Concentrate

Especially good for diabetics and those who are watching their calorie intake. It is highly concentrated in the powder form although one teaspoon contains only three calories. You will only need a few grains to sweeten a cup of tea. It doesn't have a bitter aftertaste. Use this in all baking to replace sugar.

Bee Pollen

Bee pollen is excellent for increasing strength and endurance. It is used by athletes as an endurance food with amazing results. Bee pollen is extremely nutritional and has all the necessary amino acids the body needs. It helps the immune system, builds resistance to disease and has a cleansing effect on the blood. Normal hair growth can be reduced by a deficiency of amino acids, bee pollen contains these necessary amino acids. Rich in all nutrients and enzymes, including boron which is needed for calcium absorption and brain function.

Try and purchase bee pollen within a 10 mile radius of your home. Start with a small amount, 1/2 teaspoon and increase to 1 tablespoon daily, in juices, cereals, or on top of salads.

Blackstrap Molasses

Very high in minerals and iron. Add this source of power to your diet. The iron in blackstrap molasses is easily assimilated and is good in infant formula. This and barley malt, are the two best sweeteners. Crude blackstrap molasses has been used in treatment for arthritis, states *Joe Oliver of England,* author of Herbal Health Secrets.

Blue Corn

Has a high protein content, a unique color, and an unusual flavor. It is generally ground into a meal and made into chips, muffins, pancakes, tortillas, and other baked goods.

Brewer's Yeast

A one-celled plant and a very high-powered food. It also should be incorporated into your daily diet. It is extremely high in B vitamins and can be added to cereals and other foods. The most popular way to take it is in drinks, juices, and shakes. **Do not confuse brewer's yeast from the health food store with baker's yeast. Never consume baker's yeast raw.**

Brewer's yeast consists of 50% protein, is very high in B-12 and contains selenium, and chromium, lacking in highly processed foods. Brewer's yeast comes in several forms: powdered, flakes, and tablets. It is rich in nucleic acids, including RNA, which is a necessary building block for the body.

People who suffer from gout (a form of arthritis) or yeast infections (candida albicans) should avoid brewer's yeast. These people need to avoid all types of yeast and fermented foods. If you are introducing yeast into your diet for the first time, beware of bloating and flatulence. You can minimize or avoid such discomfort if you start with just a small amount of yeast, less than a teaspoon daily. The flaked yeast dissolves instantly and is good in casseroles, baked bean dishes, nut butters, spreads, vegetables soups and other dishes. It does not require refrigeration and has a long shelf life. Store in a tightly closed container in a dark place.

Carob

A fruit from a Mediterranean evergreen tree. It is grown like a pod. It is also known as honey locust or St. John's bread. John the Baptist supposedly sustained his life in the wilderness using carob. High in calcium, B vitamins, magnesium, and pectin, it is used in place of chocolate, which is known to be high in caffeine. Use carob in place of chocolate in all recipes. It comes in a powdered form, chips or drops, liquid and candy form. Carob is low in fat, so it does not need preservatives like *BHA* and *BHT*, which are added to chocolate as a preservative for fats. Carob has little sodium and no oxalic acid and contains 8% protein.

Cayenne Pepper

Should be used in place of black pepper. We do not recommend the use of black pepper. Cayenne pepper is great for circulation, the heart and the colon. Remember, it is very hot, so use it sparingly.

Fructose

Found in fruits and honey, it contains half the calories of sugar, is extracted from fruit, but is generally more expensive than sugar. Some people with blood sugar problems can handle this form in small amounts, but most cannot. Fructose does not require digestion, but like white sugar it is absorbed directly into the bloodstream. Some claims have been made that it requires little insulin and is the ideal sugar for the diabetic or hypoglycemic patient. We do not recommend it for anyone who has blood sugar problems. This form of sugar is recommended over processed white sugar, you use half the amount of fructose. It does not work as well in bread or cookies, it absorbs the liquids and can make the baked goods dry. It is great in pies. It dissolves better in cold beverages than sugar.

Garlic

One of the most valuable miracle foods. It has the ability to lower the blood pressure and cholesterol and aid in digestion. It is used to combat many diseases and illnesses, even cancer. The Russians call it a natural antibiotic. Garlic should be consumed daily. If you are not a garlic fancier, try using garlic tablets. Kyolic is an excellent one on the market that is odorless. Also, in the recipes we have an excellent garlic oil recipe.

Garlic will keep indefinitely in a jar filled with oil, **if kept refrigerated.** Refill with garlic cloves as they dwindle down. Freshly peeled buds can be used in any recipe calling for garlic. If you feel there is too much odor from eating garlic, chew a few sprigs of parsley, mint, caraway or fennel seeds after eating it.

Ginger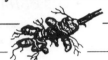

A yin root vegetable. The pulp and juice are used in many food preparations. Grated fresh ginger is preferred over powdered. It is used mostly in Oriental dishes. Try it in your stir-fry recipes.

> **Ginger is an extremely potent snail and slug repellent, it will stop snails, slugs, or ants from crossing if it were spread on the ground as a barrier around the plants. Many spicy flavors of herbal seasonings were developed by plants to protect them from insects,** *HerbalGram,* **No. 25/1991.**

Instant Nonfat Dry Milk

If you use milk in cooking, this is the product to use. It costs less, does not spoil and has a natural sweetness. It can be used in make-ahead recipes forbiscuit mix, pancake mix or any recipe that calls for milk.

In the place of bleached white flour, substitute whole wheat flour, rye flour, corn, oat, rice, or whole wheat pastry flour. Omit white flour from your diet. It loses most of the nutrients in the milling process. It clogs up the system with excess mucus. Replace boxed processed cereals with granola, whole flaked, or cracked grain, cooked or raw.

Kuzu

A root starch and excellent thickener. Similar to arrowroot or cornstarch, it must be disolved in cold liquid and the mixture stirred while it heats, thickening as it reaches the boiling point. It has an alkalizing effect. One tablespoon kuzu starch will thicken 1 cup of liquid to the consistency of Chinese vegetable sauce; 2 1/2 tablespoons kuzu to 1 cup liquid makes a pudding consistency, which cools to the consistency of soft tofu. As a remedy, kuzu can be used in two ways: (salty and runny like a thick broth or with juices such as papaya and apple and apple juice-kuzu made thick like a pudding.

Kukicha Tea

Made of the leaves and twigs of naturally grown Bancha tea bushes. Kukicha tea is a soothing beverage that aids the digestion and has been sipped with meals for centuries..

Lecithin

Good added to all diets. The elderly and the person with weight problems can benefit from daily use. It is high in choline and inositol, helps brain function, a fat emulsifier, and good for elevated cholesterol. Add to baked goods in place of part of the oil. The liquid form is much more versatile, and only a small amount is needed. Use in gravies, fudge, icings, and any recipe where you want a smooth product. It aids in mixing oil with any liquid, like gravies and dressings so the ingredients do not separate and the oil won't rise to the top.

Lecithin is available in three forms: granules, capsules, and liquids. The granules are mildly flavored and can even be eaten without any preparation. You can also sprinkle it over foods such as cereal and casseroles or mix it in soups, juices, pancake batter or baking dough. Use capsules when traveling. Liquid lecithin is an oil which should be refrigerated after the container is opened. Also, the liquid can be used to oil baking pans. Lecithin is a must in the adult diet. It aids in keeping cholesterol levels lower and protects the cardiovascular system.

Millet

This grain is "King of the Cereals." Extremely high in protein, millet is very easy to prepare; see the Grains section to prepare millet as a cereal. We suggest incorporating millet in your diet two times a week. If you have sugar problems, millet would be a great asset in your daily diet. Remember, you can cut up dried fruit in your millet, oatmeal or whatever grain you happen to be preparing for breakfast and cook it in your cereal. Dried fruits can be consumed with cereal. (This is different than fresh fruit, which needs to be digested quickly and should not be held up in the stomach with other foods.)

If you look in the recipes you will also find millet prepared as a pudding, a great snack between meals, as a dessert, and as a breakfast. Millet can also be ground into flour. It is excellent as a baby's first cereal to alternate with brown rice cereals. It is easily digested and has a very mild flavor.

Miso

A paste made from soybeans that has been aged in wooden barrels for three years. It contains living enzymes that aid digestion. There are different types of miso, such as: kome, genmai, hacho, mugi, and a light, sweet type used in desserts.

Mugi is the most popular for seasoning, it is made from soy and barley. **Hacho** is stronger and made with soybeans but without barley. **Kome** is the mildest in flavor, with brown rice used in place of barley. **Genmai** is made from brown rice and soybeans.

Miso is good added to dips, spreads, sauces, soups, and stews. It has a slightly meaty taste and makes a good seasoning.

Do not boil miso. Like tamari sauce, add it at the end of the cooking to preserve all the enzymes and nutrients. It should be stored in a cool place and generally is not refrigerated because refrigeration destroys the living enzymes. Mold sometimes forms on top of miso, but this is simply an indication of its living quality. Just cut off the mold and discard, it is not harmful.

Miso is used in macrobiotic diets. There are several good books out on this wonderful product

Rice

Should be consumed in its brown form. Never eat white rice. There are three types of brown grain rice. **Short grain** is higher in nutritional value and lower in calories than the **long grain**, but it clumps together more than the long grain variety. Use long grain when having company and short grain for yourself. There is also **sweet rice**, which is slightly softer, sweeter, and stickier than the other varieties. Sweet rice has been used traditionally in Japan to make special holiday cakes. When toasted, sweet rice puffs up like popcorn. **Rice malt syrup** is a good natural sweetener, found in health food stores. Try substituting brown rice for potatoes with meals. It's by far one of the most nutritious foods that can be found and high in the B-complex vitamins.

Sea Salt

Contains an abundance of minerals and is produced by the evaporation of sea water. If you must use a small amount of salt, use sea salt in place of iodized or white table salt. *We do not recommend adding salt.*

Spike

Can be used in nearly all cooking. It is derived mainly from dried vegetables. It is low in sodium and contains a small amount of sea salt. Once you try spike on scrambled eggs, in soups, casseroles or whatever, you will love it.

Tahini

Ground sesame seeds made into a fine paste, with all the nutrients intact. It is rich in vitamins, minerals, protein, and essential fatty acids. Tahini is also very high in calcium. It is wonderful in sauces, salad dressings, use it on crackers or whole grain bread and top with sesame seeds or jam. You can purchase it at health food stores. Blend it with cooked chick peas, add lemon juice, a crushed clove of garlic, and olive oil and you have a highly nutrition dip or spread. Excellent as a butter substitute.

Tamari Sauce

Use in place of soy sauce. Derived from the soybean, it is an excellent source of protein. You can purchase tamari sauce at health food stores. Use it in dishes like soups, casseroles, nutburgers and stir-fried vegetables. Always add tamari at the end of the cooking to add enzymes and nutrient content. There is also a wheat-free tamari. Omit sea salt altogether when using this sauce because it has a salty flavor.

There is also a white tiger tofu sauce by Westbrae. It is bottled like soy sauce with a wonderful Oriental flavor, that is good on chicken, tofu, rice, and vegetables. *We recommend it because it is naturally fermented and preserved, whereas commercial soy sauce has preservatives added, including MSG.*

Tempeh

Pronounced tem-pay. A staple food in Indonesia, produced by fermenting pre-soaked and cooked soybeans and sometimes a grain with culture called rhizopus (a starter culture grown on hibiscus leaves is innoculated with hulled soybeans). Tempeh is high in protein. If grey or dark spots appear on the tempeh it is not a sign of spoilage. Tempeh is good sauteed in a little oil or tamari sauce. It is often mixed in with vegetable dishes, grains and casseroles.

Tofu

Derived from soybeans, it is known as bean curd. It is white, cheese-like in texture and very high in protein, B vitamins and bland in taste, but takes on the flavor of any food that is combined with it. It will keep approximately two weeks when stored covered with water in a bowl or jar in the refrigerator. After opening, drain off the water and cover with fresh water. Before using tofu in recipes like cream cheese frosting or tofu cheesecake, always drain it and pat dry. Tofu is also excellent sliced, patted, dry, dipped in tamari sauce, and soaked a few minutes, then dipped in sesame seeds and sauteed. It will take the place of a burger, it is a good meat substitute with any meal.

Umeboshi Plum

Prepared by the Japanese they are salted, pickled and aged for several years and are good in salad dressings, spreads, dips and cooked with grains, beans, and vegetable dishes. The plums are pickled in salt for two about months, sometimes with beefsteak (chiso) leaves, which give them a bright color. They taste salty-sour. Make sure that they have not been doctored up with other ingredients: Only plums, water, salt, and perhaps chiso or beefsteak leaves should be listed. This plum reduces excess acidity or alkalinity in the body. Some of the symptoms are upset stomach, burning anus, degenerative diseases.

Wheat and Corn Germ

If you choose to buy wheat germ separated from flour, make sure the product is fresh. Wheat germ rapidly turns rancid. In fact, it is almost impossible to purchase wheat germ that has not become rancid. The product should be vacuum packed. If not, it should be refrigerated and have either a packing or "use by date" on the label. When you can buy it toasted, it has a longer shelf life. Use wheat germ oil capsules or germ that has been sealed and toasted. Surprisingly, corn germ is very high in nutrients, some even higher than wheat germ. Try using corn germ in recipes like corn bread, breading for chicken and fish.

Yeast

Microscopic fungi that feeds on sugar and starches in the batter of your baked goods. It produces a carbon dioxide gas as a result, which causes batter or dough to rise. Active dry yeast, rapid yeasts, and compressed yeast cakes are all made up of similar strains of yeast. When purchasing yeast check to make sure it does not contain preservatives, like BHA. BHA has been found to cause cancer in tests done on laboratory animals. **Do not confuse baker's yeast with brewer's yeast, these are very different products.**

Yogurt

Made from milk, it has a custard-like consistency and a slight sour taste. It has a list of health benefits too long to mention and is important in the daily diet helping digestion and reducing bloating and gas. Yogurt is very high in the B-vitamins. It replenishes friendly bacteria in the intestinal tract that are vital to good health. Antibiotics destroy the good bacteria allowing the bad bacteria to take over, resulting in all types of health problems. Candidiasis is an example of a health problem that can result when the good bacteria are destroyed. Be sure to include this product in your diet, but do not consume yogurt that is laced with sugar and chemicals. Soured dairy products are better for you: buttermilk, cottage cheese, yogurt, etc. Yogurt can be used in place of sour cream in recipes. It can be mixed with fruit and granola and used in making dressings and power shakes.

White sugar, corn syrup, sucrose, dextrose, and glucose should be omitted from the diet and replaced with uncooked, unfiltered raw honey, using 1/2 cup honey instead of one cup sugar and reduce the liquid called for in the recipes by 1/4 cup. If no liquid is called for in the recipes, add three tablespoons of flour. Use pure maple syrup, unsulphured molasses, fruit juices, purees and juice concentrate. You can use undiluted apple juice concentrate in a lot of recipes where sweetener is called for, like cobblers and pies, but it is also good in other dishes and baked goods.

Omit baking soda and replace with Rumford's low-sodium baking powder which is aluminum free, using two parts baking powder in place of one part soda.

Never consume white distilled vinegar. Use pure apple cider vinegar or rice vinegar.

In place of white pasta, spaghetti, macaroni shells, noodles, use whole grain pastas.

Instead of soda pop, use fruit juices, mineral water, herb teas, real soda pop with real flavorings, sweetened with fructose or honey. These can be found in health food stores. Omit coffee, Chinese teas (except for green tea) and other caffeinated teas. Replace with herb teas and cereal beverages. Replace commercial peanut butter with your own fresh ground nut butters or make sure it is unhydrogenated peanut butter that can be purchased at your health food store. The same applies to cashew, sesame, or almond butter. Buy unsulphured organically grown dried foods without preservatives, if possible.

When browning onions or mushrooms, try using tamari sauce instead of oil or butter if you are on a fat-free diet. The flavor is excellent.

Use more sesame, sunflower and pumpkin seeds. Be careful when purchasing sesame seeds. Be sure they have been kept under refrigeration and have not become rancid. Or they should be in nitrogen packed containers. All nuts and seeds should be under refrigeration or nitrogen packed. You do not want to consume rancid nuts, seeds, or oils. They deplete the body of many vital nutrients and stress the liver.

Remember, in almost all recipes you can substitute unprocessed whole grain and natural sugars in place of white flour, white sugar, salt, etc. We recommend throwing out all white, processed products. Once you learn how to cook the dishes in this book you will want to take all your old recipe books and convert them to natural recipes (or give them away).

The foods that can be eaten plentifully are fresh fruits and vegetables, steamed vegetables, nuts (except peanuts), seeds, beans, legumes, and whole grains. The whole grains are good soaked overnight and a light cooking in the morning with a little honey added, or seasoning and herbs. The nutrients are not lost from hard boiling in this manner.

To regenerate your body or if your body is producing too much mucus, avoid sugar, salt, milk, and dairy products, red meat, white flour products, caffeine drinks, and eggs.

Do not use aluminum cookware. Some doctors believe Alzheimer's disease is caused by the accumulation of aluminum in the brain. Do not use coated pans. Cook with only stainless steel, iron, glass or Corningware ®.

Do not peel vegetables or fruits. Eat the whole fruit or vegetable when you can. Make applesauce in your food processor. Core apples, leave skins on and cut up into the processor. Add a little honey if you like it sweeter, cinnamon, and serve. It is really delicious. You can add a little lemon juice and it will keep longer. We do tomatoes the same way skins and all, for sauces, soups, etc. they can be frozen in this form.

Use potatoes with skins on, even for potato salad.

Make apple butter the same way as the applesauce, using cinnamon sticks. Put them in the roasting pan and bake at 250° all day (at least 6 - 9 hours), until desired thickness is reached. Put in a jar and you have delicious homemade apple butter.

Try cooking with more stems and leaves. Use some of the celery leaves, outer leaves of lettuce and

Things to remember for quality foods:

1. Avoid white foods (except cauliflower) as much as possible.

Do not discard edible outer green leaves of vegetables like cabbage, broccoli, and lettuce. Encourage your grocer to leave the outer, green leaves on. The outer leaves have been kissed with sunlight and filled with vitamins and minerals. Avoid bleached celery and bleached endive. Choose yellow turnips over white, dark green to light. Use sweet potatoes more frequently. Color in food is a sign of vitamin content. Use a mixture of colors to get a variety of nutrients.

2. Avoid stale food. Buy the freshest food your market has, ask what days they receive the fresh produce. If possible, grow your own.

3. Eat raw food. Select and serve raw food once or twice a day, fruits and vegetables.

4. Choose cooking methods carefully. Select cooking methods that will minimize vitamin and mineral loss. Avoid frying entirely, use steaming instead. Always remember that every cooking method has its faults and may destroy vitamin value to a certain extent.

5. Undercook rather than overcook vegetables, except dried peas and beans. Vegetables taste better and keep their color when not overcooked and undercooking saves the nutrients.

6. Do not use soda when cooking vegetables, as it destroys vitamins.

7. Save all cooking juices and vegetable water for soup stock so you use all the nutrients dissolved in the water.

8. Food combinations are important. Do not combine fresh fruits with another food; eat fruit alone. Do not consume liquids, including water, with your meals. Starches and protein are a poor combination.

9. Cook in covered pots, not aluminum or coated pots.

10. Use as little water as possible and steam vegetables.

11. Avoid overcooking.

12. Avoid fried foods and processed foods.

13. Eat fresh raw fruits and vegetables twice daily.

14. Do not fry foods in hydrogenated oils.

15. Use foods in their natural state as much as possible.

16. Wash all melons before cutting, they may contain dangerous bacteria. Do not juice the rinds.

17. Store grains in a cool dry place.

18. Place bay leaves in containers to deter insects, but learn to accept the fact that food without insecticides might have a few bugs. I would rather eat a healthy bug than poisonous chemicals. After many years in the retail business I have never seen insects in foods with preservatives. They seem to always pick the organically grown grains over the ones where pesticides where used. We should pay more attention to insects and all life forms. They can tell us a lot. If you see a bug in your grains or flours, do not panic. It means you have a quality product, worth eating.

19. Do not use the same cutting board for poultry or meat as you use for vegetables. This is important: salmonella poisoning can be transferred. Arthritis has been thought to be connected to this food poisoning.

20. Be careful with all canned foods. If the top is not tight or bulges, do not use it.

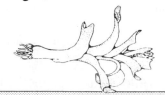

Research at the *State University of New York at Buffalo School of Medicine* points to a link between sodium and an increase risk of gastric, or stomach cancer. After interviewing 293 patients with gastric cancer, researchers found that high sodium diets are associated with high rates of gastric cancer.

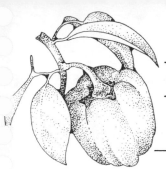

Nightshade Vegetables

Are these healthy for you to eat?

What are nightshades? As a botanical family, the *Solanaceae* comprise some ninety-two genera with over two thousand species. Its members include many stimulating, medicinal, or poisonous plants, such as tobacco, henbane, mandrake, and belladonna (also known as the deadly nightshade). The food plants of the nightshade family include some of our most popular vegetables: tomatoes, potatoes, eggplant, and peppers of all kinds (green, red, chili, paprika, cayenne, hot and sweet, except for black and white pepper.) **Research has found that when people with joint pains stopped consuming all varieties of nightshades, their condition improved dramatically.**

It turns out that nightshades are high in *alkaloids,* chemical substances with a strong physiological effects. In the case of potatoes, storage conditions after harvest that include light and heat, may over time increase the content of the alkaloid *solanine* to toxic limits. Improperly stored old potatoes have been know to cause symptoms severe enough to require hospitalization, including gastrointestinal inflammation, nausea, diarrhea, and dizziness.

Earl Mindell in his book, <u>Unsafe at Any Meal</u>, stated the following concerning potatoes, "Solanine, present in and around these green patches and in the eyes that have sprouted, can interfere with the transmission of nerve impulses, and cause jaundice, abdominal pain, vomiting, and diarrhea."

These alkaloids act a little like a variation of Vitamin D, in that they appear to affect the metabolism of calcium. Nightshade foods may, through a mechanism not yet understood, remove calcium from the bones and deposit it in joints, kidneys, arteries, and other areas of the body where it does not belong. Thus, they may contribute to arthritis.

Nightshades are consumed in appreciable quantities mostly in dietary systems that also include milk products. These foods often show up in pairs: tomato sauce and cheese, potatoes and sour cream, spicy Indian foods, yogurt, and eggplant parmigiana.

Nightshades, with their calcium-disturbing alkaloids, have something to do with the digestion or assimilation of milk products, which have an excessively high calcium content. Cow's milk contains four times more calcium than human mother's milk, and that may turn out to be too much for the human metabolism to handle.

In other words, when the nightshades are consumed in calcium-rich diets, they help keep the calcium from depositing in the wrong places, as long as the body is functioning properly. If it is not, then either the nightshades pull out calcium from the wrong places or the dairy calcium is improperly used by the body and collects in the joints and tissues.

Symptoms of improper storage include bone loss, tooth decay, and what is called the "naked tooth feeling" (a sensation of rawness or brittleness in the teeth). If you are avoiding dairy foods and eating a low fat diet, you may want to eliminate the nightshade vegetables from your diet.

Dr. Collin H. Dong, a San Francisco Physician created a diet called the "*Dong Diet.*" He believes **arthritis** is caused by allergic reactions to certain food and chemical additives in the food. His diet prohibits meat, fruits, tomatoes, all dairy products, all acids including vinegar, all types of peppers, hot spices, chocolate, roasted nuts, alcoholic beverages, especially wine, soft drinks, all foods containing preservatives, additives and chemicals, especially MSG (monosodium glutamate).

His diet favors fish, because fish oils appear to benefit arthritis. This diet cuts back on most of the nightshades, eggs, vitamin A and D, in supplement form, and foods fortified with these vitamins, such as margarine. The sun on the skin promotes sufficient vitamin D, the green leafy vegetables, the orange colored ones, such as carrots, sweet potatoes, and cantaloupes provide plenty of vitamin A in the diet.

Norman F. Childers, a former Professor of Horticulture, Rutgers University had severe joint pains and stiffness after consuming tomatoes in any form. He was aware of the nightshade family of plants and their toxicity. He observed livestock kneeling because their knee joints were too painful to hold them up, after eating weeds containing *solanine*. He then started to test the nightshade foods one at a time and found that each one aggravated his arthritic pain. He eliminated all of the nightshade vegetables from his diet and within months his pain vanished. He totally believes that those who are sensitive or allergic to the nightshade vegetables will cure the aches and pains of arthritis by avoiding those foods.

The macrobiotic diet, noted for its healing properties, forbids meat, eggs, dairy products, poultry, fruit juices, and nightshade vegetables.

If one has arthritis, bone loss, or aching muscles and joints, the nightshade vegetables should be omitted from their diet to see if their condition improves.

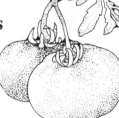

Nightshade Family Vegetables

Bell peppers (green, red, yellow, cherry)
Cayenne pepper (capsicum)
Chili peppers
Eggplant
Hot peppers (long & red, red cluster)

Paprika
Pimento
Potatoes
Tomatoes

(Black and white pepper do not fall into this category.)

Tobacco in all forms carries toxic *solanine* and *nicotine* substances into the blood and tissues. These are especially damaging to the muscles and nerves, *The Desert Arthritis Medical Clinic, Desert Hot Springs, CA.*

Dr. Collin H. Dong, a San Francisco physician who has practiced family medicine there for fifty years, has created the Dong diet. According to Dong, his diet works for arthritis because arthritis is caused by allergic reactions to certain foods and chemical additives in the food. "It's what you don't eat that counts," he says. The Dong diet excludes:

1) meat
2) fruits, including tomatoes
3) dairy products of all kinds
4) vinegar or any other acid
5) pepper of any variety
6) hot spices
7) chocolate
8) dry roasted nuts
9) alcoholic beverages, especially wine
10) soft drinks
11) all additives, preservatives, and chemicals, especially monosodium glutamate

The Dong diet is considerd a fish-centered diet. Fish oils appear to benefit arthritics.

What Your Doctor Won't Tell You, Jane Heimlich, pg. 143

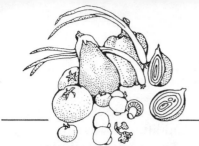

Power Foods

Artichoke

Artichokes are rich in potassium and magnesium, making them good for the heart. They also contain significant amounts of calcium, phosphorus, iron, vitamin C, and niacin. Steam this vegetable and serve with a yogurt or tofu dip. To extract the meat from the leaf, pull the lower part of the leaf through your teeth. After you've finished the leaves, remove the inedible fuzzy core, cut the remaining heart into pieces, and enjoy.

Cactus Pear

Available July through March, this fruit tastes like watermelon, it can be peeled, seeded, and pureed into a topping for frozen yogurt. One cactus pear = 42 calories, 22 mg. potassium.

Camu Camu

This fruit is slightly bigger than a cherry and has a very sour taste, because of the high vitamin C content. **There is more vitamin C in this fruit than any other plant known, up to 30 times as much as a citrus fruit.** The Camu Camu grows along the Peruvian Amazon.

Carambola

This fruit is commonly called star fruit, about the size of an avocado, it has a glossy yellow skin and 4-6 ridges. When cut crosswise the slices look like stars. The flavor tends to be similar to citrus. Carambola is a good source of potassium and vitamin C, it contains no fat and a single fruit is only about 40 calories.

Celeriac or Celery Root

Available August through May, celery root or celeriac is a knobby and often muddy root. It comes from a celery like plant of which only the root is edible. It tastes of celery and walnut, and adds a very mellow flavor to soups and stews. Try raw, peel and cut into julienne strips, coat with a vinaigrette dressing.

Look for small, hard roots with a smooth skin. One celery root is about 2/3 of a cup sliced and 39 calories, 300 mg. of potassium, and no fat. It is high in phosphorus, and is beneficial to the nervous, lymphatic, and urinary systems.

Chayote

This fruit tastes of cucumber and apple, and can be sauteed, boiled, or steamed, 3/4 of a cup chunked is 24 calories, 150 mg. potassium and 18% of the RDA for vitamin C.

Fennel

Sweet fennel or anise is a vegetable related to the celery family. It has a firm, crisp white bulb and green fronds. The fronds are similar to those on the dill plant. The lower part of the plant is a large white bulb that is much larger than a celery bunch. The flavor is a sweet, pleasant, licorice flavor. Try it raw, in salads or with a dip. High in vitamins A and C. To prepare, remove the outer leaves, chop off the top, split the bulb lengthwise. Remove the thick inner core at the bottom of the vegetable, this can be cooked and added to stews.

Try fennel sauted in 1 tablespoon of oil until tender, but crisp. Add 1/2 inch of water and simmer for 20 minutes. You can also chop and steam it for 8-10 minutes. Another method for cooking fennel is to slice the bulb in half and boil it for about 15 minutes.

Heart of Palm

A dieter's dream, contains only 21 calories per cup, what other food can compare? Because they perish so quickly they are found canned most of the time. Hearts of palm are very rich in vitamin A. Because of their delicate flavor they can be added to countless dishes, seafood, soups, gumbos, and salads.

> "Genetic engineers are taking genes from bacteria, viruses and insects and adding them to fruits, grains and vegetables," said *Dr. Rebecca Goldberg, a Senior Scientist with the Environmental Defense Fund, New York Times,* **June 17, 1992. Your only defense is to eat organic grains and produce. PB**

Horned Melon

This melon tastes like lime, cucumber, and banana. It can be cut into wedges, or eaten straight from the rind.

Jerusalem Artichoke

Available October through June, this tuber can be scrubbed, sliced and stir fried. There is no need to peel it. Three fourths of a cup sliced, is 76 calories, 19% of the RDA for iron, 13% for vitamin B1.

Jicama

This is a brown rough-skinned root, white inside. Jicama, pronounced hee-keh-mah, should be peeled and sliced as it is sweet and crunchy and can be eaten raw or cooked. Try it in a stir fry. One equals 3/4 of a cup sliced, is 41 calories, 175 mg. potassium, meets 33% of the RDA for vitamin C.

Kiwi

This fruit is slightly tart, tasting like a cross between strawberries and green grapes, and is known in China as the Chinese gooseberry. The fruit can be peeled and sliced or scooped from its peel. Look for kiwis that are slightly soft and plump. If a kiwi is not yet ripe, keep it in a paper bag with an apple or banana for a few days. Ripened fruit can be kept in a refrigerator for up to three weeks. The Chinese used kiwi in an experiment for esophageal cancer. They found high levels of nitrites in their patients and those who ate kiwi fruit were found to have a dramatic decrease in their nitrite readings. Do not use kiwi in Jello, it will keep it from jelling because of the enzyme content. One kiwi is 46 calories and supplies more than twice the RDA for vitamin C, vitamin K, and potassium, making them good for high blood pressure.

Kiwicha (Amaranth)

Kiwicha is high in protein, particularly the amino acid lysine, normally not found in plants. Amaranth is eaten like a granola bar. It is popped like popcorn and held together with honey. This food is native to Central and South America.

Mangoes

A tropic treat. Few fruits contain as much vitamin A as the mangoes, in addition to having a high content of vitamin C. The tender flesh contains insoluble fiber. Pick ripe ones that are grass green with touches of yellow. Most are also freckled. A ripe one will give slightly to gentle pressure. Peel the skin as you would a banana and enjoy after chilling. Good baked in custards, pies, breads, muffins, or stewed with other fruits and used as toppings.

Mesquite Pod

Mesquite grows in pods, much like that of the carob in Argentina. The flavor of this fruit is sweet and spicy, the pods can be made into mesquite honey or brewed into tea. They are rich in compounds that may help control blood sugar.

North American Indian Groundnut

This is a tuber that has three times the protein of potatoes and is thought to contain anti-cancer agents. It is edible when cooked, it can be made into a flour for bread or fried into hash browns.

Nuna

This food is also called pop beans, because it puffs and bursts in half when heated. It is higher in protein and fiber than popcorn. This food is grown in the Andes of Peru and Bolivia, and not presently available in the U.S.

Passion Fruit

This fruit is tart and lemony, it lends a tropical flavor to a fruit salad. Three fruits equal 54 calories, 189 mg. potassium, 27% RDA for vitamin C.

Plantain

It looks like a banana but is very different. Plantains have higher amounts of vitamin A and potassium than bananas, but are similar in their low fat content and sodium. They are rich in fiber. Plantains are too starchy to eat raw, they must be cooked. You can steam, boil, bake, or peel and place on fish before baking for a different treat. Good sliced and sauteed in garlic oil, with a dash of cinnamon, ginger, and/or Spike seasoning and served as a side dish.

Quince

Quince is a bumpy yellow or green fruit, similar to an apple in shape and size. The fruit should be hard.

Raw, quince is so sour and dry it is almost inedible. Cooking alters this fruit into a food of the gods. It is similar to a baked apple when cooked, only it tastes even better. The flavor is tart, yet sweet. firm but still pliant, and very juicy. It is free of fat, high in vitamin C, and contains minerals and B vitamins.

Quinoa

This is the grain of the future. It was the staple food of the Inca Empire, referred to as the Mother Grain and revered as sacred. Quinoa (pronounced keen-wah) provides ALL the essential amino acids, including lysine a scarce amino acid in vegetables and methionine and cystine in an almost perfect profile. These are especially important for vegetarians because most plant sources have inadequate amounts. Compared to other grains it is not only high in protein but also iron, thiamine, B-6 and phosphorus. Its time is here! A modern, highly nutritious convenient food, it is quick and easy to prepare as a side dish, hot cereal, in soups, and salads.

Red Banana

This banana is sweeter than the yellow variety, it is especially good in bread. One banana is 118 calories, 22% of the RDA for Vitamin C, 10% for Vitamin A.

Tamarind

Inside the pod of this fruit is a pulp that is date and apricot flavored. It can be pureed and added to chutneys and curries, 1/2 cup of pulp is 144 calories, 377 mg. potassium, 17% of the RDA for Vitamin B-1.

Taro

Tastes like a combination of potato and water chestnut, it is good used to thicken stews and soups, 1 cup is 107 calories, 591 mg. of potassium.

Tepary Bean

These beans are white and golden brown, and only about half the size of a navy bean, although they are much higher in fiber and protein, and thought to contain a substance that controls blood sugar. The tepary bean makes a delicious rich, and nutty flavored soup and is a North American bean.

Green Power Food in Pill Form

Wheatgrass, barley grass, and *spirulina* are the best sources of *beta-carotene*, chlorophyll and minerals -- good for all *colon disorders, AIDS, cancer* and all illnesses. *Wheatgrass* is best when juiced fresh and combined with other vegetables. *Powdered barleygrass* can be added to quality water. *Spirulina* is high in protein beta-carotene, gamma linolenic acid (GLA) and a nutrient essential for the formation of hormones. Good for vegetarians because it contains B-12, lacking in most vegetarian diets. It is also rich in calcium, iron, RNA, DNA, and trace minerals. *Kazuko Iwata, Kagawa Nutrition College,* found that inclusion of spirulina in the diet increased the activity of the enzyme, lipoprotein lipasi, which is involved in fat metabolism. *Iwata, K., et al. 1990. Journal of Nutritional Science & Vitaminology* 36:165-171.

Wheatgrass, barley grass, and *spirulina* will be main foods of the future. They contain everything that is currently known to build a *healthy immune system,* all found in powdered and tablet forms NOW!

A Japanese study detailed the effects of spirulina added to the diet of rats with serum cholesterol problems induced by fructose. A high-fructose diet increases the level of cholesterol and triglycerides in the blood, but spirulina added to the diet consistently reduced levels of both cholesterol and triglycerides.

Kazuko Iwata, *et al.,* from *Kagawa Nutrition College,* found that inclusion of spirulina in the diet increased the activity of the enzyme, lipoprotein lipase, which is involved in fat metabolism. *Iwata, K., et al. 1990. Journal of Nutritional Science & Vitaminology* 36:165-171.

Winged Bean

The leaves of this plant are like spinach, the pods are similar to green beans, and the tendrils like lacy asparagus. Everything in the plant is edible, even the roots are nutty tasting tubers with four times the protein of potatoes. The seeds contain up to 42% protein, and the Vitamin A content is one of the highest recorded. This bean is from Southeast Asia, and the pods grow up to 10 inches.

The Raw Foods Story

Shred your vegetables in a food processor or by hand, fresh for each meal. Do not store them for later use. All of the following raw foods recipes are excellent for raw juice therapies. See the Magnificent 12 section and the Green & Leafy section then add the vegetables to juices or salads that will benefit you.

Raw foods contain live enzymes needed for healing and many nutrients, proteins and substances to speed the healing process. Use only freshly made juices, never canned.

Do not go overboard on spinach greens and Swiss chard because they contain oxalic acid, which inhibits the absorption of calcium, zinc, and magnesium, but do not omit them entirely because these foods also contain other important nutrients. Do not eat more than one beet and its top daily. Use parsley sparingly, it is a strong diuretic.

Prepare ahead for use on these salads, the following dressing:

Salad Dressing

1 cup pure virgin olive or canola oil
1/4 cup pure apple cider vinegar
Dash of garlic powder
Dash of onion powder and kelp
1 teaspoon chopped parsley
1/4 teaspoon barley malt concentrate
    or brown rice syrup
1/4 cup water

Combine ingredients in a jar. Shake well

If on a **weight loss** program omit the dressings and instead squeeze the juice of a fresh lemon on salads, it brings out the flavor of the vegetables. Lemons are a great blood cleanser and healer.

Add grated fresh horseradish to each serving for chronic **lung disorders, bronchitis** and **asthma**. Add onion to the recipes for sinus conditions and colds.

Grated raw potatoes are good for **peptic ulcers, diabetes** and **heart disorders**. High in potassium, cut out the center of the potato and discard it, cut slices about one inch thick, including the peel.

Soak all but organic vegetables in 1 teaspoon Clorox and a gallon of water. Scrub root vegetables well.

This is good for treatment of **gall bladder trouble, cancer, liver disorders, heartburn, indigestion,** and **all colon disorders.**

Shred the following:
1 beet
1 carrot
1/4 head of cabbage

This is good **after surgery.** For **infection** and **inflammation of the colon, skin disorders** and as a treatment for **tuberculosis of the bones and lungs**. Onions are highly recommended for **diabetes.**

Grate or shred the following:
1/4 head of cabbage
1 turnip
1/2 onion
1 stalk celery
1 carrot

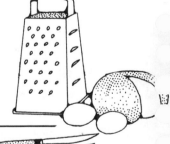

Vegetable Benefits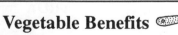

Leafy greens are essential in the diet. Add these to all salads. Studies have shown a cut in caloric consumption extends one's life. Vegetables are excellent sources of all vitamins, minerals, proteins, rich in fiber, and low in calories.

Helps rid the body of **toxins**, in **intestinal disorders** by elimination of the uric acid, in **heart disorders**, and in **high blood pressure**. Onions **build muscle, calms the nerves, improve the skin, nails and hair.**

Chop:
1 green pepper
1 stalk celery
1/4 cucumber
1/4 onion
1/4 jicama
1/4 crushed raw garlic

Very effective in reducing **hemorrhoid**s and a good general **tonic**. Use some of the turnip tops in the juice.

Chop & tear:
1/4 bunch spinach or chicory
1/4 bunch watercress
1 turnip
2 carrots

Use as a juice and in salads for **anemia** and **blood disorders**.

Chop & tear:
Kale or mustard greens
Dandelion greens
Turnips
Beet tops
1 clove garlic, mashed

This **improves kidney function** by reducing water retention. Aids in **weight loss**, in **vitamin deficiency** and in **digestion**. **Cleanses** the **system** and the **liver**.

Chop finely:
1/4 bunch parsley
1/2 jicama
1/4 bunch watercress
1/2 bunch dandelions (8 leaves)
1/2 turnip or one stalk of celery
1/4 cucumber

This is good for chronic **liver disorders**, **blood disorders**, **gall bladder**, and all **glandular problems.**

Grate:
medium beets
1/4 black radish
1/4 head red cabbage
1 apple

Good for **growing children** and anyone suffering from **bone softening**, in any form. High in usable calcium and magnesium plus potassium. Turnips are high in vitamins A, B-complex, C, and sulfur, iron, copper, iodine, as well as magnesium.

Chop & tear:
Large kale leaves
1 turnip, with 2 of the leaves, chopped
Handful of dandelions, torn
1 carrot, shredded

Good for water retention, colon disorders, vitamin deficiencies, cancer and digestion.

Shred & tear:
1 stalk celery and leaves, chopped
1/2 bunch spinach
1/8 bunch parsley
1/2 cucumber, chopped
1 carrot, chopped
3 radishes, sliced

Power Fruit Salad

1/4 papaya, fresh
1/4 cup pineapple, fresh
1/2 cup seedless grapes
1/2 sliced banana

Excellent for **digestion, colon disorders, enzyme dificiencies, heart disorders**, and **body detoxifier.**

Use for all **chronic diseases, blood disorders, colon cancer, colon disorders,** and **obesity**. This combination **cleanses all the glands and the blood stream**. Also good for the **lungs, asthma** (add raw, grated horseradish) and **bronchitis**.

Tear:
Romaine lettuce
Watercress
Beet greens
Turnip greens
Carrot, shredded
Chopped wheat grass (*optional*)

Good for colon cancer and polyps, ulcers, digestion, glandular function, bone formation, premature aging, skin disorders, osteoporosis, arthritis, and eye disorders.

Add grated raw garlic to salads, or use garlic oil for all heart disorders, high blood pressure, candidiasis (yeast and fungus infections). Garlic is beneficial in combating all degenerative diseases.

Good for all types of **cancer, heart disorders, high blood pressure, viral disorders,** and any type of illness. If very sick you can steam these slightly and use fresh lemon juices in place of salad dressing.

Chop & shred:
1/2 cup cauliflower, chopped
1/2 cup broccoli, chopped
1/4 cup onion, chopped
1/2-1 parsnips, shredded
1/2 carrot, shredded

President Bush's Thyroid Tonic. Excellent for **Thyroid function, mineral disfunctions,** also good for **cancer**.

Tear & chop:
1/8 bunch watercress
1 cup broccoli
1/2 cup cauliflower
1/4 bunch chopped parsley
6 drops liquid kelp

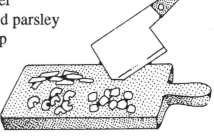

Parsley
Add a small amount of parsley for genito-urinarytract disorders, stones in the kidneys and bladder, nephritis and other types of kidney disorders. Good for the adrenal and thyroid glands. Also good for dieters because of its strong diuretic properties. Use parsley sparingly because it is very powerful.

Our Temperment Is Greatly Affected By The Food We Eat

Research into brain function reveals evidence that the emotions of love, faith, joy, fear, depression, and even our sense of purpose in life, are not merely attitudes created through our mind's thought processes. They are actually produced and reinforced by biochemical activity within the brain.

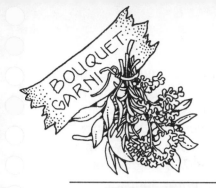

Sea Vegetables

Power-packed Ocean Foods

The ocean contains rich sources of many nourishing substances that are high in essential minerals, the 43 trace minerals, chlorophyll, iodine, protein, essential fatty acids, vitamins and much more. Iodine is essential for the thyroid gland. It stimulates the parathyroid glands making it easier to absorb the calcium in seaweed needed to nourish bones and leg joints. This is one reason kelp is good for arthritis sufferers.

The darker sea vegetables contain *alginic acid* which converts heavy metals in the body into harmless salts that are easily discharged. Kombo, wakame, hijuki and kelp are the dark sea vegetables.

Research at *McGill University, Canada* has found that the dark sea vegetables can even remove radioactive *Strontium-90* from the body.

Medical doctors in Nagasaki, Japan, in attempting to treat radiation-poisoned victims, following the dropping of the atomic bomb in 1945, saved many of their patients by administering a diet of miso soup, brown rice, and **sea vegetables**.

The *Canadian Medical Association Journal* also reported the importance of different marine algae in preventing absorption of radioactive products, as well as in their use as possible natural decontaminators.

Kelp comes in tablet, powdered and liquid forms and is recommended for arthritis and thyroid malfunction, and is good in aiding in protection from chemotherapy, radiation, and x-rays.

Seaweed contains calcium phosphate making it good for brittle bones common in osteoporosis.

The calcium, iodine, and sodium alginate in seaweed also serve as buffers against cancer.

Seaweed may also be an important factor in the low rates of certain cancers in Japan. In 1974, the *Japanese Journal of Experimental Medicine* reported scientists had found several varieties of kombu that were effective in the treatment of tumors. Ten years later, a *Harvard University Medical Center* researcher reported that eating a diet of 5% kombu, significantly delayed the inducement of breast cancer in animals. Other experiments on mice with leukemia, in which sea vegetables were used in the treatment regimen, showed great promise.

The high content of potassium in seaweed is good for the heart, kidneys, and in weight loss. The iodine needed by thyroid glands aid in weight loss also.

Seaweed nourishes membranes making it good for nervous disorders, colds, constipation, and skin disorders.

The edible seaweed, dulse, is one of the most nutritious and is harvested off the shores of Nova Scotia and California. All 43 trace minerals are found in dulse. Dulse is good to use in soups, stews, casseroles and any dish you are preparing. Kelp is another popular seaweed and may be the most used. Kelp is used in place of salt because of its salty taste. It contains concentrated amounts of calcium, potassium, sodium, silicon, zinc, chromium, selenium, barium and vitamins A, B, D, and E, and iodine.

Since seaweed is also high in protein, it should become a dietary staple. Nothing can compare to it as a rich source of minerals, essential to maintaining and improving one's health.

Seaweed Varieties

Seaweed should be added to everyone's diet in some form. It is a natural source of trace minerals. It is rich in calcium, iron, magnesium, zinc and all minerals. Hiziki, nori, arame, and kombu are used the most. Start with small amounts until you get used to the taste in soups and other foods. Seaweed is also a dietary aid for obesity and heavy meat eaters. All seaweeds are rich in calcium, iron, potassium, phosphorus, manganese, sodium, zinc, iodine and the vitamins A, C, and B-complex, including B-12 which is rare in plant foods.

Agar Agar

This is a Japanese vegetable gelatin derived from seaweed and used as a thickener. It can replace gelatin which is derived from animal protein. You do not need to boil agar agar to make it thicken, this preserves additional nutrients. It is good in fruit pies, jello, jellies, jams, and soups. It comes in flakes, bar form and granulated. Use two tablespoons of flakes to three cups liquid, one tablespoon granulated to three cups liquid, and use seven inches of the bar to three cups liquid. Always soak agar agar in one cup of liquid for five minutes before adding the rest of the liquid. If it is not as thick as you like, remember that it thickens when it cools. Agar agar is also used for constipation, and as additional fiber.

Alaria

Alaria is seaweed with a wild taste, it needs to cook longer than wakame. Cook at least 20 minutes to bring out the sweet, mild taste and chewy texture. It is rich in vitamin A, the B vitamins, and calcium.

Algin

Algin is derived from Pacific kelp. It has the ability to draw harmful pollutants, like lead, from the body. It is high in nutrients and minerals from the sea.

Arame

A black seaweed with a stringy texture, it has a mild taste and odor. It must be cooked for seven hours to make it tender, then it is dried in the sun.

Dulse

Dulse has a strong and distinctive flavor, a chewy texture and can be eaten as a snack directly from the bag. Use it in a variety of ways; in soups, salads, and sandwiches. It is rich in protein, fluoride, and iron. Check for occasional tiny brine shrimp and shells in the folds.

Preparation: Rinse lightly to tenderize for salads, sandwiches. The more soaking, the more tender and the more mineral loss. It cooks very quickly, in 5 minutes, in any juicy dish like soups, pastas, casseroles, stir-fries. You can pan fry it in a medium skillet or oven roast at 250 degrees until crisp. Then crumble over pastas, pizza, soups, salads or it can be served as a chewy snack but must be kept slightly moist, so as not to be tough.

Hijiki

Hijiki is a black colored Japanese seaweed, rich in vitamins, minerals and protein. It will cook to a firm texture, and swell 5 - 6 times its original size after cooking. Use it as another vegetable to add to soups, casseroles, and stews.

Kelp

Kelp is native to the Atlantic, and harvested in early spring. This seaweed is rich in potassium, iodine, mannitol, and calcium. Kelp contains glutamic acid which acts as a tenderizer for cooking beans. It dissolves quickly in soups, beans, and stews. It can also be eaten raw. Granulated or powdered kelp is used as a condiment or a flavoring. It is high in the major minerals: calcium, potassium, magnesium, and iron. It has been used in the treatment of thyroid problems. Try it as a substitute for salt. We recommend using kelp daily in the diet. It can be purchased in a health food store in tablet form if you do not like the flavor. Use kelp sparingly.

Kelp (Atlantic Kombu)

Thinner and "sweeter" than Japanese kombu. It provides mega-minerals, glutamic acid (a natural flavor enhancer), and more dietary fiber than oat bran.

Preparation: A must for soup stocks. Leave it to "dissolve" for 15-30 minutes. It swells to twice the volume and the minerals stay in.

The white powder on its surface is a beneficial mineral precipitate, not mold.

A portion of kelp in any bean-based dish will enrich, improve digestibility and shorten cooking time.

Marinate it in vinegar or soy sauce to tenderize it or pickle.

Roast bite-sized pieces of kelp in light oil until crisp and greenish for delicious "chips."

Kombu

Kombu is a sea vegetable, high in iodine and trace minerals. It has been used for thousands of years for flavoring stock and as a vegetable seasoning.

Kuzu

Kuzu can be used as a thickener in gravies, sauces and desserts. It is sometimes used in the macrobiotic diet to soothe the stomach and strengthen the intestines. It is a good source of quick energy.

Nori

Nori is a dark Japanese sea vegetable rich in minerals. It comes in sheets and is toasted above a flame and torn into desired sizes to garnish noodles, vegetables, rice and so on. It is said to be good for prostate and thyroid problems. Nori is high in protein, B-1, B-2, B-6, B-12, and vitamins C and E.

Sea Palm

A sea vegetable high in minerals and trace elements. Use it in soups, salads, and sautes.

Raw oysters, raw clams, and raw mussels can cause serious illness in persons with liver, stomach, blood or immune disorders.

Wakame

Wakame is a long, dark green sea leaf. It can be used in salads, eaten raw (soak in water first), and soups.

Wild Nori

It grows on rock beds along the northern coast of California. It is greenish purple, but dries a dark brown color. It is rich in vitamin C, and contains up to 25% protein by weight. It also contains vitamin B, complex, carbohydrates and trace minerals.

Zucchini Dulse Julienne

12 small zucchinis
1-1/2 cups diced dulse
1/2 cup olive oil
1-1/8 cups red wine vinegar or apple cider vinegar
1-1/2 teaspoon kelp granules Sea Seasonings
3 chopped scallions
3 teaspoons each oregano, basil, and parsley
3 cloves crushed garlic

Cut the zucchini into matchstick pieces, place in a bowl and add all of the above. Toss lightly and chill. Add carrots or peppers for color.

Sea vegetables aid in the growth of nails, hair, bones, and teeth, reduce blood cholesterol levels, and aid in the functioning of all endocrine glands, especially the thyroid.

Most people suffer from a deficiency of iodine, found in all sea vegetables. Thyroid function is improved by eating kelp and other sea vegetables.

There are cases of excess iodine in the diet if one consumes large amounts of iodized salt. Early symptoms of excess iodine include rough skin, hyperactivity, mental and emotional imbalances and poor concentration. If you consider the high percentage of salt found in fast-food hamburgers, french fries, and so forth, malnutrition-related problems may be on the rise because of the iodized salt.

With sea vegetables, the iodine is balanced with other nutrients, so do not be afraid of consuming them. Most Americans need the added minerals, and vegetarians need the B-12 content found in sea vegetables.

Be aware that there is a difference between eating sea vegetables and taking nutritional supplements. While sea vegetables can be eaten as frequently as desired, supplement intake should be carefully monitored.

Downeast Squash Soup

24" piece of dry kelp
3 large onions
12-16 cups winter squash, cubed
1-1/2 cup parsley, chopped
Miso or tamari to taste.

Cover kelp with water and simmer 10 minutes. Remove, cut into bite size pieces and combine with onion, squash, add water to cover. Simmer until squash is soft. Add the parsley at the end, along with the miso or tamari.

Recipes compliments of Maine Coast Sea Vegetables, Franklin, Maine.

Also see the following in the Soups section:

Carrot onion Miso soup
Mushroom Soup
Tofu Soup

Lung Protectors

Carrots, yams and squash protect the lungs from environmental pollutants when at least one of these is consumed daily. These foods are especially important for those who live in polluted cities or work in occupations involving toxic fumes like metal workers and anyone handling chemicals. Smokers and those exposed to second-hand smoke should also consume these foods.

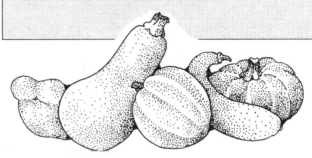

Protein Content in a One-Cup Serving of Vegan Foods		
Food	Protein grams per cup	Protein grams per 100 cal
Tempeh	31	9.4
Soybeans, cooked	29	9.7
Lentils, cooked	18	7.8
Kidney beans, lima beans, black beans and chickpeas (all cooked)	15	5.6-6.9
Pinto beans, cooked	14	6
Black-eyed peas, cooked	13	6.6
Soy milk, plain	10	6.5
Quinoa, cooked	11	4.7
Peas, cooked	8	6.4
Bulgur, cooked	6	3.9
Spinach, cooked	5	12.2
Broccoli, cooked	5	11.4
Brown rice, cooked	5	2.4

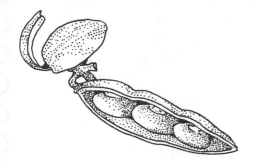

Growing Your Own
Sprouts

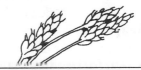

Sprouts should be an important part of your diet. They supply fresh greens year round when grocery bins are filled with vegetables from faraway places which may have been chemically treated to retain freshness and appearance.

Alfalfa is the most popular raw sprout. **Wheatgrass** is also best served raw. You should cook all large sprouts.

Avoid supermarket sprouts, they contain mold, and are rarely fresh. Sprouts should be fresh and kept for only 2-3 days. Grow your own! *Sprouting directions:*

Use a quart or half-gallon jar for sprouting. If using the larger size, double the amount of seeds used.

1) Purchase only high quality untreated organic seeds, grains or legumes which have been tested for germination. Rinse the seeds in lukewarm water.

2) Place two tablespoonfuls of seeds (1/2 cup of legumes or grains) in the sprouting jar with three times as much water as seeds. Soak overnight. Many small seeds require four hours of soaking, while some require none. Seeds with very hard coats, such as guar beans, require longer soaking, as long as two days.

3) After soaking, drain the water from the jar. Rinse seeds in fresh lukewarm water and drain again. Lay the jar at an angle (about 70 degrees) in a warm, dark place so the seeds can drain. Cover with a dishcloth or similar cloth.

4) **It is important to rinse and drain seeds twice a day.** If they dry out, the seeds are ruined. In hot, dry weather you may need to rinse them three times a day. Drain the seeds/sprouts in a dish rack over the sink. In very humid weather, the sprouts should be kept wrapped in a towel near a sunny window. All sprouts do better wrapped or kept in the dark until ready to "green." Take care to turn the jar over gently. Rapid movement of the jar may cause awkward shifting of the sprouting seeds, breaking the tender shoots and causing spoilage.

Suggestions

1) Do not presoak **chia**, **alfalfa**, **cress**, **oat** or **mustard seeds.**

2) Wire mesh screening is best for draining small seeds. Switch to screening with larger openings for better drainage of bigger sprouts. Screens with lids can be found in health food stores, or you can use cheesecloth secured with a rubber band around the top of the jar.

3) Rinse water drained from sprouts is nutritious and can be used in soups or to water your plants.

4) When the sprouts reach their full height, place them on a window sill in direct sunlight to develop the chlorophyll; the tiny leaves will turn green within a day.

5) On the fourth day, rinse the hulls from **alfalfa** sprouts to prevent premature spoilage. Fill the sink with cold water and soak the sprouts. As the hulls float to the top, skim them off with a strainer .

6) Gelatinous seeds such as **guar**, **flax** and **chia** may not sprout well in a jar.

7) Use sprouts with seeds attached. Sprouts should not be overcooked, which destroys their crispness. Cooking time should be only long enough to remove the raw flavor. We recommend cooking all sprouts except alfalfa.

8) Sprouts may be cooked and served as a plain vegetable. To saute, place a small amount of oil in a pan, add sprouts and a small amount of water or tamari sauce. Cover and cook 10 minutes. (Some people prefer to cook sprouts only 5 to 8 minutes.) Minced onion or mushrooms browned in the oil add flavor, as do shredded carrots, turnips and cabbage.

9) You can steam sprouts before eating in two tablespoons of oil, then cover with butter or you can brown them in a small amount of oil.

10) Cooked sprouts can be added to any vegetable combination for casserole dishes and are popular in stir-fry vegetables. They are a good addition to salads

and scrambled eggs or omelets.
  11) Add to potato salad.
  12) Mix sprouts in sandwich spreads.
  13) Mix them with soft cheese, to make a dip.
  14) Try them in rice dishes.

Wheat grass is the most highly nutritious food on this planet and it is easy to grow. Fill a large tray (the type used for bedding plants) with soil and plant the seeds. Cover with plastic and place them on a window sill until the first sign of green appears. Remove the plastic, water as needed and watch your fresh greens grow. Wheat grass juice is used throughout the world for healing many diseases and is excellent for all intestinal disorders.

Sprouts are alive, they are highly nutritious, no one food offers more. They contain concentrated nutrients.

Sprouts contain protein, vitamins A, B complex, C, D, and E, iron, enzymes, potassium and magnesium, calcium and phosphorus, trace elements like zinc and chromium, and essential amino and fatty acids.

Sprout and Bean Salad

16 ounces cooked red kidney beans
Juice of 1 lemon
8 ounces chopped bean sprouts
6 tablespoons olive or canola oil
2 stalks chopped celery
Dash of barley malt sweetener or your choice
1/2 diced green pepper
Dash of Spike seasoning
1/2 finely chopped onion

Stir together the beans, sprouts, celery, pepper, and onion. Make the dressing, blending the lemon, oil and sweetener together. Season to taste. Pour dressing over salad and top with fresh sprouts.

> **LIFE SPROUTS**
> **P.O. Box 150**
> **PARADISE, UT 84328**
> **1-800-241-1516**
>
> have a full line of sprouters and high-quality seeds

Sprouting Chart - Daily Growth					
Seed	Quantity	Yield	Rinses	Time	Height
Adzuki	1/2 cup	2 cups	4	6 days	1 inch
Alfalfa (salads)	2 tbsp	1 quart	2	4 days	1-2 inches
Alfalfa (baking)	1/4 cup	1-1/2 cups	2	2 hours	1/8 inch
Beans (Kidney, Lima, Fava, Green, Pinto)	1 cup	4 cups	4	6 days	2 inches
Chia	2 tbsps	3 cups	1	4 days	1-1/2 inches
Cress	1 tbsp	1-1/2 cups	2	4 days	1-1/2 inches
Fenugreek (salad)	1/4 cup	4 cups	2	5 days	3 inches
Garbanzo (chick pea)	1 cup	3 cups	5	4 days	1/2-1 inch
Guar beans (soak for 36 hours)	1 cup	4 cups	4	5 days	2-3 inches
Lentils	1 cup	6 cups	2	4 days	1 inch
Millet	1 cup	2 cups	3	3 days	1/4 inch
Mung beans	1 cup	4 cups	4	4 days	2-3 inches
Peas	1-1/2 cups	4 cups	2	4 days	1/2-1 inch
Radish	1 tbsp	2 cups	2	5 days	1/2-1 inch
Red Clover	3 tbsp	1 quart	2	5 days	Green
Soybeans	1 cup	5 cups	8	5 days	1/2-3/4 inch
Sunflower	1 cup	3 cups	2	2 days	1/2 inch
Wheat	1cup	4 cups	3	4 days	1/2 inch

Squash

A diet high in squash consumption can **lower the risk of cancer, particularly in the lungs.** Studies show that foods with high potassium content can reduce **hypertension** and the risk of **stroke.** Ethiopians chew the seeds of the squash plant for **purgatives** and **laxatives.** The use of the pumpkin and squash seeds to **expel worms**, including the tapeworm, is a common practice around the world. The seeds contain *protease trypsin inhibitors* which keep **viruses** and **cancer** causing chemicals from becoming active in the intestinal tract. The deep orange winter squash, like butternut and hubbard, are packed with *carotenoids*, including *beta-carotene*, which is a known anti-cancer substance.

Squash also helps to heal **inflammation, relieves pain** and soothes the **stomach** and protects the **spleen.** The Chinese use the seeds to combat tape worms and round worms.

A study was done on a group of men from New Jersey, many who had smoked for years, according to the *National Cancer Institute.* Those who ate the least of the vegetables had nearly double the chances of getting lung cancer. The men with the lowest risk ate two and one half servings of some type of vegetable daily. **Carrots and other deep orange vegetables slow the cancer promotion process in the body, which can continue in damaged cells for years.** Even nonsmokers, exposed to passive smoke, would benefit from the protective qualities these vegetables provide.

Squash are good used in casseroles, breads, cookies, muffins, omelets, sauces, salads, soups, pancakes, cakes, pies, puddings, pickles and relishes. They can be cooked many different ways, baked, sauteed, steamed, scalloped, stuffed, or mashed. The seeds can be dried, to provide a good source of protein, phosphorus, and vitamin A.

All winter squash are good baked. They can be topped with a little honey and soft safflower margarine and seasoning.

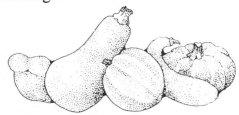

Spaghetti Squash

Spaghetti squash resembles an oval, yellow pumpkin without ridges. It is not a true squash but an edible gourd and a good source of vitamin A and potassium. It should be stored in a cool, dry place.

To cook, cut off the stem and split the squash lengthwise. Scoop the seeds out. Pierce the cleaned squash in a couple places and bake the squash for 1 hour, at 350 degrees, open side down on a cookie sheet. Turn the squash and bake an additional 45 minutes, or until tender. Then, loosen the flesh of the squash with a fork, and it will come off in spaghetti-like strands. Top with your favorite sauce.

Summer Squash

Very high in vitamin A, and low in calories, they are best eaten as soon as they are picked. Some common types of summer squash are: caserta, chayote, cocozelle, cymling, yellow or golden crookneck, yellow straightneck, vegetable marrow, and zucchini.

Winter Squash

High in vitamin A, also supplies potassium, and generally higher in carbohydrates. Winter squash should be picked when it is mature, and kept at a cool temperature (no lower than 40 degrees) for several months. Some common types of winter squash includes acorn, banana, buttercup, butternut, delicata, delicious, gold nugget, hubbard, marblehead, pumpkin, and spaghetti.

Fresh or canned pumpkin is rich in beta carotene (nearly four times as much as a large carrot), an antioxidant and precursor of vitamin A in the body. Researchers at the *National Cancer Institute* and *the U.S. Department of Agriculture*, singled out pumpkin for its beta carotene content for cancer of the lung, mouth, throat, gastrointestinal tract, and prostate.

Squash-Nut-Raisin Bread

2-1/4 cups whole wheat flour
2 teaspoons Rumford's aluminum free baking
   powder
1 teaspoon cinnamon
1/2 cup soy milk
1 tablespoon arrowroot powder or egg substitute
   or 2 eggs
1/4 cup canola or safflower oil
1/2 cup honey, maple syrup, or barley malt
   syrup
1/2 teaspoon nutmeg
1 cup chopped walnuts or nuts of your choice
1/2 cup raisins or any dried chopped fruit
1 cup pureed cooked winter squash

Mix flour, baking powder, salt, and spices. Combine squash, oil, honey, and soy milk with egg substitute, mix with the dry ingredients. Stir in nuts and raisins. Pour into a oiled loaf pan and bake at 350 ° for 30 - 40 minutes. Test by sticking a toothpick into it, when it comes out clean, the bread is done.

Pumpkin can be used in place of the squash, if pumpkin-nut bread is preferred.

Carrot and Butternut Squash Casserole

1-1/2 pounds butternut squash, peeled, seeded,
   and diced
3 cups sliced carrots
1 cup vegetable stock or water
3/4 cup low-fat plain yogurt
6 tablespoons sesame oil
Dash of sea salt or Spike and cayenne pepper
Minced parsley for garnish

In a large saucepan cook vegetables covered with water or vegetable stock, until almost tender. Drain, add yogurt and seasonings and blend until ingredients are all combined, but not pureed. Fill oiled casserole dish and bake for 15 minutes at 350°. Sprinkle with parsley and serve.

Squash Coleslaw

2 cucumbers
1 yellowneck squash
1 zuchini
1 carrot
1/2-3/4 cup plain yogurt
1/2 cup tofu mayonnaise or your choice
Dash of spike seasoning or salt
1/2 honey teaspoon to taste
Shread first 4 ingredients, place in a large bowl and add the rest of the ingredients. Toss together, chill and serve.

Zucchini Casserole

1 pound zucchini, sliced or cubed
1 pound yellowneck squash, diced or cubed
1 quart (4 cups) cut-up and skinned
   fresh tomatoes or home canned
1/2 teaspoon barley malt sweetener
   or 2 tablespoons honey
3 cloves garlic, minced
1 medium onion, chopped
3 tablespoons vegetable oil
1 teaspoon Italian seasoning mix
1/4 teaspoon sea salt or Spike seasoning

Saute all vegetables and garlic in oil, until partially cooked and still crisp. Add tomatoes and seasonings, simmer for 1/2-1 hour. Good with cooked pasta, for variety.

Pumpkin Soup

Vegetables of your choice (can include):
   onions, celery, carrots
2 cups water
1 can pumpkin (or fresh cooked)
2 cups soy milk (or your choice)
Dash curry powder, cummin, thyme, and
   Spike seasoning

Mix vegetables, water and pumpkin in pan and simmer until soft. Place all in a blender with milk and seasonings. Puree until smooth.

Substitutes

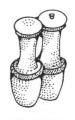

Here are a few alternatives to salt that will add zip to your cooking without the dangers of salt.

Naturally Salt Free   All purpose seasoning by *Modern Products, Inc.* Contains: Sesame seeds, red and green bell peppers, lemon and orange peels, onion, garlic, paprika, basil, white pepper, tomato, celery seed, oregano, thyme, mustard, cumin seed, and cayenne pepper.

Vegit   All purpose seasoning by *Modern Products, Inc.* Contains: Special yeast grown on blackstrap molasses, kelp, hydrolyzed vegetable protein, toasted onion, dillseed, ripe white pepper, celery, parsley flakes, papain enzyme, mushroom powder, orange and lemon peel, plus a delightful herbal bouquet of oregano, sweet basil, marjoram, rosemary and thyme.

Make your own   Mix 1 tablespoon each of the following crushed, dried herbs: kelp, basil, green pepper, curry powder, celery seed, dried onion, parsley, sage, majoram, green onion. Mix all together and store in a tight fitting shaker jar.

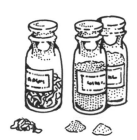

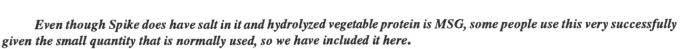

Instead of Salt

Saltless (*McCormick*)
Mrs. Dash (*Alberto-Culver*)
Seasoned Saltless (*McCormick*)
Seasoned Salt-Free (*Lowry's*)
No Salt (*RCN Products*)
Bernard Jensen's Broth or Seasoning

American Health, May 1992 pg. 97

Even though Spike does have salt in it and hydrolyzed vegetable protein is MSG, some people use this very successfully given the small quantity that is normally used, so we have included it here.

Spike   All purpose instant seasoning by *Modern Products, Inc.* Contains: Salt crystals, hydrolyzed vegetable protein, mellow toasted onion, onion powder, orange powder, soyflower, special high-flavor yeast, celery leaf powder, celery root powder, garlic powder, dill, kelp, Indian curry, horseradish, ripe white pepper, orange and lemon peel, summer savory, mustard flour, sweet green and red bell peppers, parsley flakes, tarragon, rosehips, saffron, mushroom powder, parsley powder, spinach powder, tomato powder, sweet Hungarian paprika, celery powder, cayenne pepper, plus a delightful herbal bouquet of the best oregano, sweet basil, marjoram, rosemary and thyme.

171

Healthy Substitutions

ORIGINAL INGREDIENT	SUBSTITUTE
Baking chocolate square	3 tablespoons carob powder + 2 tablespoons water = 3 tablespoons carob chips
Baking powder or baking soda - 1 teaspoon	1 teaspoon Rumford's Aluminum-Free Baking Powder = 1 teaspoon cream of tartar = 1/2 teaspoon baking soda + 1 teaspoon baking powder = 2 teaspoons arrowroot powder
Butter or margarine	Equal amounts of sesame oil or a vegetable oil of your choice, tahini butter (ground sesame seeds that Near Eastern people often use in place of butter)
Buttermilk or sour cream- 1 cup	1 cup low-fat plain yogurt = 1 cup sweet milk plus 1 tablespoon lemon juice or vinegar = 1/2 cup tofu and 1/2 cup plain yogurt, blended = 1 cup cottage cheese, blended until smooth
Canned fruits and vegetables	Fresh fruits and vegetables. If fruits and vegetables are not in season, use only frozen or home canned.
Cereals, processed or boxed	Whole grains, flaked or cracked grains, granola, millet, barley, brown rice, and buckwheat (found in health food stores)
Cocoa	Powdered carob in equal amounts
Coffee, black tea	Cereal beverages and herb teas, Ovaltine, Horlicks (a carbonated drink, sweetened with barley malt), Instant Dandylion Blend, Instant Dandelion Kofy, Bambu (made of chicory, figs, wheat, malted barley, and acorns), Inca (roasted barley malt, barley, and chicory) and Pero
Cornstarch	Arrowroot (thickens when cool), agar agar, instant tapioca , kudzu. For casseroles try potato flakes or potato powder.
Cottage cheese	Use equal amounts of tofu

Healthy Substitutions

ORIGINAL INGREDIENT	SUBSTITUTE
Beef Boullion, 1 cup	One tablespoon miso in one cup water = 1 cup vegetable broth = 1 package Hain's Dry Onion or Vegetable Soup mix in one cup of water − 1 cup Vege X, all vegetable bouillon = 1 cup Morga Vegetable Broth Mix
Ground beef	Use the same quantity of ground nuts, soy granules, miso, tofu, textured vegetable protein as the beef and flavor with tamari sauce. Use in place of meat for seasoning in soups, casseroles, etc. miso, tamari sauce, vegetable bouillon, Spike, Hain'sDry Soup mixes. If a soy sauce has MSG, use tamari sauce instead; a wheat-free variety of tamari sauce is available.
Dried fruit, sulphured	Organic, unsulphured fruit without sugar or preservatives.
Egg, 1 in baking recipe	2 egg whites = 1/2 teaspoon baking powder + 2 tablespoons soy flou = 1 tablespoon arrowroot powder = 3 tablespoons Jolly Joan Egg Substitute
Egg whites, 2	Two tablespoons unflavored gelatin dissolved in 2 tablespoons water, whip, chill and whip again
Flour, 1 tablespoon all-purpose (to thicken sauces)	1-1/2 teaspoons cornstarch =1-1/2 teaspoons arrowroot = 1 tablespoon quick-cooking tapioca = 2-1/2 teaspoons whole grain flours = 1 tablespoon oat or soy flour
Flour, white or cake	Whole wheat flour, unbleached flour, can use part oat flour, triticale, rice, rye or cornmeal in some recipes
Garlic powder 1/4 teaspoon	1 clove fresh garlic

Avocado

Avocados are excellent added to the diet of those who have low blood sugar (Hypoglycemia) problems. The good fats will aid in stabilizing the blood sugar. Diabetics should limit their intake of avocados.

Try mashed avocado on a baked potato instead of butter. When baking muffins and nut bread, try substituting avocado for some of the oil. Instead of sour cream use mashed avocado in dips and on tacos, or mix with mayonnaise for potato salad, etc.

173

Healthy Substitutions

ORIGINAL INGREDIENT	SUBSTITUTE
Hydrogenated fats, lard, shortening and refined oils	Cold-pressed, expeller-pressed, and unrefined oils. (No palm or palm kernel or cottonseed oils)
Milk, 1 cup in baking (for milk-free diets)	4 tablespoons powdered soy milk in one cup water = 1 cup almond milk or nut milk, soy milk or coconut milk = 1 cup juice = 1 cup Rice Dream Milk
Pasta and spaghetti made from white flour	Whole wheat, spinach, corn pasta (found in health food stores)
Peanut butter (Commercial)	100% nut butters that are unhydrogenated, like sesame, almond, cashew, sunflower, pecan
Salt	Spike, herb seasonings, sea salt or Bronner's salt substitute
Sour cream or buttermilk- 1 cup	One cup tofu, blend until smooth, = 1 cup yogurt = 1 cup cottage cheese
Sugar-1 cup	One-half cup honey =1 cup raw sugar = 3/4 cup honey and 1/4 cup less liquid (if no liquid is used in recipe, add 1/4 cup flour for each 3/4 cup honey) = 1 cup date sugar = 1/2 cup maple syrup = 1/2 cup purees like apple juice concentrate, barley malt concentrate, rice or barley malt syrup=1/4 cup raisin juice (soaked and blended) = two mashed and blended bananas
Vegetable shortening in baking, 1 cup	One cup cold-pressed, or expeller-pressed vegetable oil
Vinegar	Unpasteurized apple cider vinegar, brown rice vinegar, lemon or lime juice to be used in salad dressing or any recipe calling for vinegar
White bread	Wheat-free rye, brown rice, millet, corn bread (from health food stores), oil-free macrobiotic bread. There are many yeast-free products and breads in health food stores. You will also find crackers, rolls, breads which are wheat-free, oil-free, sugar-free, and contain no preservatives.

Sugar

By any other name...

Every American consumes an average of 135 pounds of sugar each year. This accounts for 500-600 calories a day, amounting to over two pounds per week. The only benefit sugar offers is quick energy.

Sugar is the number one additive in the food industry. Manufacturers list many ingredients on their labels that most people do not understand. Stay away from foods that have a long list of ingredient names that are not recognizable foods; these are chemicals, artificial colorings, preservatives, isolated substances and additives. It means they are not in a form natural to the body and put a heavy strain on the liver and digestion.

Natural sugars are carbohydrates, that are important sources of energy for us. Carbohydrates can be divided into three categories: monosaccharides (simple sugars), disaccharides (double sugars), and polysaccharides (starches and fibers, including breads and potatoes). A study published in the *Journal of Reproductive Medicine*, 1984 issue, found that the intake of sugar, dairy, and artificial sweeteners correlated positively with the incidence of candida vulvovaginitis.

When the diet omitted those elements, more than 90% of the patients were found to be free of yeast infections for over a year. One of the major drawbacks of sugar is that it raises the insulin level, inhibiting the release of growth hormones which in turn depresses the immune function. People who consume high amounts of sugar and low fiber diets are more prone to cancer, *Science News*, November 10,1990.

Many sources of sugar and sweeteners have different names, which include:

Acesulfame K

Also known as Sunette and Sweet One. This is a sweetener of white, odorless crystals made from acetoacetic acid.

Aspartame

More commonly known as NutraSweet and Equal. This sweetener is made up of a combination of aspartic acid, amino acids, and phenylalanine. Aspartame loses its sweetness when used in cooking or baking. **Do not use if you have phenylketonuria and are pregnant or lactating. Do not give to child**

Sweet, but not Sugar

Acesulfame-K: Gained FDA approval in 1988 under brand name Sunette it leaves no aftertaste and is 200 times sweeter than sugar. It is not metabolized, so it has no calories. Used in chewing gum, instant coffee, tea, dry beverage mixes, gelatins, and nondairy creamers. The *Center for Science in the Public Interest* objects to acesulfame-K, saying that Sunette caused tumors in rats. The FDA concluded that the tumors had occurred spontaneously.

Aspartame: Approved in 1981, sold under the brand name Equal. It is found in thousands of goods, from colas to breath mints, under the name NutraSweet.

Since its approval, critics have charged that aspartame causes myriad adverse health effects, ranging from headaches and dizziness to seizures.

Saccharin: Available for nearly one century, this is truly an artificial sweetener—it comes from petroleum. About 300 times sweeter than sugar it is noncaloric. Although the FDA proposed a ban on saccharin after studies suggested a link between it and bladder tumors in rats, it was saved by public demand, to be left on the market. Federal regulations require that products containing saccharin must be labeled.

Barley Malt

Comes in a powder and syrup concentrate, very good for those on diets and suffering from **diabetes** or **hypoglycemia**. *Dr. Bronner's* Barleymalt is an excellent sugar substitute. It tastes just like sugar, without the after-taste often associated with sugar substitutes. In cooking and baking, barleymalt can be substituted for sugar. It is highly concentrated, a dash (1/8 teaspoon) has only three calories and replaces two teaspoons of sugar.

Brown Rice Syrup

This is derived from brown rice, it is also a good form of sugar for those with **diabetes**.

Fructose or Levulose

Another monosaccharide, this form of sugar is found in fruit (though not grapes) and honey. Other names for it are corn fructose, high fructose, fruit fructose, fruit sugar, invert sugar syrup (in a mixture of glucose and fructose), beet sugar, brown sugar, turbinado sugar, raw sugar, tupelo honey, honey, and unpasteurized honey. When consumed, fructose may aggravate high blood levels of triglycerides.

Glucose

Also a monosaccharide, known as grape sugar, dextrose, corn syrup, corn sweetener or glucose syrup. This sugar occurs naturally in the body and is needed for **brain function**. Complex carbohydrates and starches found in food such as greens, vegetables and fruits are broken down into glucose during digestion. In some circumstances glucose can be derived from the breakdown of protein and fat.

When glucose is consumed in the forms mentioned and not broken down by the body from complex carbohydrates, it causes the blood sugar to rise quickly and drop as quickly.

Honey

This is a natural syrup made up of glucose, fructose, and water.

Lactose

A disaccharide, found in milk. Approximately 80% of the adult population in the world do not have the enzyme needed to digest lactose.

Maltose

Manufactured from starch. A disaccharide, found in malted syrup, maltodextrin, dextrins, and dextrose. Maltose is found in germinating seeds.

Rice Syrup

A sweetener made by fermenting rice and boiling the resulting until it becomes a thick syrup. Similar in texture to honey.

Saccharin

Most commonly known as Sweet n'Low, Sprinkle Sweet, Twin, and Sweet 10. It is made of a chemical similar to acesulfame K. Saccharin does not taste good when used in baking. It has a bitter aftertaste, and its safety when consumed, is under review.

Do not use if pregnant or lactating. Do not give to children.

Sorbitol, Mannitol & Xylitol

These are naturally occurring sugar alcohols. They can cause diarrhea, can be used by individuals with a blood-sugar sensitivity.

Sorghum

Sorghum molasses and whey are forms of sugar.

Dr. Bronner's Barleymalt Sweetner **contains: Barleymalt, orange juice solids, calcium-magnesium-phosphate, parsley, chia seed, calcium-saccharate balanced with soya-bean-hydrolyzed-vegetable-protein (HVP), dulse sea lettuce, lemon juice solids, potassium salt, rosehips, anise and mint.**

Sucanat Evaporated Cane Juice

100% evaporated sugar cane juice, organically grown, without the use of synthetic pesticides, contains no preservatives or additives. Naturally brown in color, contains all the nutrients from the sugar cane.

Sucrose

A disaccharide, containing equal parts fructose and glucose. Also known as cane, sucrose, beet, unrefined, raw, turbinado, confectioner's, and powdered sugar, as well as sugar syrup, brown sugar, and glaze. This sugar is produced from sugar cane or sugar beets. When consumed, it adds empty calories, and causes the blood sugar to rise high and fast.

There are sweeteners used in place of those listed above such as, barley malt, rice syrup, barley syrup, blackstrap molasses, and herbal sweeteners found in health food stores. Blackstrap molasses is rich in iron and minerals and lacks none of the essential nutrients that other sugar forms often are deficient in.

When whole foods containing any of these sugars are consumed, the foods also provide vitamins, minerals, and proteins stabilizing the blood sugar and aiding digestion. When fruit is eaten, the fructose is diluted by large portions of water contained in the fruit.

Sugar consumption is thought to be the cause of many Western health problems, including tooth decay, diabetes, and obesity. If a craving for something sweet were satisfied by a piece of fruit or chewing on cane sugar, as is done in other parts of the world, these diseases would not be so widespread. **Refined sugars missing these nutrients, create problems for the body in the process of sugar metabolism.** The vitamins and minerals are used from the body's stores to digest sugar, so instead of feeling energetic from sugar, the body quickly feels weak and fatigued.

When you consume as little as two teaspoons of sugar a change occurs in your blood chemistry and the body is no longer in homeostasis the balanced state where our body functions best. After the body digests sugar, the mineral balance will change, for example, calcium may increase and phosphorus decrease. When a mineral in our blood stream increases dramatically it can become toxic, this is because minerals only function efficiently in balance with each other. Kidney stones, gall bladder stones, arthritis, hardening of the arteries, and cataracts of the eyes can be caused by toxic calcium. When minerals in the blood stream decrease, the body does not have enough to work synergistically with enzymes, since enzymes are mineral dependent.

Enzymes are needed to digest food, when food goes undigested it putrefies. The undigested, putrefied food then irritates the gastrointestinal tract and can get into the blood stream. This can cause headaches, dizziness, fatigue, anger or depression if it goes to the brain. It can go to the bones, joints, and tissues and cause stiffness and arthritis. If the putrefied food goes to the skin, via the blood, it can cause acne, psoriasis, or other skin problems. The white blood cells become overworked and exhausted when the body consumes abusive food continuously.

A high sugar intake may lead to all sorts of behavioral changes from aggressiveness in adults to

Other Names For Sugar

Barley malt	Date Sugar	Herbal Sweetener	Polydextrose
Beet Sugar	Demerar Sugar	High fructose Corn Syrup	Raw Sugar
Blackstrap Molasses	Dextrin	Honey	Sorbitol
Brown Sugar	Dextrose	Invert Sugar	Sorghum
Cane Sugar	Fructose	Lactose	Sucanat
Carmel	Fruit Fructose	Maltose	Sucrose
Corn Fructose	Glucose	Manitol	Sugar
Corn Sweetener	Grape Sugar	Maple Syrup	Turbinado
Corn Syrup	Grape Sweetener	Molasses	

hyperactivity in children.

Sugar can raise blood-cholesterol levels in most individuals, however, a task force of scientists with the FDA concluded in 1986 that there was not any conclusive evidence that a high sugar intake is a risk factor in heart disease. Some researchers suggest that a small number of carbohydrate-sensitive individuals with high insulin or triglyceride levels may be particularly sensitive to sugar, especially fructose. The body reacts to sugars by increasing cholesterol and triglyceride levels. If sugar consumers have cholesterol problems, it could be the company they keep; cakes, cookies, candy bars, and pies all combine sugar with fat.

Common table sugar has recently joined the ranks of those food additives that contribute to high blood pressure. Researchers, at *Georgetown University Medical Center in Washington, D.C.*, found in tests performed on animals, that sugar was just as likely as salt to produce a dangerous increase in blood pressure.

To diminish cravings for sugar, consume more whole grains, squash, sweet potatoes, apples, and frozen bananas (see recipes.) Use desserts sweetened with barley malt or rice syrup or powdered barley concentrate. Dried fruit, apricots, dates, figs, and raisins make good sweeteners for whole grain cereals. Chop and cook them with the cereal or mash and puree them for baking and use in recipes calling for sugar. (All dried fruits should be rehydrated by soaking in boiling water to soften and to destroy the bacteria.)

Remember, sugar is found in almost all processed foods like sodas, fruit drinks, frozen dinners, breads, cereals and canned foods. High-fructose corn sweetener is the most popular with food processors because it is inexpensive. So learn to read labels and be familiar with the different names for sugar to know how much you are really consuming.

Sugar Content of Some Popular Foods		
Food	Serving Size	Teaspoons of sugar
Canned Applesauce, sweetened	1/2 cup	4.3
Chocolate Chiffon Pie	4.6 oz.	7.8
Cranberry Sauce	94% cal. from sugar	
Coca Cola	12 oz.	9.8
Dannon Frozen Yogurt, fruit	8 oz.	7.4
Gatorade	8 oz.	3.5
Ice Cream Sundae	1 cup	19
Jello	1/2 cup	4.2
Jelly Beans	10	6.6
Ketchup	64% cal. from sugar	
Milky Way Candy Bar	1 oz.	3.9
Nature's Valley Granola Bar	1 oz.	3.3
Pecan Pie	4.6 oz.	12
Quaker Instant Oatmeal, Cinn.	1.5 oz.	4.3
Sara Lee Chocolate Cake	3.2 oz.	7.9
Sherbet	1/2 cup	6.7
Sponge Cake with Icing	3.2 oz.	10.7

We can't emphasize enough how important it is to omit sugar from the diet or at least cut it way back. It can cause sleepless nights, anger, mood changes, depression, fear, anxiety, obesity; and it overworks the organs of the body. The next time a television commercial tries to tell you to buy a candy bar for that sudden burst of energy, consider this: the liver can only store about 150 grams of glycogen, derived from food sugar, and the excess becomes fat globules. While fat globules might not sound particularly bad, they are what we call ''a spare tire,'' ''heavy thighs'' and ''flabby forearms.''

Tofu

The most versatile protein

Tofu, also known as bean curd, is fast becoming a popular staple. It is made by curdling soybean milk. It can be found in the supermarket produce section, in health food stores, and in oriental food shops.

Tofu is an excellent baby food, good for growing children, vegetarians and the elderly, because it has a high protein content and is easily digested. It is good for healing and for sensitive **stomachs**. Tofu is low in calories, fats, and carbohydrates and is rich in calcium and potassium. It is a good source of protein when trying to lower cholesterol levels as it contains no cholesterol, and is low in fats.

Tofu, having no flavor of its own, can become whatever flavor you want when it is prepared. No other food can substitute for mayonnaise, sour cream, cream cheese in cheesecake, dips, low calorie dressings, meat, cheese, sandwich spreads, and much more.

Buy fresh tofu, unless it is vacuum packed, change the water as soon as you get home. Fresh, clean water should be used to rinse and soak the tofu each day. Use distilled water to store it in, tofu is best used in one week to ten days after opening.

Frozen tofu has a meaty texture that resembles ground beef in recipes, such as chili, spaghetti, sloppy joes, etc. You must freeze it properly. Drain the chunk of tofu well and take a paper towel and squeeze out all the excess liquid. Let it set a few minutes and pat dry again. Cut into 1/2 inch chunks and spread on a cookie sheet and freeze for three to four hours. Then store the tofu in a freezer bag. To use, thaw and crumble. Add to your recipe and it will resemble meat in texture and take on the flavor of the food you are cooking with it.

Remember tofu has no flavor, as you cook with it in recipes, taste the dish because it may need more flavorings than usual.

For baby foods add tofu to a blender along with other foods you are preparing like fresh fruit, vegetables or canned baby foods. This will assure you that your baby is getting enough protein and calcium.

The type of bean used will determine the nutritional content of the tofu. Approximately 1/2 cup or 1/2 pound of tofu contains the following:

Protein	**9.4 gm**
Calcium	**154.0 mg**
Potassium	**50.0 mg**
Fat	**5.0 gm**
Iron	**2.0 mg**
Sodium	**8.0 mg**
Calories	**86**

Forms of Tofu

Silken tofu - softest form to medium soft (Japanese style)

Chinese style - medium firm to dense firm cheese - hard pressed

Tofu comes packed in water. Fresh tofu has a delicate scent with little smell to it. Each package should have an expiration date, so be sure to check this date before buying. **If it smells a little sour do not use it, unless you boil it for 20 minutes, otherwise return it.** Remember, the medium-firm tofu is good for slicing, freezing, and cubing. The softer form may be used the same way but it has to be drained, squeezed dry, and does not hold its shape as well. You can make it even firmer by placing paper towels on the top and bottom of the tofu and placing a heavy chopping board on it for fifteen minutes or longer. The soft tofu is best for blending in recipes like mayonnaise, cheese cake, etc. Marinading tofu gives it the flavor you desire. Always marinate tofu in a stainless steel or glass container. If you are marinating cubes, use a flat dish and turn several times. If using frozen tofu, press the marinade into the tofu every so often. Do not let it stand out at room temperature longer than an hour, if you need more time, place in the refrigerator.

Tofu makes great dips, just add a *Hain's* dry soup mix into 1 pound of blended soft tofu and refrigerate a few hours. Onion, mushroom, vegetable and even the cheese soup mix is easy and delicious

179

Tofu

with tofu. If you like you can use dried minced onion or chopped chives, or dried vegetables and season with garlic granules, a little Spike, cayenne pepper, dried parsley, and a little miso or vegetable bouillon granules. Remember to use tofu in place of sour cream, cream cheese and other similar dairy products. If you want a guacamole dip, blend the tofu, ripe avocados, salsa sauce, a touch of garlic powder, and a little lemon juice.

For jalapeno dip omit the avocados and add chopped onion and jalapeno peppers and a tablespoon of oil. Always chill before serving, to flavor the whole dish. Experiment and create your own dips the way you like them. All you need is blended tofu and seasoning and the flavor you desire like dill, chive, curry, or garlic.

You can also make sandwich spreads using blended tofu and adding chopped nuts, pimento (red peppers), pickle relish, and a sweetener, if desired. To cut down on nut butters for children, add half mashed tofu to a nut butter and/or jelly for a healthier sandwich.

Tofu is very versatile. As you become familiar wth it, you will love its many uses.

Tofu, fish oil, fiber, vitamin D, and a low fat diet, may lower the risk of developing **breast cancer**, the major cancer killer of American women. In 1987, one in every eleven women developed breast cancer, now its one in nine.

The *National Cancer Institute* estimates that about 1.5 million women will be diagnosed with the disease over the next decade and that about 30% of them will die.

At an *American Cancer Society* seminar in Daytona Beach, Flodida, *Dr. Stephen Barnes, Biochemist, University of Alabama* said, "Experimental studies involving 30 rats indicated that *isoflavones*, naturally occurring substances found in soybeans and tofu, seemed to reduce the rate of mammary cancer by half." The active soybean agents were also referred to as *phytoestrogens* because they counter cancer-inducing estrogen (female hormone), in much the same way as the synthetic drug Tamoxifen (a synthetic hormone) does. These substances are found in regular soybeans, tofu (soybean curd), soy milk, soy flour, and miso (soybean paste) sold at health food and Asian food stores.

Also this spring, *Dr. Rashida Karmali, Associate Professor of Nutrition, Rutgers University,*

announced findings that supplements of fish oil equal to what Japanese women commonly eat in fish, suppressed biological signs of developing cancer in breast-cancer-prone women.

For those with an egg allergy try *Tofu Scramble*, an all natural, eggless mix. Low in calories, no cholesterol, quick and easy to fix and incredibly good.

Vegetarian Health Society

DeliciousGravy

1/2 cup mashed tofu
1-1/2 cup water
Package *Hain's* Brown Gravy mix

Blend tofu with water in a pan, add Hain's brown gravy mix and cook on medium heat, stirring constantly, until thickened.

Good over browned, sliced tofu patties, mashed or baked potatoes and brown rice. It's a delicious brown gravy packed with protein. You can also saute sliced mushrooms and onions and add to the gravy one cup plain yogurt, and place over noodles as a Stroganoff.

Grilled Tofu Sandwiches

8 ounces drained, sliced tofu
2 tablespoons miso or tamari sauce
1 tablespoon expeller-pressed vegetable oil
4 slices whole grain bread
Green onions, finely chopped

Mix oil and miso together, spread on tofu slices. If you are using tamari, marinate for one hour in the sauce. Broil on an oiled cooking sheet, without turning, for about 8-10 minutes, until hot. Spread mayonnaise on bread, sprinkle with green onions, or add a thick slice of onion and tomato. Top with broiled tofu slices.

Variation: prepare open-faced sandwiches topped with sliced, sauteed mushrooms, and onions with barbecue sauce or Hain's prepared dry gravy mix.

No-Cook Fruit Pudding

2 cups tofu
2 cups fresh fruit or mashed bananas
1/4 cup expeller-pressed vegetable oil
1 tablespoon lemon juice
1 teaspoon vanilla
1 teaspoon barley malt sweetener or 1/2 cup honey (omit sweetener if using bananas, sweetener to taste).

Blend all the ingredients in a blender or food processor, until smooth.

Chill for a couple of hours in a pie shell, may use crumbled cookies or graham crackers on bottom or place in pudding cups. Top with sliced fresh strawberries or fruit of your choice.

Tofu Mayonnaise

6 ounces of drained tofu, patted dry
1 tablespoon of lemon juice
2 tablespoons canola or safflower oil
1/2 teaspoon sea salt *(optional)*
Puree all ingredients until smooth.

Variation: add pickle relish, fennel, chopped onion, a dash of horseradish, or fresh-grated horseradish. You now have a tasty sauce. Tofu mayonnaise has 1,422 fewer calories, 15 grams more protein, and 165 grams less fat than regular mayonnaise.

Creamy Italian Dressing

Combine in blender:
1/2 pound drained tofu
4 tablespoons virgin olive oil
2 tablespoons apple cider vinegar
1 teaspoon sea salt or Spike seasoning
1/2 teaspoon dried onion flakes or diced fresh
   onion *(optional)*
Fold in:
4 cloves garlic, minced or 1/2 teaspoon garlic
   powder (not garlic salt)
2 tablespoons honey or sweet pickle relish
1 teaspoon Italian seasoning or 1 pack Hain's
   Italian seasoning mix
1/4 teaspoon barley malt sweetener *(optional)*

Cucumber Tomato Salad

3 cups sliced tomato
4 cups cucumber, sliced
1/2 large onion, sliced
1 cup celery, sliced
1/2 cup chopped parsley or 1 tbls. dried parsley

Mix together.
Dressing:
1/2 pound drained tofu, mashed
3 tablespoon lime or lemon juice
2 tablespoons olive oil
1 teaspoon barley malt sweetener or your choice
1/2 teaspoon Spike or a dash of sea salt
1 clove minced garlic
1/4 teaspoon cayenne pepper *(optional)*

Blend together until smooth. Mix together the dressing and vegetables. Serve chilled.

Cottage Tofu Salad

1 pound drained tofu, crumbled
1 tablespoon fresh parsley, chopped
1-1/2 teaspoon dried chives
1/4 teaspoon dill weed

Blend until smooth and creamy:
1/2 cup of the above tofu
2 tablespoons olive oil
1-1/2 teaspoons apple cider vinegar
1-1/2 teaspoons lemon juice
1 teaspoon sea salt

Pour this over the crumbled tofu mixture and mix. Serve as a sandwich spread or on a bed of lettuce and tomato as a salad.

Tofu Whipped Cream

1 pound soft tofu
1/4 cup expeller-pressed vegetable oil
4 tablespoons honey
1/2 tablespoon lemon juice
1/2 teaspoon vanilla

Blend until light and fluffy. Chill.

Tofu Whipped Cream II

2 firm cakes, drained tofu, patted dry
6 ounces soy or cow's milk
6 tablespoons rice or barley malt syrup or
   honey

Mix tofu, soy milk, and sweetener in blender until soft peaks develop. Chill until ready to serve as whipped cream topping, for fresh fruits or pies.

Scrambled Tofu

A fast breakfast, or a quick hot protein dish for any meal.

1 tablespoon expeller-pressed vegetable oil
1/2 cup chopped onion
1/2 cup chopped green pepper
1/2 cup sliced mushrooms
Saute and add:
1 pound drained, crumbled tofu
1 tablespoon tamari
1/4 teaspoon Spike or a dash of sea salt
1 teaspoon basil
1/4 teaspoon garlic powder

Saute until tofu starts to brown. Serve hot with whole grain toast.

Tofu and Broccoli in Garlic Sauce

2 pounds cubed tofu
1/2 cup tamari or soy sauce
1/2 pound fresh sliced mushrooms
1 pound broccoli florets
3 cloves garlic, crushed
1 tablespoon prepared mustard
3 tablespoons honey
1/2 chopped sweet red pepper
1/4 teaspoon ginger or 1 teaspoon fresh ginger,
   peeled and grated

Marinate the tofu in tamari, turning occasionally. Mix together and set aside: 2 cups boiling water with 2 cubes vegetable bouillon or 1 tablespoon miso.

Drain the tofu, save the liquid. Brown both sides of the tofu in 3 tablespoons olive oil. Remove when done. Saute onions and mushrooms until soft, in 1 tablespoon olive oil. Stir together garlic, miso mixture, mustard, honey, red pepper, and ginger. Add to sauteed vegetables. Add tofu and reserve liquid. Simmer over medium heat for 1 minute. Add broccoli. Simmer 3 more minutes, remove from heat and let sit for 5 minutes. Serve over brown rice or noodles.

Tofu recipes from Tofu Rella by Sharon.

Food from the Soybean

Miso	Soybeans fermented into a paste, excellent for seasonings, a meaty taste.
Natto	A bacterially fermented soybean.
Soy Flour	Soybeans ground into flour, substitute by using for part of the wheat flour in a recipe and to increase protein content.
Soy Grits	The oil is extracted from the soybeans, the residue is coarsely ground.
Soy Milk	A liquid extracted from the soybean and made to taste like milk.
Soy Oil	The oil is extracted from the bean.
Tamari	Naturally aged and fermented soy sauce.
Tempeh	A mold-fermented soy patty.
Tofu	Curdled soy milk, using a mineral coagulant, and pressed into a cake.

Cool, Clear & Clean

Water

As we age we loose our desire for thirst. This is one reason why we should make it a habit to drink water even when we are not thirsty. We cannot stress enough how important drinking 8 or more glasses of quality water a day can be. You would probably eliminate bowel, bladder problems, and headaches by drinking water. Toxins build up in the system causing headaches, if not enough water is consumed to flush these toxins out. The bladder functions better with plenty of water. Anxiety attacks, food tolerance reactions, burning in the stomach from too much acid, headaches, colitis pain, hot flashes, and many other disorders have been relieved by drinking a full glass of water. This flushes the system, relieving these symptoms quicker than any herb, drug, or food. Nothing on our planet can take the place of quality water.

An epidimec of chronic fatigue syndrome (CFS) is on the rise and it is one of the disorders that requires at least 8 glasses of water daily. Toxins and chemicals that cause muscle aches, headaches, and extreme fatigue, very common complaints, are flushed out by water. We would poison ourselves with our own metabolic waste products and toxins without water. The kidneys remove wastes like uric acid, urea, and lactic acid that must be dissolved in water. If not enough water is present, these substances are not removed effectively, and may cause damage to the kidneys. Digestion and metabolism also rely on water for certain enzymatic and chemical reactions in the body. Water carries nutrients and oxygen to cells through the blood, and regulates body temperature through persperation. Water is even more important if you have arthritis, musculoskeletal problems or are athletic, as it lubricates the joints. Is this too simple to be true? When will man realize the simple things that God created are always our best medicine. Man has gotten away from the natural substances provided for healing. If the system could profit from charging a high price for water as an aid in healing, they would.

Man is still unaware of the benefits of water. The aging process can be slowed down by consuming water. Arthritis, kidney stones, constipation, arteriosclerosis, obesity, glaucoma, cataracts, diabetes, hypoglycemia, and many other diseases can be prevented and/or improved by consuming quality water. Just give it a try and you will feel the difference quickly. It is not expensive and certainly worth trying, but you must drink 8-10 glasses of water daily.

We strongly believe quality water is the best treatment for all disorders on our planet. The average amount of water in a human body is 65%, but varies considerably from person to person and even from one body part to another. The lowering of the water content in the blood triggers the hypothalamus, which is the brain's thirst center, to send out the demand for a drink.

As inorganic minerals, mainly from faucet drinking water, enter the bloodstream, traces of these minerals adhere to the artery walls. Cholesterol sticks to them, causing the arteries to narrow risking possible blockage. Other deposits from inorganic minerals occur where blood flow is slowest including:

• joints	• arthritis
• small veins	• varicose
• small arteries	• hardening
• inner ear	• hearing loss
• eye lens	• cataracts
• lungs	• emphysema

Peter F. Morgan-Good News About Drinking Water

Fresh clean air and quality fresh foods that add fiber to the diet are the other important things that will prevent and cure almost all disease. Without air, life would cease in 6-10 minutes. Without water life would end in 3-5 days, but man can go without food for 30-40 days. **WATER-WATER-WATER**, fresh air and quality fresh foods are the most important ingredients for a long, healthy disease-free life. In the Hunza Valley, people who live well into their 100s raise their fruits and vegetables in organic soil and eat most of their foods raw. These fruits and vegetables are 90% naturally purified water.

183

Stress release, daily exercise, and a positive mind-set are also important. Since there are so many things to avoid in our world today, heed the revelations above and avoid everything else, and you have the secrets to a healthy life.

A drop in your body's water content is actually reflected as a decline in a blood volume. This causes a slight rise in the concentration of sodium in blood. These changes quickly trigger a sensation of thirst. People often consume only enough liquid to quench a dry or parched throat but not enough to cover all their water loss. You can become dehydrated quickly, as an adult you have a lower percentage of reserve body water than when you were younger. Drink more water than you think you need.

There are several kinds of water: hard, boiled, soft, filtered, well, faucet, mineral, deionized and distilled. There is only one water that is clean, steam-distilled water. With minerals added, this is as perfect as we can get in today's polluted world.

Distillation is the process of converting liquids into a vapor state by heating. The vapor cools and is condensed back into a liquid and stored. This removes solids and other impurities, producing pure drinking water. Steam-distilled water is preferred (be sure the bottle states steamed), with Trace Mineral Drops from Utah's great Salt Lake by *Trace Mineral Research*, added back to the water. The concentrated Trace Mineral Drops are inexpensive and can be purchased at a health food store. No other substance on our planet does so much to keep us healthy and get us well as water does, and the price is right. **Boiling** water does not work the same because all the harmful chemicals are left concentrated in the water.

Faucet water is full of harmful chemicals and inorganic minerals that the body cannot use. Faucet water is not clean or pure enough for consumption. Parkinson's disease sufferers are more likely to have drunk well water and lived in rural areas than people without the disease. Risk of Parkinson's may be linked to an overload of environmental toxins. *William Koller, M.D., Neurologist at the University of Kansas*, believes toxins are the cause of this disease, but which toxins specifically are unknown.

More than 20,000 cases of giardiasis, caused by an intestinal parasite from drinking water, have been reported in the United States.

More than one-third of all community water systems have been cited for failure to meet the EPA's water safety standards. **More than 700 contaminants have been found in water supplies nationwide and 200 are toxic chemicals**. The EPA only monitors 38.

Thirteen million Americans were exposed to potentially dangerous contaminants because 36,000 public water supplies were in violation of the federal water standards in 1987.

Pesticides and agricultural chemicals invade our nation's water supply, as well. **Well** water near an agricultural area should be tested for nitrates that can cause a serious blood disorder in infants and adults. Nitrates are present when nitrogen in chemical fertilizers and manure work down into the soil and eventually into the water that feeds the local wells.

Radon, a gas formed in the earth's crust, migrates in to water systems and may cause lung cancer. The EPA estimates 8 million Americans have high levels of radon in their water, which is then air-borne when the water is run in the home. The most likely place for radon to be present is in private wells and other underground water sources. Areas known to contain radon include: New Jersey, North Carolina, New England, and Arizona, but it's not limited to these areas alone.

Government agencies and environmental organizations have reported that lead is a potential hazard and 42 million Americans (1 in 6), are drinking water contaminated with high levels of lead. Water testing is advised especially if the household includes children under age 6, pregnant woman or a woman likely to become pregnant. Small children and fetuses are vulnerable to the brain damaging effects of lead. Lead may also cause liver and kidney problems, and harm the cardiovascular, immune, and gastrointestinal systems of the body.

Water is essential for breathing, the lungs must be moistened by water to facilitate oxygen intake and carbon dioxide excretion. Approximately one pint of liquid is lost each day from exhaling. If not enough water is taken in for fluid balance, every body function could be impaired. The more you exercise, the more water must be consumed to keep your body's water level in balance.

Excess body fat, poor muscle tone, digestive problems, organ malfunction, joint and muscle soreness and water retention may be due to not enough water intake. The way to eliminate fluid retention is to drink more water. Proper water intake is the answer to weight loss or the body cannot metabolize fat and water is retained, which adds to one's weight, if not enough water is consumed.

Spring water flows from the earth on its own from a particular spot, then it's bottled near that source. There are no added or deleted minerals.

Purified or distilled water is completely demineralized. This involves boiling the water, converting it to steam, and then condensing it. Metals including lead, cadmium, mercury, aluminum, and other toxins are removed.

Mineral water is basically any water that is not distilled. It contains at least 500 parts per million total dissolved solids. The more minerals or solids, the stronger the taste.

Reverse osmosis forces the water through a semipermeable membrane while charged particles and larger molecules are repelled in this high-tech system of purifying water. It is the best system for treating water that is brackish (high in salt), high in nitrates, and loaded with inorganic heavy metals such as iron and lead.

Club soda is water that's been artificially carbonated with carbon dioxide and contains added minerals and salts.

Seltzer water also has added carbon dioxide, but no salts.

Grapefruit seed extract is ideal as a safe and simple way to disinfect drinking water when camping, back packing or in any emergency situation where safe drinking water is not obtainable, and boiling is not possible.

Available water should first be filtered, (at the least, let suspended water particles settle). Retain the clear water and add 10 drops of grapefruit seed extract per each gallon of water. Shake or stir vigorously and let sit for a few minutes. A slightly bitter taste may be noticed. This is just the inherit taste of the grapefruit seed extract.

Safe and easy to carry with you, grapefruit seed extract is actually a first aid in many uses.

The Third Opinion Report, June 1990, pg.7

Testing Your Tap Water

The Environmental Protection Agency supplies a phone number to help you locate the office or lab near your area that does certified water testing. Call the EPA's toll-free number:

Safe Drinking Water Hotline 1-800-426-4971

A number of labs send a self-addressed container that allows you to put the filled bottle into a local mailbox. Tests cost start as low as $15 to $20 a tap and results are usually available in 2-3 weeks.

National Testing Labs 1-800-458-3330
Suburban Water Testing Labs 1-800-433-6595
Water Test 1-800-426-8378

There are EPA "Recommended Maximum Contaminant Levels." To recieve information on this and other educational material, contact:

National Sanitation Foundation
P.O. Box 1468
Ann Arbor, MI 48106
313-769-8010

Water Quality Association
4151 Naperville Road
Lisle, IL 60532
708-505-0160

Other water treatment systems that remove various contaminants include distillers, water softeners, and ultraviolet treatment units. Before you purchase one of these units, write or call the National Sanitation Foundation listed above. This nonprofit testing and certification organization verifies manufacturer's claims, certifies that the materials used are non-toxic and structurally sound. Periodic unannounced audits of products are conducted to insure compliance with standards.

For a comparison of various water filtering systems for in-home use, please refer to the chart on the next page.

Water Filter Comparisons

Filter Type	Cost	How They Work	What They Reduce
Activated Carbon	$20-$60 for faucet or pour-through model $89-$200 for countertop $75-$600 for under sink $499-$1,250 for whole house system	Water is filtered through a carbon trap that absorbs the contaminants.	Chlorine, color, herbicides, lead, hydrogen sulfide, turbidity, and volatile organic chemicals (VOCs)
Reverse Osmosis	$150-$250 for countertop $530-$1,500 for under sink	Forces pressurized water through a contamination-rejecting membrane; sends improved water to holding tank.	Arsenic, cadium, chromium, iron, chlorine, color, lead, giardia, giardia cysts, nitrate, radium, sulfate, turbidity
Distillation	$99-$995 for countertop model $599-$1,020 for free-standing unit $799-$4,500 for entire house system	Raises water temperature to boiling, leaving contaminants behind. Purified water vapor condensed to liquid.	Arsenic, cadmium, chromium, iron, lead, giardia cysts, nitrate, sulfate, and turbidity
Water Softener	$950-$3,500 for whole house system	Replaces calcium and magnesium with sodium to "soften" the water.	Calcium, iron, radium
Carbon Filtration	$25 for faucet mounted $300 and up for under counter systems	Passes water through carbon (charcoal or a solid carbon block) and captures contaminants. When carbon sites fill up the filter cartridge is replaced.	Bad taste, odors, chlorine, organic chemicals and pesticides

Your cooking and herb teas deserve pure water.

There are many good herbs that can be taken alone or in combination. A number of distributors, such as, *Celestial Seasonings, Inc., Alvita,* and *Select Harvest* offer herb teas in a variety of forms and flavors.

In addition, a specific blend of herbs, called Daily Detox, is now available; it is designed to detoxify the system and certain organs. This blend contains: yellow dock, milk thistle, burdock root, echinacea, dandelion, fenugreek, sarsaparilla, ginger, cascara sagranda, red clover and hibiscus, which are combined to detoxify the bowels, blood, liver, skin, kidneys and lungs.

Yogurt

Also known as kefir, yahourt, leban, and acidophilus milk.

Plain yogurt is basically milk with the "friendly bacteria" added. These bacteria produce lactase, an enzyme, that attacks the natural milk sugar lactose, producing lactic acid that curdles the milk and gives yogurt its tart flavor.

Yogurt is nutritionally superior to milk in many different ways. Each eight-ounce serving contains 30-45% of your daily calcium requirement. Yogurt has more digestible milk protein than milk. Even those who cannot tolerate milk because they lack the enzyme to break down lactose can eat yogurt without discomfort. Yogurt is an outstanding source of protein, calcium, potassium, phosphorus, vitamin B-6, B-12, niacin, and folic acid. It contains just as much potassium as a banana does. The *Long Island Jewish Medical Center* reports that eating a cup of yogurt a day can significantly cut the incidence of **vaginal yeast infections**. The yogurt used in the study contained live cultures of lactobacillus acidophilus.

Also, yogurt has been found to boost the **immune function** of animal and human cells, causing these cells to make more antibodies and other disease fighting cells. Yogurt fights infections with two separate mechanisms, boosting the immune system and killing off harmful bacteria.

Yogurt contains high levels of natural fatty hormonal substances called prostaglandins E2 that are known to antagonize hormones. These substances also protect the lining of the **stomach** from toxins. Another benefit derived from yogurt is its ability to lower blood cholesterol. As a result there are few foods that have this many healthful benefits.

According to the *Food and Drug Administra-*tion, each 110 grams of non-fat yogurt contains less than 0.5 grams of milk fat, and low-fat yogurt contains between 0.5-2.0 grams of milk fat, while whole milk yogurt has approximately 3.5 grams of fat per 100 grams. An eight ounce (1 cup) serving of skim non-fat yogurt contains only 110 calories, a very healthful addition to any diet.

Despite its low fat content not all yogurts are equal. Yogurt that is good for you must be sugar-free. Yogurt produced by heat processing is required by the FDA to be labeled "heat-treated" after culturing. Manufacturers are also required to add either lactobacillus bulgaricus or steptococcus thermophilus bacteria, but are not required to list if these cultures are living or active. Some makers heat the yogurt to add tartness and extend the shelf life of the product. Destroying most of the active cultures (friendly bacteria), and the healthy benefits. Make sure the label reads "active yogurt cultures." "living yogurt cultures" or "contains active cultures." Remember to purchase "live" yogurt that does not contain added sugars, preservatives, or thickeners.

Lactobacillus acidophilus is not destroyed by the acidic gastric juices of the stomach, unlike two other forms of bacteria used for yogurt. The lactobacillus acidophilus resides on the intestinal walls where it can destroy disease-causing bacteria, providing a deadly environment for salmonella, listeria, and other forms of bacteria that cause **food poisoning**. Research carried out in Japan and the United States shows that you can prevent and sometimes cure diarrhea and dysentery with yogurt and it is particularly effective for **infant diarrhea**. Children given yogurt have also been shown to have greater resistance to **flu** infections.

Dr. Khem Shami, from the University of Nebraska, finds yogurt to be more effective as a preventative than a cure for diarrhea and dysentery. He says, "By ingesting lactobacilli in food form after diarrheal stress, one can reduce diarrheal incidence."

> **For vegans, there are many soy yogurts on the market that can be found in health food stores.**

There is evidence that yogurt may help prevent **cancer**, primarily in the **colon**. A top researcher in Boston has found that acidophilus culture can help suppress activity in the colon that converts harmless chemicals into carcinogenic agents. *In 1986, the Journal of the National Cancer Institute* published a French study that found women who ate high levels of dairy fat, like that in cheese, had a higher risk of **breast cancer**. Through the same study it was found that those who ate the most yogurt had the least risk.

> If you have a severe allergy to milk products, even yogurt, there is a soy yogurt and non-dairy acidophilus. This is particulary important if you have the yeast infection, candidiasis, or if you are on antibiotics. The acidophilus bacteria is a natural enemy to yeast.

The benefits from homemade yogurt are numerous. It aids in **neutralizing uric acid** in the body. It helps prevent and combat **digestive tract infections**. Live yogurt cultures flourish in the digestive tract and have a natural antibiotic effect. Yogurt is essential in our world of excessive antibiotic treatments that destroy the "friendly bacteria" in the body. Many doctors recommend acidophilus yogurt for patients on antibiotics; it replenishes the good bacteria and helps prevent diarrhea and yeast infections, which then require more antibiotics and set up a reoccuring cycle. Antibiotics disrupt the balance of good and bad bacteria, killing off the helpful organisms and allowing the others to prevail. Yogurt can also help boost the **immune system**, an effect observed in animal studies. Some scientists believe that live yogurt cultures help lower **cholesterol** levels in the body and live yogurt has been used to treat certain cancers.

The University of Nebraska conducted research with mice that showed yogurt bacteria slowed the growth of bacteria as much as 75%. The bacteria contained in active yogurt cultures suppresses the

> When taking antibiotics, wait at least an hour before eating yogurt or any other dairy product. The calcium in yogurt and other dairy products may interfere with the drug's actions.

growth of deadly **cancer** cells. These effects are found only in fresh yogurt. The bacteria in frozen yogurt do not have the same effect on cancer.

In Poland, **bowel cancer** patients were fed a quart of yogurt every day for two months. This resulted in a reduction of cancer in ten of the patients. The bacteria in yogurt can also lower **cholesterol** levels in the blood, which will reduce the chance of strokes and heart attacks. The bacteria helps fight **dysentery, cholera, diarrhea,** and **other infections**.

> The National Cancer Institute has determined that malignant tumors shrink in patients who consumed a steady diet of yogurt. Studies at the *Harvard Medical School and the University of Chicago Medical School* show that yogurt is especially effective against vaginal cancer.

The enzymes in yogurt supress the putrefactive organisms in incompletely digested foods, such as those seen in food **allergies**. Yogurt enzymes also prevent gas and bloating. The eldery, with insufficient digestive enzymes, need to supplement their diets with plain yogurt.

To reduce calories and fat use 1/2 mayonnaise and 1/2 plain yogurt for salad dressing, potato salad, bean salad, cole slaw, pasta salads, tuna and other sandwiches. Plain yogurt makes a good substitute in recipes calling for sour cream and is great for baked potatoes. Plain yogurt also can be substituted for buttermilk in waffles, pancakes, breads, muffins, biscuits, and in many other food dishes. Experiment and try your own recipes. Do not substitute yogurt in cakes without adjusting the amount of leavening.

Dennis Savaiano, a *nutrition Professor at the University of Minnesota,* conducted a study of 16 lactose-intolerant men. Frozen yogurt caused gas and bloating due to the **lactose intolerance**. Frozen yogurt is often made by small companies that buy commercial yogurt and then pasteurize it. When the yogurt is pasteurized a second time or frozen, the beneficial bacteria that produce lactase are killed. Frozen yogurt is generally high in fat and has added sugar. Yogurt advertised as low-fat and no-sugar may be loaded with chemicals. Plain yogurt is the most digestible form.

188

Yogurt is very easy to make at home. Fresh yogurt contains bulgaricus and thermophilus cultures in high amounts, it tastes smooth and has a mild, non-tangy flavor.

Making your own yogurt

Yogurt will have a soft consistency, if skim milk, low-fat or non-fat milk is used. If the yogurt is too soft, add 1/3-1/2 cup of non-fat dry milk in powder form directly to your quart of milk before heating it. This will make your yogurt not only thicker but creamier. The longer the yogurt remains in the machine the firmer and more tart it will become and separation of curd and whey may occur.

Only unpasteurized, unflavored yogurt contains the live culture. Make sure your yogurt starter is fresh with an expiration date months ahead. If you use commercial yogurt as your starter, make sure the product has not been entirely pasteurized to prolong the shelf life.

• Heating the milk for too long or on too high a temperature will produce a poor quality yogurt

• Flavor yogurt after several hours of refrigeration or right before eating

• Watery substances on the top of your yogurt after refrigeration may be mixed in or poured off

The company, *Yogurt Plus*, will soon be filling the market with a new idea for yogurt. Their yogurt is filled with vegetables! Varieties will include cucumber and mixed vegetables with spices and herbs. All varities contain only 2 grams of fat.

Add yogurt to fruit snacks. For a refreshing healing beverage, replace ice cream shakes with mashed bananas and fresh berries in yogurt. Children love it!

Yogurt Flavors

Add 1 tablespoon of 1 or more of these to 8 ounces of fresh yogurt:

Frozen juice concentrate --apple, orange, pine apple or your favorite
Dietetic or all fruit jam, preserves, or jelly
Juice nectar -- pear, apricot, or peach
Molasses or maple syrup
Applesauce with a dash of cinnamon and raisins
Natural cereal
Honey with a teaspoon of vanilla
Barley malt sweetener to taste

Yogurt Hints

(1) Always keep 4 tablespoons of plain yogurt set back for the next batch. Yogurt takes 8-10 hours to develop with yogurt culture, only 3-5 hours using some of the fresh yogurt from your last batch. The freeze-dried yogurt starter, *Yogourmet* makes a firm yogurt and is found in health food stores.

(2) Never use an electric mixer. If the yogurt turns out too liquid because the culture used in the beginning were not strong enough or there were antibiotics in the milk, then try using this liquid yogurt for better results.

(3) Your health food store should carry yogurt thermometers, needed for accurate temperature control, as well as automatic yogurt makers. Some automatic yogurt makers are very inexpensive.

(4) When ready to place in jars, **fill to the rim** before placing in the refrigerator, no room for excess air will preserve the yogurt for a longer period of time. Strain the yogurt, before refrigeration, through a white cotton cloth for thicker and smoother yogurt.

(5) If you must purchase yogurt, read labels carefully and buy the ones that contain no sugar. Be sure the label states "live cultures." Purchase only plain low-fat yogurt that has an expiration date at least 10 days ahead on the carton. If there is no date do not purchase. To increase the benefits of yogurt, mix in 2 capsules of acidophilus before consuming.

Non-Dairy Yogurt

Of special intrest to vegans and those with dairy allergies, yogurts made from soy milk are getting better all the time. White Waves Dairyless, made by *White Wave, Inc.*, Boulder Colorado is the tastiest and creamiest non-dairy yogurt. The product is sweetened with juices and comes in a variety of flavors. Soy Latte is a non-dairy yogurt sweetened with honey, it also comes in several fruit flavors.

189

Yogurt Recipes

Yogurt Dressing

The following is good as a dressing for salads, such as potato, bean and coleslaw.
   1/2 cup yogurt
   1/2 cup soy or eggless mayonnaise
   Lemon juice or vinegar to taste
   Barley malt sweetener to taste
   1 tablespoon chili sauce or hot sauce
   1 finely mashed clove garlic

Mix all together
Good as a dip with nachos.

Mashed Low-Fat Potatoes

6 large baking potatoes
1 cup plain low-fat homemade yogurt
Dash of Spike seasoning *(optional)* or sea salt
Chopped chives

Scrub and boil potatoes in water until tender, then drain. Mash potatoes until smooth, add yogurt and season with Spike to your liking. Top with more yogurt and chives or chopped parsley. Reheat in oven.

Fresh-Fruit Yogurt

1 quart yogurt
2 slices canned or fresh pineapple
4 tablespoons unsweetened pineapple preserves

Pour yogurt into container, add preserves. Blend in chopped pineapples and refrigerate about an hour. You may use any kind of fresh fruit, and omit the preserves for less calories.

Vegetable Dip

Steam 3 carrots, mash and mix with one pint of yogurt. Serve with raw vegetables. This is a healing summer snack.

Yogurt Avocado Dressings

Good for low blood-sugar.

1 cup yogurt
1 mashed avocado
1/2 teaspoon finely mashed clove garlic or
   sprinkle of garlic powder
1 teaspoon fresh lemon juice
Dash of Spike seasoning *(optional)*

Mash the avocado in a small bowl, add the other ingredients and beat until thick. Serve over crisp lettuce or use as a dip. Also good on baked potatoes.

Fruit Sherbet

2 cups yogurt
1 small can unsweetened frozen concentrated
   fruit juice
2 teaspoons vanilla *(optional)*

Mix all ingredients together, place in a freezer tray and freeze. Serve topped with fresh fruit.

Health Drink

Juice three medium carrots. Add to one pint sugar-free plain low-fat yogurt and mix

Cool Fruit Salad

Great for digestive disorders.

3 cups fresh pineapple
1 cup melon balls
1 cup diced papaya or fresh peaches
3 cups yogurt
3 tablespoons honey or sweetener of your choice
2 cups sliced strawberries
4 sprigs fresh mint (*optional*)

Cut pineapple in quarters, remove core, cut pineapple from shell and cube. Refrigerate shell until serving time. Stir together 1 cup of pineapple with mango and papaya. Chill. Spoon 1/3 cup yogurt in each pineapple shell, cover with mixed fruit. Spoon a layer of the remaining honey-sweetened yogurt on top, cover with sliced strawberries. Garnish with whole strawberries and a sprig of mint.

Currant Nut Dessert

High in the essential fatty acids found in walnuts or pecans.

1 cup yogurt
1/4 cup currants or raisins
1/4 cup chopped raw walnuts or pecans
1 teaspoon vanilla
1 pinch cinnamon
Touch of barley malt sweetener (*optional*)

Mix ingredients and chill.

A Bit of Yogurt Culture

In the Soviet Republics of Georgia and Armenia there are herdsmen who live to be more than 120 years old. They eat large quantities of yogurt every day, and the incidence of cancer in this group is very low.

Fresh Cucumbers in Yogurt

Good for the dieter.

4 cucumbers
2 cups yogurt
1 tablespoon finely chopped chives or onion
Dash of Spike seasoning or sea salt
2 tablespoons red pepper (*optional*)

Split peeled cucumbers lengthwise, scoop out seeds, slice very thin. Sprinkle with salt, blend, and chill for one hour. Press cucumbers between dry towels until free of water. Return to bowl, add yogurt, and seasoning. Blend well. Sprinkle with chives.

Yogurt Cream Cheese

A low-fat substitute for cream cheese and sour cream.

Line a strainer with three layers of cheesecloth and fill with a quart of homemade nonfat plain yogurt. Place in a bowl in the refrigerator to drain overnight. The next morning you will have a creamy, textured cheese to use as you would cream cheese. Good mixed with *Hain's* Dry Onion Soup Mix as a dip or on top of baked potatoes. Also use this creamy cheese mixed with fruit, chopped nuts, raisin, or herbs as a spread.

The Stopper

Good for diarrhea in infants and adults.

1 pint plain homemade yogurt
3 bananas
1 tablespoon ground flaxseed, rice or oat bran

Blend bananas and mix with yogurt and fiber. *Pureed carrots in place of the bananas works wonders also.*

191

Once you have tasted homemade yogurt you will never buy yogurt again. It is creamier, lighter, and is not tart. I love my homemade yogurt and make a gallon a week. I eat mine plain because I love the cool creamy taste. If using it for a health reason, consume it first thing in the morning and a couple hours after dinner. It works best on an empty stomach.

Homemade Yogurt

1 quart raw, skim, goat, cow, or 2% homogenized milk (*Use 1 cup 2% to 3 cups skim for a richer taste.*)
4 tablespoons unflavored, unpasteurized yogurt from your last batch
  (or a packaged yogurt culture, follow instructions on the package)
3-4 tablespoons non-instant, non-fat dried milk powder for a firmer yogurt (*optional*)

Make a paste from a small amount of milk and the milk powder, add to the rest of the milk. Put in a heavy pan over low heat. Scald the milk to the boiling point. **It should be steaming with bubbles on top, but not boiling.**
Your health food store carries yogurt thermometers and automatic yogurt makers.

Keep milk at 140-150° for 10 minutes to destroy any unwanted organisms in the milk. Remove from heat and let cool to 100° (lukewarm) or warm to the touch. Mix your yogurt culture into the milk. Make sure it is smooth and without lumps, do not beat but mix gently. Put into clean jars (scald them first) and cover. Keep the jars at 110°. *If kept too hot or too cold, it will not thicken.*

Places to Keep Yogurt at 110°

In a heavy skillet with a few inches of water
  over a pilot light.
In a preheated oven of 110° (use an oven
  thermometer).
An electric frying pan with the water as high
  as possible, kept on lowest heat.
Test with a thermometer before using.

When the yogurt is left in a yogurt maker too long (over-incubation) the whey and the curd will separate. The whey is a watery layer on top of the thick, solid layer, the curds. Once this separation has occured, it can not be reversed.

The yogurt will thicken more after it is refrigerated. One tablespoon of unsweetened gelatin can be added in place of dry milk for thicker yogurt and increased protein.

Proper Food Handling

Listeria bacteria do not change the taste or smell of a food. *CDC, FDA, FSIS,* and the *National Advisory Committee on Microbiological Criteria for Foods* (which includes food scientists from federal health agencies, universities, and private industry) have developed food handler advice for preventing listeriosis.

Although most people are at very low risk for listeriosis and other food-borne illnesses, they can be reduced by following these tips:
  • Keep raw and cooked foods separate when shopping and preparing, cooking and storing foods or bacteria
  in juices from raw meat, poultry or fish might contaminate a cooked food
  • Wash hands, knives, and cutting boards after handling uncooked foods
  • Wash raw vegetables thoroughly before eating
  • Thoroughly cook and reheat all foods of animal origin, including eggs
  • Read and follow label instructions to "keep refrigerated" and "use by" a certain date
  • Keep your refrigerator clean and the temperature at 34F to 40F

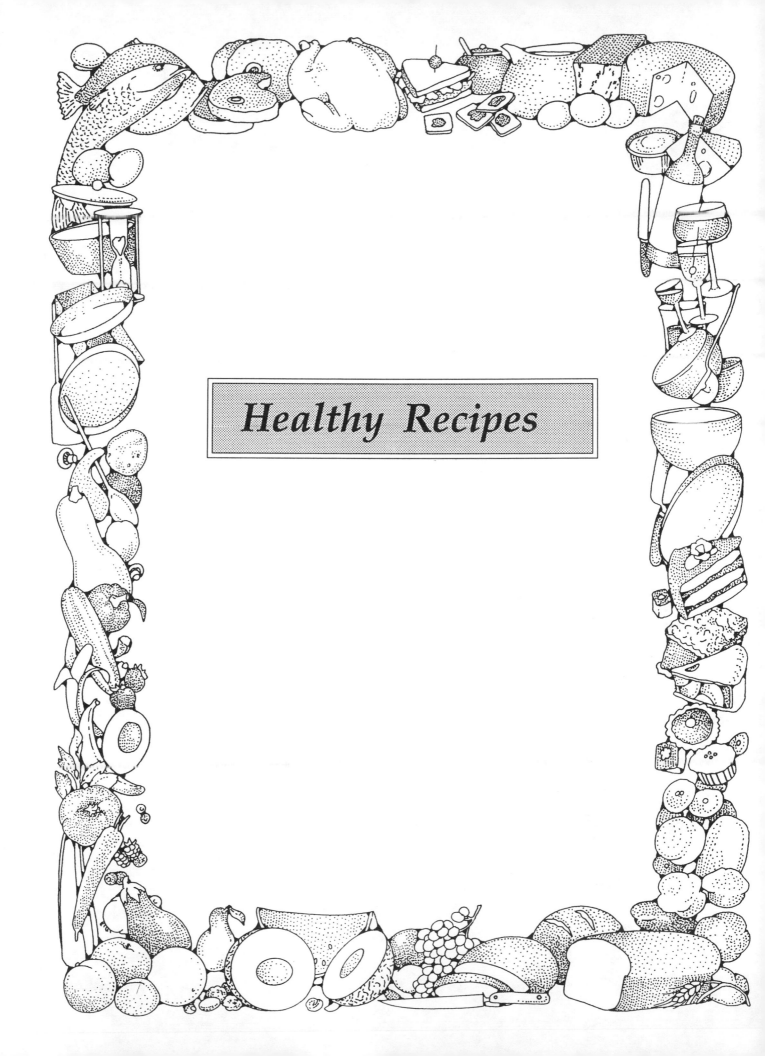

Healthy Recipes

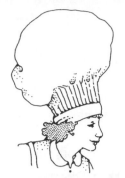

Hints for the Cook

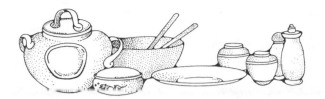

Use vegetable broth or bouillon for sauteing in place of oil.

When browning onions or mushrooms, try using tamari sauce instead of oil or butter, if you are on a fat-free diet. The flavor is excellent.

Add dry soup mix to cooking water before adding brown rice for a delicious flavor.

Thicken soups, gravies, and stews with potato slices or add cubed, fresh potatoes to the pot and as it cooks, the starch will thicken the liquid.

For greaseless gravy, pour pan drippings into a tall glass. The grease will rise to the top in minutes and can be easily removed.

Wash dirt and dust from the lids of cans and your can opener before you open them to remove bacteria.

Lay a large spoon or spatula across the top of a pot to prevent the contents from boiling over and splashing during cooking.

Do not use aluminum cookware. Some doctors believe **Alzheimer's disease** is caused by the accumulation of aluminum in the brain. Do not use coated pans. Cook with only stainless steel, iron, glass or Corningware®.

Use a glass or metal mixing bowl, not plastic, when beating egg whites. Plastic tends to retain grease, which can prevent whites from whipping.

Use only glass containers for storing herbs and spices. Some of the chemicals leach out into herbs and spices stored in plastic containers. The same applies to storing leftovers, use only glass containers.

Never keep spices close to the stove top, they lose their flavor and color from the heat.

When using herbs which are to be removed from broth after cooking, place them in a stainless steel tea ball or tie them in several layers of cheese cloth, attaching the tied ends to the pot handle.

Fresh herbs may be chopped and frozen for future use in cooked dishes. Use frozen, no need to defrost.

Parsley, onions, celery, and garlic go with just about everything, keep them on hand.

Grow fresh herbs all year in flower pots in your window sill.

To remove the skin of garlic before chopping, press the side of a knife or a bottle on the clove, the skin will split and is easily taken off.

Do not burn garlic, it will spoil the taste of the whole dish.

To avoid tears when cutting up onions, store them in the refrigerator for several hours. Chop the bottom of the bulb off last, limiting exposure to the irritating sulphur compounds.

Lemon effectively removes garlic and onion odors from the hands.

Submerge lemons in hot water 15 minutes before squeezing to yield almost twice the amount of juice.

Freeze fresh lemon juice in ice cube trays and store in plastic bags as cubes to add to herb teas and in cooking, on fish and any other way that fresh lemon would be used.

Frozen orange or grapefruit juices will have a fresh-squeezed flavor if you add the juice of two fresh oranges to the reconstituted frozen juice.

Do not peel vegetables or fruits. Eat the whole food. Use potatoes with skins on, even for potato salad.

Do not discard edible outer green leaves of vegetables such as cabbage, broccoli, and lettuce. Encourage your grocer to leave outer, green leaves on. The outer leaves have been kissed with sunlight and filled with vitamins and minerals. Avoid colorless celery and endive. Choose yellow turnips over white, dark green vegetables over light. Use sweet potatoes more frequently. A rich color in food is a sign of high vitamin content. Mix your colors to get a variety of nutrients.

Try cooking with more stems and leaves. Use some of the celery leaves, outer leaves of lettuce and cabbage.

Unflavored gelatin mixed with *Knudsen* Very Veggie Juice makes a good low calorie and low fat dressing for salads.

Improve the taste of a large can of tomato juice by pouring it into a glass bottle and adding one green onion and a stalk of celery cut into small pieces. After it stands for a while it tastes like the more expensive, already seasoned juice.

Freeze tomatoes whole for cooking. Skins will slip off easily when the tomatoes are defrosted.

When canning, use rubber gloves (the sort used to wash dishes with) to remove the skins from tomatoes and other vegetables or fruits that need their skins removed. The thick gloves will protect your hands from the heat and the textured surface on the fingers will make the task go much quicker.

If the stem of a cantaloupe is still attached or if the scar is jagged, it was taken from the vine too early. If the melon is fully ripe the stem scar will be smooth. Wash melons well before cutting, to avoid salmonella poisoning.

Peaches ripen quickly if you put them in a box covered with newspaper.

Store cheese in a tightly covered container with some sugar cubes, to prevent mold.

To soften hardened cheese, soak in a little yogurt.

Brush a little oil on a grater before you start grating cheese. the cheese will wash off easily.

Use a potato peeler to cut cheese into strips for salads and other garnishes.

Skinless turkey contains about 1/3 less fat than skinless chicken.

Debone turkey and chicken with a pair of kitchen scissors. It is much easier than working with a knife.

Chicken will be juicier if you use tongs to turn it during cooking. Using a fork will pierce the meat and let the juices run out.

Do not use the same cutting board for poultry or meat that you use for vegetables. **Salmonella poisoning can be transferred.** Arthritis has been thought to be connected to this food poison. Be careful with all canned foods. If the top is not tight or it bulges, do not use it.

Truss up poultry with unwaxed dental floss, it does not burn and is very strong.

Thaw frozen fish in milk. The milk draws out the frozen taste and provides a fresh-caught flavor.

Poached fish will be firmer and whiter if you add a bit of lemon juice to the cooking liquid.

In the place of bleached white flour, substitute whole wheat flour, rye flour, corn, oat, rice, or whole wheat pastry flour. Omit white flour from your diet. It loses most of the nutrients in the milling process and clogs up your system with excess mucus. Replace boxed processed cereals with granola, whole flaked, or cracked grain, cooked or raw.

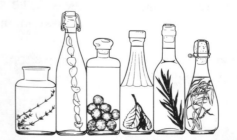

Store grains in a cool dry place. Place bay leaves in containers to deter insects, but learn to accept the fact that food grown without insecticides might have a few bugs. I would rather eat a healthy bug than poisonous chemicals. After many years in the retail business, I have never seen insects in foods with preservatives. They seem to always pick the organically grown grains over the ones where pesticides where used. We should pay more attention to insects and all life forms. They can tell us a lot. If you see a bug in your grains or flours, do not panic. It means you have a quality product worth eating.

White sugar, corn syrup, sucrose, dextrose, and glucose should be omitted from the diet and replaced with uncooked, unfiltered raw honey, using 1/2 cup honey instead of one cup sugar and reduce the liquid called for in the recipes by 1/4 cup. If no liquid is called for in the recipes, add three tablespoons of flour. Use pure maple syrup, unsulphured molasses, fruit juices, purees and juice concentrates. You can use apple juice concentrate (undiluted) in a lot of recipes where sweetener is called for, primarily in cobblers and pies, but it is also good in other dishes and baked goods.

Omit baking soda and replace it with low-sodium baking powder which is aluminum free, using two parts baking powder in place of one part soda.

If your cake recipe calls for oil and you have run out you can substitute an equal amount of mayonnaise.

Use liquid lecithin in place of oil in recipes that require the baking dish to be coated with oil to avoid sticking food. Lecithin is much healthier to use.

Use more sesame, sunflower and pumpkin seeds. Be careful when purchasing sesame seeds. Be sure they have been kept under refrigeration and have not become rancid. All nuts and seeds should be under refrigeration or nitrogen packed. You do not want to consume rancid nuts, seeds, or oils. They deplete the body of many vital nutrients and stress the liver.

Use a clean coffee grinder or a seed grinder for pulverizing seeds and nuts.

To avoid pasty pasta, allow at least 5 quarts of rapidly boiling water per pound of pasta.

When preparing pasta, throw chopped vegetables in the boiling water with the pasta, drain when done, add seasonings, and serve.

When done, run cooked spaghetti under hot, not cold water before draining, to prevent stickiness.

In place of white pasta, spaghetti, macaroni shells, noodles, and so on, use whole wheat pastas.

To regenerate your body or if your body is producing too much mucus, avoid sugar, salt, milk, and dairy products, red meat, white flour products, caffeine drinks, and eggs.

Never consume white distilled vinegar. Use pure apple cider vinegar or rice vinegar.

Instead of soda pop, use fruit juices, mineral water, herb teas, real soda pop made with fruit juice concentrates added to sparkling water sweetened with fructose or honey, or sodas found in health food stores. Omit coffee, Chinese teas and other caffeinated teas. Replace with herb teas and cereal beverages. Replace commercial peanut butter with your own fresh ground, or make sure it is unhydrogenated peanut butter which can be purchased at your health food store. The same applies to cashew, sesame, or almond butter. Buy unsulphured organically grown dried foods without preservatives, if possible.

To soften nut butters, add 1 teaspoon of hot water and stir.

Remember, in almost all recipes you can substitute unprocessed whole grain and natural sugars in place of white flour, white sugar, salt, etc. We recommend throwing out all the white processed products. Once you learn how to cook the dishes in this book you will want to take all your old recipe books and convert them to natural recipes (or give them away).

The foods that can be eaten plentifully are fresh fruits and vegetables, steamed vegetables, beans legumes, nuts (except peanuts), seeds, and whole grains. Soak whole grains overnight and lightly cook in the morning with a little honey or a bit of seasoning and herbs. The nutrients are not lost from boiling in this manner. Or pour boiling water into a Thermos[R] over your grain, place the lid on it and let it sit overnight; in the morning, your hot cereal will be ready to eat.

Things to remember for a quality diet:

1. Avoid white foods, except cauliflower, as much as possible.

2. Avoid stale food. Buy the freshest food your market has, shop on the days they receive the fresh produce. Or better yet, grow your own.

3. Eat raw food. Select and serve raw fruits and vegetables, once or twice a day.

4. Choose cooking methods carefully. Select cooking methods that will minimize vitamin and mineral loss. Avoid frying entirely, steam instead. Always remember that every cooking method has its faults and may destroy vitamins to a certain extent.

5. Undercook rather than overcook vegetables, except dried peas and beans. Vegetables taste better and keep their color when not overcooked and it saves nutrients.

6. Do not use soda when cooking vegetables. The use of soda destroys vitamins.

7. Save all cooking juices and water for soup stock, to use the nutrients dissolved in the water.

8. Cook in covered pots, not aluminum or coated pots.

9. Use as little water as possible and steam vegetables.

10. Avoid overcooking.

11. Avoid fried foods and processed foods.

12. Do not fry foods in hydrogenated oils.

13. Use foods in their natural state as much as possible.

14. Wash all melons before cutting, they may contain dangerous bacteria and mold.

15. Broiling and frying produce 50 times as many potential carcinogens as boiling or baking.

16. Frying increases the fat content in most foods. Fat is implicated in **colon, breast, and prostate cancers**.

17. Cured, smoked, and pickled foods are high in nitrites and nitrates, which react to produce *nitrosamines* during digestion. Consumption of these foods may increase the risk of **liver, stomach**, and **esophageal cancers**.

Nutrient Sources for Vegetarians

Vegetarians who eat no meat, fish, poultry, or dairy foods face the greatest risk of nutritional deficiency. Nutrients most likely to be lacking and some non-animal sources are:

- *vitamin B₁₂*--fortified soy milk and cereals
- *vitamin D*--fortified margarine and sunshine
- *calcium*--tofu, broccoli, seeds, nuts, kale, bok, choy, legumes (peas and beans), greens calcium-enriched grain products, and lime-processed tortillas
- *iron*--legumes, tofu, green leafy vegetables, dried fruit, whole grains, and iron fortified cereals and breads, especially whole-wheat (absorption is improved by vitamin C, found in citrus fruits and juices, tomatoes, strawberries, broccoli, peppers, dark-green leafy vegetables, and potatoes with skins)
- *zinc*--whole grains (especially the germ and bran), whole -wheat bread, legumes, nuts, and tofu.

As all plant foods--including fruit--contain some protein, by eating a variety of fruits, vegetables and grains, even vegans probably can get enough of this nutrient.

Combine legumes such as black-eyed peas, chickpeas, peas, peanuts, lentils, sprouts, and black, broad, kidney, lima, mung, navy, pea, and soy beans *with* grains such as rice, wheat, corn, rye, bulgar, oats, millet, barley, and buckwheat. There are also food protein analogs made to look like meats, such as hot dogs, sausage, and bacon available in your health food store.

Is Microwaving Safe?

There have been many concerns about microwaves since they have been on the market. Within the microwave are parts called heat susceptors. These are discs or strips that heat up and brown microwaved foods. The susceptors are a source of hazardous chemicals, and materials around them also break down in the intense heat creating more toxins that can get into the food.

The packaging of the food products to be used in the microwave must also be considered. Plastics, glasses, and metals can leach dangerous heat-activated elements into the foods. Plastic wrap specifically designed for microwave ovens for example, can be hazardous. One additive, diadipate (2-ethylhexyl), or DEHA was found by the *British Government* to leach into fatty foods at room temperature, as well as at cooking temperatures. Vegetables that had been cooked in containers with the plastic wrap as a covering were found to have low levels of DEHA, even when the wrap did not touch the food directly.

According to researchers in London, bacteria like salmonella and listeria can survive the cooking process in the microwave. These bacteria are especially likely to survive if the food is salted before it is cooked. The salt appears to prevent the microwaves from penetrating into the center of the food, by absorbing the microwave energy, and the resulting **cold spots** can harbor dangerous bacteria. The study, conducted at *Leeds University in England*, microwaved two dishes of mashed potatoes, one without salt, the other with high amounts of salt. **The core temperature of the dish with the salt was 64 degrees lower than that of the salt-free potatoes.** when the packaged food was cooked according to the

The researchers then cooked refrigerated dinners with 200-1000 mg. of salt added, and they found that when packaged food was cooked according to the instructions centers did not become hot enough to kill the bacteria.

To avoid cold spots when cooking with a microwave, be sure to cover the food you are cooking, but not with plastic wrap. Use a paper towel or paper plate over the food or the specially designed lids that come with microwave cooking dishes. Put a little water on the dish and arrange the food to be of uniform density, then cover and cook. The cover will hold in the steam killing any bacteria. Rotate and stir the food. In all ovens there are areas that do not get strong microwaves. If the food is stirred up it will not remain in one of those areas. If you leave the food in the microwave a few minutes after the cooking is completed it will continue cooking. The heat will continue to spread throughout the food. When heating leftovers, heat them up on medium-high or high heat. This will be hot enough to kill bacteria. Warming them only to eating temperature is not hot enough. Make sure they are steamy and hot, then let them cool down to eating temperature. Cutting the food into small pieces also will help the microwaves to penetrate the food most effectively. This will aid in cooking the food completely and killing the bacteria. Debone meats when cooking them in the microwave. The bone can impede the cooking process of the meat around it.

Poultry should not be cooked in microwave ovens. The meat may not get fully cooked, thus allowing dangerous bacteria to survive. We don't recommend cooking any type of meat in a microwave oven. Red meat is also highly contaminated with bacteria. Meat should always be thoroughly cooked. *We use our microwave only for heating leftovers.*

MSG
Monosodium Glutamate

MSG (monosodium glutamate), as *George Schwartz,* the eminent crusading physician has emphasized, could be responsible for ailments seemingly far removed from digestive distress. He contends that it has been **implicated in damage to the central nervous system, endocrine organ disorders, cardiac distress, and illness in other parts of the body.**

Conventional wisdom used to suggest that MSG was found only in Chinese foods and canned soups, but *Alfred Scopp, of the Northern California Headache Clinic* warns that, " MSG has spread to soups, sauces and salad dressings in restaurants, as well as many canned, frozen and prepared foods found in local supermarkets. Worse still, MSG masquerades under a variety of names, such as hydrolyzed vegetable protein, hydrolyzed plant protein, natural flavor and Kombu extract ," *The Edell Health Letter,* Vol. 10, No. 19, October 1991.

It is not easy to avoid MSG when it shows up in so many different foods under many different names. MSG and its derivatives, hydrolyzed proteins and autolyzed yeast, have no nutritional value or preservative value. They are used solely to enhance food flavors. Food companies use MSG to flavor, to hide unwelcome tastes, and to cover inferior ingredients used in products.

One form of MSG is autolyzed yeast. Unfortunately, the label of a product containing this ingredient can list it as "yeast extract" or "natural flavoring." Small comfort for the uninformed consumer who is also sensitive to MSG. When autolyzed yeast and hydrolyzed protein are listed on a label of a product as flavorings, their protein source need not be identified.

Hydrolyzed protein is a natural flavoring from animal blood or other decaying protein sources. This substance is then subjected to acid hydrolysis, normally concentrated hydrochloric acid, at temperatures from 200-220° Farenheit for 4-6 hours. Sodium hydroxide (which is sold commercially as Drano) is then added to neutralize the solution.

"Reported effects from MSG ingestion include **headaches, nausea, diarrhea, mood changes, sleep problems, flushing of the skin, excessive sweating, chest pain, facial pressure, and hyperactivity**. People with asthma, those susceptible to migraines, infants, and children are more likely to be sensitive to synthetic MSG and can become hyperactive or develop learning disorders, *Bonnie Liebman , Let's Live,* April 1992.

Other sources of MSG include hydrolyzed milk proteins that may be labeled as sodium caseinate or calcium caseinate. These additives are often found in frozen dairy products, like ice cream and yogurt, without being identified. They can also be found in hot chocolate mixes, breads, and processed meats. **MSG should be avoided by nursing mothers and their infants.**

However, you must be aware that MSG, a compound of sodium and glutamic acid, an amino acid, is also found in many natural foods, including peas, tomatoes, mushrooms, and cheese. In fact, every time you eat a food containing protein you are certain to ingest glutamate, according to the *Tufts University Diet & Nutritional Letter,* Vol. 9, No. 12. The natural form found in foods is not the problem, it's the pure synthetic crystalline MSG that many companies add to their product as a flavor enhancer that creates havoc.

Companies add 45 million pounds of HVP, most often pegged as containing MSG, to processed foods each year and that should scare all of us natural-foods people. Its a staggering amount and many people do not realize that there are hundreds of different hydrolyzed vegetable proteins, most containing the synthetic MSG. If you are eating out and you seem to feel worse than when you eat at home even though you order all the right foods, suspect MSG. Ask your pharmacist for test strips to insert into your foods to see if MSG is present. The strip changes color if MSG is present in its synthetic form.

For more information, read the book, *In Bad Taste: The MSG Syndrome,* by *George R. Schwartz, M.D.,* internationally known physician and toxicologist.

Breakfast & Energy Bars

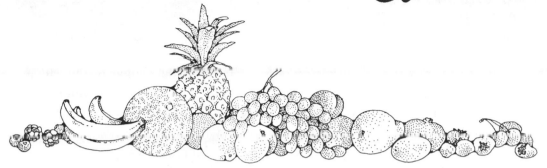

Breakfast Apricot Bar

No eggs, no wheat, no dairy.

Top and bottom mixture:
1/2 cup apricot juice (from health food store)
1 box crispy rice cereal
1/2-3/4 cup honey or pure maple syrup
1 cup quick cooking oats
Mix all together, press half the mixture on bottom of 9x13" oiled pan.

Filling:

1 pound dried, diced apricots	1 teaspoons cinnamon
2 cups apricot juice	1 teaspoons ginger
1 cup honey	1/2 ginger
1 tablespoon arrowroot powder	1/2 teaspoons cloves

Blend all in a saucepan and bring to a boil, turn down the heat and simmer to thicken, about 20 minutes. Pour over bottom mixture in the pan. Put the top mixture over all and pat down. Bake at 375° for 20-25 minutes. Cool and cut into bars.

Carob Pecan Balls

1 cup expeller-pressed vegetable oil	1 cup oat flour (make your own by putting oats in a blender)
1/2 cup honey or fructose	
1 teaspoon vanilla	1 cup finely chopped pecans
1 cup whole wheat flour	1/2 cup carob chips

Cream oil, honey and vanilla. Add flours slowly, while stirring. Fold in nuts and carob. Form into balls. Bake at 325° for 10 minutes. Sprinkle with fine coconut or powdered milk.

Energy Granola Bars

No cooking required.

1-1/2 cups granola
1/4 teaspoon sea salt
1/2 cup wheat or corn germ
1/2 cup finely shredded coconut
1/2 cup chopped dates or raisins

1 cup powdered soy or skim milk
1/4 cup fruit juice
1 cup date sugar or raw sugar
2-1/2 cups crunchy nut butter
1 cup sesame seeds (*topping*)

Mix fruit juice with dry sweetener to moisten. Mix all ingredients together, except sesame seeds, adding nut butters last. Knead in butters; you may need a little liquid for the mixture to hold together. Add honey or fruit juice, a tablespoon at a time, until you can press into a long or square pan about an inch or more thick. Press sesame seeds or chopped dried fruit on top. Chill and cut into bars and wrap each separately in plastic or waxed paper. Store in the refrigerator.

Granola Bars

2 cups honey, or maple syrup or part molasses
   or juice concentrate
2/3 cup expeller-pressed vegetable oil
2 cups oats
1 cup finely shredded coconut
1 cup chopped dates

1 cup raisins
1 cup finely toasted wheat germ
1/2 cup oat bran
1/2 cup oat flour
1 cup whole raw almonds or any nut

Melt honey and oil together, set aside. Mix the rest of the ingredients and pour honey-oil mixture over it and stir until well coated. Press the mixture densely into oiled cake pans, 1" high. Bake in 300° oven for 45 minutes. Cool slightly and slice into squares before completely cool.
Variation: Substitute diced dried apples, in place of dates and add a little cinnamon for a different bar.

Protein Oatmeal Bars

1 cup fructose or raw sugar or honey (if using
   honey, increase flour 1/2 cup)
1/2 cup expeller-pressed vegetable oil
1 teaspoon vanilla
2 eggs or equivalent egg substitute

1/2 cup whole wheat flour
1/4 teaspoon sea salt
1/2 cup protein powder or soy powder
1 cup quick cooking oats
1 cup chopped walnuts or nuts of your choice

Cream sugar, oil, eggs and vanilla, mix well. Mix together dry ingredients and add to creamed mixture. Spread in oiled 9x12" pan. Bake for 30-40 minutes at 350°. Cool and cut into bars

Peanut Butter Fingers

Lots of B vitamins and protein, no cooking required.

1/2 cup peanut butter or almond butter (better for you)
1/2 cup rice polishings
1/2 cup expeller-pressed vegetable oil

1/2 cup honey or maple syrup or rice syrup
1/2 cup puffed rice or rice crisp
3 heaping teaspoons soy protein powder
2 tablespoons carob powder *(optional)*

Mix oil and honey, add nut butter, mix well. Add rice polishings (sifted) and protein powder and mix well. Add puffed rice and fold in. Form into small finger shapes and roll in finely chopped nuts or coconut. Try different nuts and seeds.

Polynesian Oat Bars

Sugar free, dairy free.

Filling:
2 cups chopped dates
20 ounce can crushed pineapple with juice
3 cups oats or quick cooking oats
1 cup oat or millet flour

1 cup dried coconut
1/2 cup chopped nuts
1-1/2 cups pineapple juice or any fruit juice
1/2 teaspoon sea salt

Cook filling to a spreadable consistency.

Cover a 9x12" dish with half the mixture. Press down. Spread with the filling. Press rest of the mixture over filling. Pat down. Bake at 350° for 30 minutes. If in a hurry, use 3 cups granola tossed with 1 cup nuts and 1 cup honey. Press in baking dish. You may use any chopped dried fruit and preserves topped with nuts.

Notes

Butter
That's Good For You

Good Things Honey Butter

This will cut down on saturated fat, and is delicious.

> 1-1/2 pounds *Hain's* soft safflower or soy margarine (cut up in small chunks)

Blend until smooth, adding:
> 1 cup cold-pressed or expeller pressed safflower oil or canola oil
> 1 tablespoon liquid lecithin
> 1/4 cup honey *(optional)*

Purchase the margarine from a health food store without food coloring and high amounts of hardened oils.

Soy Honey Butter

Use in place of butter.

1 tablespoon honey
1/2 cup soy oil

1 tablespoon liquid lecithin
1 cup soy flour

Blend together in processor or blender.
Use over vegetables or as a baste for meats.
(Good for cholesterol problems, heart disorders, breast cancer, and all illnesses, use in place of butter and cream sauces.)

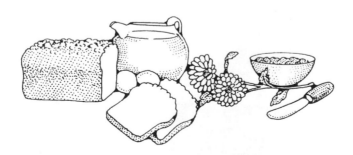

Cakes and Toppings

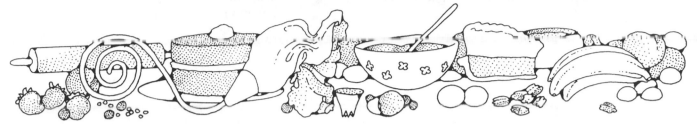

Blueberry Cake

The best, very rich and moist.

3-4 cups fresh or frozen blueberries
2 cups honey
1 cup date sugar or raw sugar or fructose
5 eggs slightly beaten or egg substitute (eggs
  make this very moist)
1 1/2 teaspoon vanilla
2-1/2 teaspoons cinnamon

1 bottle *R.W. Knudsen* blueberry syrup or
  increase the honey 1 cup
2-1/2 cups expeller-pressed safflower oil
2 cups whole wheat flour plus 2 cups unbleached
  flour or pastry flour
1-1/2 teaspoons aluminum-free baking powder
1/2 teaspoon sea salt

Blend 1/2 the blueberries in your processor or blender, set aside. Mix the dry ingredients, mix the wet ingredients, then combine. Fold in the whole blueberries, and the processed ones. Pour into oiled cake pans and bake at 350⁰ for 35-45 minutes. Frost with cream cheese frosting or cook 1 cup of the blended blueberries and honey until thick and pour over the top, or use *Knudsen's* Blueberry Syrup as a topping. If using the egg substitute, add one mashed banana for moistness.

Fresh Fruit Shortcake

2 cups unbleached or whole wheat flour or 1
  cup of each
1 tablespoon aluminum-free baking powder
1/2 cup expeller-pressed vegetable oil

2/3 cup almond or soy milk or yogurt
4 cups fresh or frozen fruit of your choice
1/4 teaspoon sea salt *(optional)*

Combine all dry ingredients. In a processor or by hand, add expeller-pressed vegetable oil until mixture resembles coarse, well-mixed crumbs. Stir in milk with a fork. Divide dough in half, roll out each half between waxed paper until it fits the cake pans. Brush with oil and top with the second half (do not press!), place it on lightly. Bake in preheated oven for 20-25 minutes at 425°. Cool and invert cake on plate and gently pull apart. Brush each half inside with butter and sprinkle with favorite fresh fruit.

You may toss and soak 4 cups of strawberries, blueberries and/or peaches in 1/2 cup fructose or barley sweetener.

High Protein Soy Spice Cake

1 cup expeller-pressed safflower oil
1 cup raw sugar and 1 cup date sugar or 2 cups
    other sugar
1-1/2 cups cooked pureed soy beans
4 eggs or egg substitute
1-1/2 cups milk of your choice
2 cups whole wheat flour

1 cup soy flour
2-1/2 teaspoons aluminum-free baking powder
2-1/2 teaspoons cinnamon
1/4 teaspoon each nutmeg, ginger, mace and
    salt
1/2 cup chopped dates
1 cup chopped walnuts or pecans

Preheat oven to 350°. Combine sweeteners, oil and pureed soybeans, beat until well mixed. Add one egg at a time, beating well after each. Stir in milk. Mix all dry ingredients and combine them both. Fold in dates and nuts. Bake in a oiled long cake pan or bread pan. Bake for 55 minutes before opening door and checking for doneness. Toothpick should come out clean and cake should spring back at a light touch.

Great warm and topped with vanilla honey ice cream or tofu whipped cream. Try orange icing on top.

Apple Five-Layer Cake

1 cup honey or pure maple syrup
1 cup expeller-pressed vegetable oil
1 cup blackstrap molasses
3 eggs or egg substitute
2 cups whole wheat flour
2 cups unbleached flour
1 cup soy or oat flour
2 teaspoons aluminum-free baking powder
1 teaspoon sea salt

2 teaspoons pumpkin pie spice or 1 teaspoon
    ginger and 1 teaspoon cinnamon
1/4 teaspoon nutmeg
1/2 teaspoon ground cloves
1 teaspoon cinnamon
3/4 cup milk (soy, almond, or your choice)
2 cups applesauce
2 cups sugar-free apple butter

In a processor or blender or by hand, blend oil, honey, eggs and molasses, beat well. Combine all the dry ingredients, add the flour mixture to the honey alternating with the milk, mix well.

Divide into five 9" cake pans. Bake at 375° for 20-25 minutes or until toothpick comes out clean.

Alternate applesauce and apple butter between layers and you may add nuts or coconut. End with the top bare or put your favorite topping on. Try the Sugar-free Apple Pie recipe for filling, sliced apples and apple juice concentrate thickened with arrowroot and a dash of cinnamon. Cook until thick and let it run down the sides. You may also use the topping between the layers.

Healthy Tip

Sucanat is organically grown, evaporated cane juice, referred to as ''raw sugar.'' All the vitamins, minerals and other nutrients of the cane juice are retained — nothing is added and only the water is removed. It is much healthier for you than chemically treated, bleached white sugar.

Baked Rich Cheesecake

Needs dairy to be rich, but substitute blended tofu in place of the cream cheese. Not for those on a low-fat diet, unless using tofu.

Filling:
16 ounces cream cheese, tofu or drained yogurt
1/2 cup fructose
2 teaspoons lemon juice
3 eggs, slightly beaten or egg substitute
1-1/4 cups plain yogurt or tofu
1 tablespoon unbleached flour or oat flour

Topping:
1 cup plain drained yogurt, see Yogurt Section
   on how to make or use cream cheese
3 tablespoons fructose
2 teaspoons vanilla

For filling, combine cream cheese, fructose and lemon juice in processor or blender, add slightly beaten eggs and yogurt. Pour into desired crust (see different kinds of crusts that follow). Bake at 350° for about 45 minutes. Combine topping ingredients and spread over baked cheesecake and bake 15 minutes longer. Chill before serving. Add sliced fresh strawberries or fruit of your choice. Fruit preserves may also be used.

Carob Tofu Cheesecake

Everybody loves this one!

3 cups tofu or 1-1/2 cups tofu and 1-1/2 cups
   cream cheese
1/2 cup liquid fructose or honey
2 bananas

1 tablespoon lemon juice
2 teaspoons vanilla
1/2 to 1 cup carob powder depending on your
   desired taste and darkness

Blend in processor until smooth. If you like it firmer, add 1/3 cup non-fat powdered soy or cow's milk. (Mixture will not be real firm until frozen.) Line a pan with sugar-free crumbled cookies, pour mixture into the pan. You may top it with carob chips and/or nuts. Put in freezer and remove half an hour before serving time.

Or you may omit the carob and top with fruit topping made from preserves or cooked down fruit and honey. Fresh fruit like strawberries, blueberries and peaches always tastes great. Blend in preserves in place of carob and sweetener. Try using half tofu in the recipe, it cuts down on the fat content.

Learn to use tofu, it's inexpensive, good for you and doesn't alter the taste.

Healthy Tip
Throughout this cookbook, expeller-pressed oil is used in place of butter or margarine. This same substitution can be used with most other recipes, because the amounts called for are the same whether it's butter or its much healthier counterpart, expeller-pressed oil. See the section on Facts on Fats and Butter That's Good For You in the recipe section, for more information on this healthy substitute for artery-clogging butter.

Good Things Fruit or Carrot Cake

Use whole eggs.

4 cups honey
2 cups date sugar or *Sucant*
10 eggs or egg replacement plus
  one mashed banana
1-1/2 teaspoons vanilla
5 cups expeller-pressed vegetable oil

8-1/4 cups whole wheat flour
8 teaspoons cinnamon
1 teaspoon sea salt
3 tablespoons aluminum-free baking powder
4 cups nuts
12 cups shredded carrots or whole fresh fruit

Mix wet ingredients together. In another bowl combine dry ingredients. Put wet and dry mixtures together. Fold in nuts, carrots or fruit. Pour into oiled cake pans and bake at 350° for about 50 minutes, less for muffins. Makes 3 large cakes and freezes well.

Carob Peanut Butter Cheesecake

No cooking required. Kids and grown-ups will love this one.

1 cup carob powder
16 ounces cream cheese or yogurt cheese or
  low-fat cottage cheese or all tofu
2 pounds drained tofu
2 bananas

2 cups honey or sweetener of your choice (if
  dry, add a little water)
16 ounces peanut butter
1 teaspoon vanilla

Blend well in processor or by hand till smooth. Pour into your favorite pie crust. Chill. *Crumbled cookies make a yummy crust for this filling.*

Yogurt Pecan Coffee Cake

1 cup whole wheat pastry flour
1 cup unbleached white flour
1 teaspoon baking powder
1 teaspoon baking powder
1 teaspoon baking soda
1/4 teaspoon salt

1/2 cup maple syrup
1/3 cup canola oil
2 eggs or egg replacement
1 cup plain nonfat yogurt
1 teaspoon vanilla

Preheat oven to 350°. Sift together first five ingredients. Beat maple syrup and canola oil together until smooth. Beat in eggs. Stir in the yogurt and vanilla. Combine the wet and dry ingredients and stir just until evenly moistened.

Spread half the batter in an oiled 9-inch pan and sprinkle half the pecan topping evenly over it. Spread the remaining batter on top and let cook 40-45 minutes. Let cool. See Pecan Topping in Cakes section.

Toppings to use over cakes, puddings, pancakes, muffins, cupcakes, ice cream, custards, yogurt, and as fillings.

Banana Crunch Topping

1 cup crushed honey-banana chips
3/4 cup quick-cooking oats
1/2 cup date sugar or raw sugar

3-4 tablespoons expeller-pressed vegeatble oil
1/4 cup chopped nuts
3/4 teaspoon cinnamon

Combine all ingredients mixing well. Put on top of cakes and bake in preheated oven at 350° for 45 minutes or until a toothpick comes out clean.

Carrot Cake Icing

16 ounces cream cheese or yogurt cheese
  (see Yogurt Section)
1 teaspoon lemon juice
1/2 cup honey

1 teaspoon barley malt
1 heaping teaspoon dry milk or soy powder
2 bananas
1-1/2 teaspoon vanilla

For two 9x12" or four round cakes. Blend in a processor or by hand until smooth.
Variation: For a chocolate flavor, add carob powder.

Sugarless Orange Cream Icing

1 package (8ounces) cream cheese or yogurt or
  soy cream cheese or blended drained tofu
1/4 dry soy or cow's milk
1 teaspoon barley malt sweetener or 1/2 cup
  honey

1/4 cup orange juice concentrate or fresh
  squeezed with 2 teaspoons grated orange
  peel

Blend all together. Top with coconut and chopped nuts. Always chill this one.
Variation: Use any juice concentrate, try apple or raspberry, any fruit preserves or bananas and carob or *Knudsen* Cranberry Juice in place of the orange, for an attractive pink color icing.

Honey Vanilla Icing

24 ounces cream cheese or 12 ounces each of
  cream cheese and tofu or all tofu
3 teaspoons vanilla
1 cup honey

3/4 cup expeller-pressed vegetable oil or *Hain's*
  Margarine
1/2 cup powdered milk or almond soy powder
1 tablespoon lemon juice (*optional*)

Cream the ingredients together by blender or by hand with a fork. If using tofu, drain and blend it until smooth
Variations: Adding powdered carob or fruit preserves, or a mashed banana is great.

207

Carob Frosting

Requires egg whites.

1 cup honey
1/4 cup plus 2 tablespoons water
1 cup dry carob powder

6 egg whites
1 teaspoon vanilla

Combine ingredients and bring to a boil, turn down heat and simmer. Meanwhile, beat egg whites until stiff. Pour the boiling mixture over the egg whites and beat hard. Beat in 1 teaspoon vanilla. More than enough to frost a two layer cake.

Stabilized Whipped Cream

1 teaspoon unflavored gelatin soaked in 2
   tablespoons cold water.

2 cups whipping cream

Whip the cream until just barely getting stiff (don't overwhip). Add the gelatin all at once to the cream, beating at the same time (do not overwhip).
This will keep nicely without separating or melting quickly.

Fruit Frosting

Use any fruit juice concentrate. Thicken with non-fat dry milk or soy powder or bring juice concentrate to a boil and add enough arrowroot powder or agar agar for desired thickness, stir constantly.
Variation: You may add chopped apple (dried) to thicken apple juice or raisins and nuts for a topping for ice cream or yogurt. Also good for fillings.

Fast Carob Frosting

1/2 cup carob powder
8 tablespoons honey
6 tablespoons expeller-pressed vegetable oil
2 teaspoons vanilla

2 tablespoons acidophilus milk or soy milk
   or yogurt
4 tablespoons milk or soy powder *(optional)*

Heat oil, milk, and honey, and add carob. Remove from heat, add vanilla. Pour over your cake and sprinkle with chopped nuts, if desired,

Pecan Topping

1 cup lightly toasted pecans, finely chopped
1/3 cup Sucant

1 teaspoon cinnamon
4 tablespoons canola oil

In a small bowl stir the pecans, Succant, and cinnamon together. Stir in the oil.

Almond Butter Frosting

3/4 smooth almond butter (purchase at health food store or make fresh)
1 cup honey or maple or fructose sugar
1 teaspoon almond extract or vanilla

1/2 cup cream cheese or blended, drained tofu
1-2 cups soy or cow's or almond powder milk

Soften almond butter, sweetener and cream cheese (may use tofu) in blender or processor. Add almond extract and the milk powder to desired thickness.

Strawberry preserves are delicious between the layers of a cake and almond butter on top and sides.

Carob Frosting

No eggs, milk or wheat--allergy-free.

3 tablespoons expeller-pressed vegetable oil
1/2 cup soy or non-fat cow's milk powder
3/4 cup carob powder
1 teaspoon vanilla
1 banana, mashed

3-4 tablespoon yogurt, if needed for spreadable consistency
1/2 cup pure maple syrup or honey or barley malt sweetener

Mix all ingredients in processor or beat by hand until well mixed and smooth.

Butterscotch Sauce

4 tablespoons expeller-pressed vegetable oil
4 tablespoons rice barley syrup
1 cup raw sugar or brown sugar

2 tablespoons arrowroot powder or cornstarch
1/2 cup powdered soy or cow's milk
2-1/2 cups water

Combine the expeller-pressed vegetable oil, syrup and sugar in a heavy saucepan and cook over medium heat until the mixture starts to carmelize. Add the arrowroot to 1/2 cup of the water, then add the powdered milk and the other two cups of water, mixing well. Pour the arrowroot mixture into the caramel mixture stirring constantly until it is thick.

Maple Sauce

3 tablespoons expeller-pressed vegetable oil
2 teaspoons lemon juice

1/2 cup pure maple syrup
1/4 cup date or *Sucant* raw sugar *(optional)*

Mix all together and heat until well mixed.

Carob Syrup

1/2 cup carob powder
1/2 cup honey
3 tablespoons expeller-pressed vegetable oil
1 teaspoon lemon juice

1 tablespoon arrowroot powder mixed with
 1 tablespoon water before adding
1/2 cup boiling water
1 teaspoon vanilla

Put carob and oil in pan. Add boiling water, mix. Stir in honey and arrowroot mixture. Boil 8 minutes. Remove from heat and let cool. Add vanilla and lemon juice. *Use on ice cream, pancakes or yogurt.*

Fruit Topping

Fresh berry or fruit syrup
4 cups chunks and pureed berries or peaches

1-1/2 cups honey or sweetener of your
 choice, dry sweetener add 1 cup water

Cook until desired thickness is reached. Make this thicker faster by using arrowroot powder or tapioca.

Fast Apple Maple Dessert or Topping

1 cup pure maple syrup
1 teaspoon arrowroot powder
1/2 teaspoon cinnamon
1/2 cup walnuts, broken up

1-1/2 cups dried, diced apples or 2 cups fresh
2 tablespoons expeller-pressed vegetable oil
(optional)

Heat mapple syrup and arrowroot to boiling, add oil if desired. Boil one minute, add cinnamon, butter, then apples, stirring constantly. Remove from heat, fold in nuts. *Serve topped with frozen yogurt, honey or ice cream, as filling in turnovers and on cakes.*

SHIITAKE MUSHROOMS
MORE IDEAS FOR USING DRIED SHIITAKE:

- Enhance prepared foods and mixes, such as soups, stuffing, sauces and gravies, dips and more.
- Marinate one hour in salad dressing, slice and add to tossed salad.
- Include in rice and other grain dishes for added flavor and nutrition.
- Mix with other vegetables for stir-fry, fried rice, and other Oriental dishes.

- Add to omelettes, scrambled eggs, or quiche.
- Make a shiitake sauce or gravy to dress up leftovers.
- Marinate and grill or skewer with kabobs at summer barbeques.
- Slice into spaghetti sauce or atop a pizza.
- Add to canned, frozen, or fresh vegetables during cooking.

(Maple River Company • Dayton, Ohio)
If difficult to find call: 1-800-524-4665

Casseroles

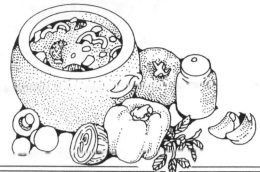

Easy Turkey Pot Roast

This is easy to prepare for company and good tasting, you can omit the meat if you are a vegetarian.

Skinless large turkey breast
1/2 head cabbage
6-8 carrots
2 stalks celery
2 onions

3 turnips
6 potatoes
1 package *Hain's* dry Onion Soup Mix
2 packs *Hain's* Brown Gravy Mix
2-1/4 cups water

Place turkey breast in roasting pan and brown lightly in oil on all sides and sprinkle with Spike. Place cabbage quartered, whole carrots, celery stalk cut in 4 pieces, onions cut in half, turnips whole, leave the skins on the potatoes and scrub well. Use whole potatoes about the size of large lemons and place around the roast. Mix the onion soup and the two packs of gravy mix together with the 2-1/4 of cups water, pour the mixture over all.

Cover and bake at 350° preheated oven for 2-3 hours, depending on size of roast, basting after 1-1/2 hours. You will have a delicious, thick gravy. Try this recipe using any kind of meat you prefer.

Zucchini Potato Casserole

2 sliced zucchinis
1/2 cup fresh sliced mushrooms
2 fresh, sliced, tomatoes
1/2 onion, sliced
2 baking potatoes, cleaned and sliced
1 green pepper, sliced

1/4 cup olive oil
Juice of 1/2 a lemon
Fresh basil
Dash of Spike seasoning
1 tablespoon dried parsley

Slice vegetables thinly, arrange in casserole, alternating slices of each vegetable. Coat with olive oil and cook for about 30 minutes at 400° until vegetables are still slightly crisp, do not overcook.

Sprinkle with fresh basil, lemon juice, salt and pepper, or Italian seasoning (used in salad dressings). Serve hot.

> **Leftover chicken or meat lasts three to four days if uncooked or cooked, without gravy or broth, but only two days if covered with a broth or gravy. Stuffing lasts one to two days and then bacteria starts to multiply.**

211

Chinese Stir Fry

Meatless, eggless, dairyfree

Dash of cayenne
2 tablespoons expeller-pressed sesame, saf
  flower or canola oil
3 tablespoons tamari sauce
1 tablespoon grated ginger root
1 tablespoon honey or 1/4 teaspoon barley malt
  sweetener

6 ounces tofu, cubed
2 cups bean sprouts
3 cups snow pea pods
1 cup carrot strips, about 2" long
2 cups Bok Choy (or celery) chopped
1 can (or fresh) sliced chestnuts *(optional)*
1 teaspoon Spike seasoning *(optional)*

Combine the oil, tamari sauce, ginger root, honey, Spike, and cayenne pepper in a heavy, large skillet or wok. Heat and add vegetables, stirring and mixing, over medium to high heat. Add cubed tofu the last two minutes. Total time, approximately 10-15 minutes. Total time, approximately 10 -15 minutes.

Serve with brown fried rice or plain rice.

Rice, Spinach & Cheese Bake

2 cups cooked brown rice
1/2 pound tofu mixed with
1 cup plain yogurt, kefir cheese, or creamed tofu
1 package spinach, steamed and drained
1/2 cup shredded carrots
1 chopped green pepper
2 teaspoons Spike seasoning or sea salt to taste

2 cups shredded cheese of your choice (reserve
  1/2 cup for top)
1/2 teaspoon garlic granules or powder
1 tablespoon Miso, mixed in small amount of
  the yogurt or kefir, then add remaining yo
  gurt or kefir.

Combine all ingredients, place in casserole or baking pan and top with reserved cheese and almonds, or put into individual dishes and bake at 350° for 30-40 minutes.

You can place in individual dishes and freeze for later use. If you learn to prepare extra for freezing, then you won't be so tempted to use store bought foods that are full of chemicals, sugar, fat, etc.

Quinoa Stir-Fry

Quinoa's unusually high quality protein has a nearly ideal amino acid balance which is difficult to obtain in the plant kingdom. It is also a good source of fiber, complex carbohydrates, calcium, phosphorous, iron and vitamins B and E.

2 cups cooked quinoa (cook like rice)
1 cup mushrooms, sliced
1/2 cup celery, sliced
1/2 cup carrot, sliced
1 onion, sliced
1/2 cup cauliflower pieces
1 red pepper, diced

2 tablespoons teriyaki or soy sauce
1 cup broccoli, chopped
3 cloves garlic, minced
1/2 cup sliced almonds
1/4 cup sunflower seeds
1 teaspoon Spike, Vegit or seasoning of your
  choice

Saute vegetables, garlic, almonds and seeds in sesame oil until vegetables are crisp. Add seasoning and quinoa. Stir until mixed and warmed through. Serve immediately. Recipe from *Alive Canadian Journal*, Oct. 1991.

Squash Casserole

4 large yellow squash, sliced
6 tomatoes, sliced
3/4 cup olive oil
1 tablespoon vegetable bouillon in 1 cup water
1/2 cup parsley, finely chopped or 2 tablespoon dried

1 tablespoon dill
1 tablespoon tarragon
1 teaspoon Spike seasoning or sea salt and dash of cayenne
3 large onions, sliced
2 cloves garlic

In a large, heavy pan saute crushed garlic in olive oil, then add squash, tomatoes and onions, and bouillon. Put in large casserole dish. Bake about 30 minutes, sprinkle top with parmesan cheese, bake 10 minutes more in a 350° oven.

Serve with garlic French bread and tossed salad. See squash section for more recipes.

Spinach Noodle Casserole

1 pound spinach noodles
3 teaspoons olive oil
1 cup Ricotta cheese or plain yogurt
1 large onion, chopped
1 teaspoon Spike seasoning or sea salt
3/4 cup eggless mayonnaise

1/2 cup grated soy cheese or cheese of your choice
2 tablespoons vegetable oil
1-1/2 cups cracker crumbs
1/4 teaspoon cayenne pepper (optional)

Cook noodles until tender, don't overcook, drain well. Add olive oil and toss. Soy or ricotta cheese, sea salt, cayenne pepper, chopped onion, grated cheese, and mayonnaise.

Put mixture in well-oiled casserole. Sprinkle cracker crumbs and Parmesan cheese or grated Swiss on top. Bake in preheated oven at 350° for 20-30 minutes.

Baked Beans

4 cups cooked beans (navy or pinto are best)
1 onion, chopped
1 onion, sliced
1/2 cup molasses
1 teaspoon dry mustard
1 cup ketchup (from health food store or home made)

2 tablespoons expeller-pressed oil
2 teaspoons Spike seasoning or 1 teaspoon sea salt
Dash cayenne pepper (optional)
1/2 cup honey or raw sugar, fructose, maple syrup, etc. (optional)

Saute chopped onion in oil, add the remaining ingredients and place in a baking dish. Top with sliced onion. Bake, uncovered, at 450° for 35-50 minutes.

> There are a number of different packaged "fast foods" in the health foods stores. Cake mixes, pancake mixes, biscuit mixes, cornbread, quick-cooking rice, and soups from *Arrowhead Mills, Fearn, Nature's Choice* and *Eden* are good, quick to prepare, and without chemicals.

Baked Creamy Potatoes

4 cups potatoes, scrub well, leave skins on, slice thinly

4 tablespoons *Hain's* soft safflower margarine contains *half the fat of other margarine or butter*

1 tablespoon chopped fresh or dried parsley

2 teaspoons Spike seasoning and dash cayenne pepper

2 cloves garlic, chopped and minced

2 cups soy milk or your choice

1 cup soy parmesan cheese or your choice, reserve 1/2 cup to place on top

Place sliced potatoes in a baking dish. Make a paste with 2 tablespoons of flour and 4 tablespoons of soy milk, mix the paste into the rest of the milk. Combine the rest of the ingredients except the margarine, pour over the potatoes, then dot with the margarine. Bake in a preheated 400° oven for about 35 minutes. Top with rest of the cheese and bake another 15 minutes until tender and lightly browned.

Scalloped Potatoes

6 sliced potatoes, with peelings on

1 cup grated soy Swiss cheese, or your choice

1 tablespoon dried parsley or fresh, chopped fine

2 tablespoons *Hain's* soft safflower margarine or your choice

1/4 cup mixed dried veggies (can omit) or use *Hain's* dry Vegetable Soup Mix

2 tablespoons vegetable bouillon (can omit)

1 cup soy, almond or cow's milk

1/2 cup plain yogurt or sour cream or tofu blended until creamy, combined with 2 table spoons flour

2 sliced onions

Dash cayenne and Spike or Vegit seasonings *(optional)*

Layer potatoes and onions in bake dish, mix rest of ingredients and pour over the potatoes and onions.

May top with tofu dogs, canned salmon, or tuna, fresh peas, broccoli or mushrooms; then top all with toasted wheat germ, cracker crumbs and grated parmesan cheese.

If you are in a hurry, pour two cans mushroom soup over sliced potatoes and onions and top with bread or cracker crumbs and cheese and bake. Bake at 350° for 1-1/2 hours or until potatoes are tender.

A recent study conducted in South Africa, by *Drs. Gregory Hussey* and *Max Klein* of *the University of Cape Town,* found a link between the value of vitamin A and beta-carotene and the prevention of a measles epidemic.
Journal of the American Dietetic Association reported that *Ronald Ross Watson, Ph.D.,* a researcher at the *University of Arizona,* suggests an intake of twelve, 500 I.U. of carotene daily for preventing cancer.

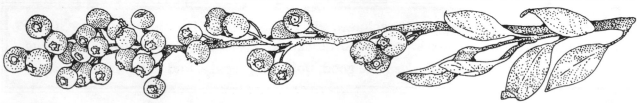

Cheesy Spinach

1 cup cheese of your choice (or cheese sauce from basic cheese) or *Hain's* dry cheese soup mix combined with 1/2 the amount of water
1/2 cup plain yogurt or sour cream
1/2 cup mashed tofu or low-fat cottage cheese
3 green onions and tops, minced

5 tablespoons *Hain's* soft safflower margarine or expeller-pressed vegetable oil
1 cup fresh sliced mushrooms
1 teaspoon Spike seasoning or sea salt and cayenne pepper

Steam the spinach lightly, drain, chop slightly. Saute the onions, mushrooms and seasonings in oil. Add the cheeses until melted, stirring constantly, add the spinach if desired.

Can serve as a side dish or over biscuits, toast or in a pita pocket, over baked potatoes, fish, chicken, noodles, cooked macaroni mixed with chopped red pepper, etc.

Cauliflower Casserole

1 large head cauliflower, broken into large flowerets
1 teaspoon expeller-pressed oil
3 green onions and tops, chopped
1 package *Hain's* dry Cheese Soup mix
1 cup shredded cheese of your choice, soy or cow's

1 cup soy milk or milk of your choice
1/2 cup plain yogurt or sour cream
1 clove garlic, chopped and minced
1 teaspoon Spike seasoning and dash cayenne pepper *(optional)*
2 tablespoons chopped or dried parsley *(op tional)*

Saute green onions and garlic in hot oil just until onions are tender. Add milk, yogurt, and soup mix, stirring constantly. Add the seasonings and cheese, stir until the cheese melts, remove from heat.

In well-oiled casserole dish, add cauliflower, pour sauce over all, top with cracker or bread crumbs, and bake at 350° for 20 minutes, covered. Uncover and bake until golden brown, about 10 more minutes.

Can add tomato slices on top before bread crumb topping.

Meatless Guide for Vegans

Protein: Grains, legumes, tofu, tempeh, soybeans, dark leafy greens, nuts and seeds
Calcium: Dark leafy greens, legumes, molasses, figs, apricots, dates, pecans, sesame seeds
Iron: Soybeans, dark leafy greens, dried fruits, whole grains, molasses, beets, grapes, carrots, parsley
Zinc: Legumes, wheat germ, whole grains, nuts, mushrooms and soybeans
B-Complex: Brewers yeast, enriched grains, sea vegetables, dark leafy greens
B-12: Sea vegetables, spirulina, kelp, dulse
Caution: Zinc, B-12, iron, and folic acid (B vitamin) may be lacking in a vegetarian diet without careful planning

215

Everyone's Shepherd Pie

8 potatoes cubed,
1 large clove garlic, minced and pressed
1 large onion, chopped
1 cup of each of the following:
  Diced carrots
  Diced celery
  Fresh or frozen each of peas and green beans
  Chopped broccoli or cauliflower
2 teaspoons Spike seasoning and dash cayenne
  pepper
1 box frozen or 2 cups fresh corn
2 tomatoes, diced
1 cup grated cheese, soy, cheddar or monterey
  jack
1 tablespoon miso, blended into 5 tablespoons
  of water

1 tablespoon butter
Dash of Spike seasoning
2/3 cup of any juice
Mix together the following:
1 package *Hain's* dry Cheese Soup Mix
1 package *Hain's* dry Onion Soup Mix
2-1/2 cups plain yogurt or 1-1/2 cup soy milk,
  you can use stock or water
2 tablespoons arrowroot or thickener of your
  choice
1 tablespoon miso blended in 5 tablespoons
  water before adding to rest

Choose crust of your choice, try potato, zucchini, rice, whole wheat etc. Only one double crust is needed for a 9"x13" baking pan, no top crust is used. Boil potatoes until barely tender, drain and mash with milk and butter and Spike. Saute onions, carrots, celery, and broccoli in hot oil for a couple minutes. Sprinkle a layer of cheese over the crust and top with half of the sauteed vegetables. Pour half of the yogurt/milk mixture over vegetables.

Sprinkle a handful of cheese on top, now layer the rest of the sauteed vegetables over the cheese. Place peas and green beans and chopped tomatoes on top, sprinkle with a dash of seasonings, pour the remaining half of the yogurt/milk mixture on top, spread a handful of the shredded cheese on top of all. Spread the top with the mashed potatoes and end with a sprinkle of shredded cheese. Bake at 350° for 40-50 minutes until top is golden.

Apple Yam Delight

16 ounces yams or sweet potatoes
2 sliced apples
16 ounces chunky applesauce
1 teaspoon cinnamon
3/4 cup instant rolled oats

1/3 cup *Hain's* Soft Safflower Margarine or
  your choice
3/4 cup date raw sugar or your choice of sweetener
4 tablespoons flour

Cut potatoes to bite size. Put oats in your blender to make oat flour. Combine oat flour, sugar, cut in the margarine until crumbly. Put half of the sliced apples in an oiled 10x6" baking dish. Mix a little cinnamon and sugar and sprinkle over the top, add the yams and the applesauce in layers and sprinkle the cinnamon-sugar mixture over it all. Top with the oat, sugar, and oil mixture. Bake at 350° for 45 minutes.

Spinach or Broccoli Bake

1 cup cooked brown rice
2 cups mashed tofu or low-fat cottage cheese or
ricotta cheese
1 package raw spinach or fresh steamed and
patted dry and/or raw broccoli

2 green peppers, chopped
2 cups grated cheese of your choice
1-1/2 teaspoons sea salt
Dash cayenne pepper
1/2 teaspoon granulated or powdered garlic

Combine all ingredients, place in baking dish, top with almonds and cheese. Bake at 350° for 30-45 minutes. Add broiled chicken, cut up, if you desire meat.

Almond Cream Green Beans

1 pound fresh or frozen green beans or home
canned
1/2 cup slivered almonds, or large pieces
1/2 teaspoon sea salt

3 tablespoons expeller-pressed oil
2 teaspoons oat or whole wheat flour
1/2 plain yogurt, sour cream, or mashed tofu
1 teaspoon Spike seasoning

Put fresh, cleaned beans in just enough water to cover, simmer for 15 minutes with sea salt. Saute almonds in 1 tablespoon oil until lightly browned, remove. Add rest of oil to the pan. Add flour to thicken, stirring constantly, add the yogurt and mix until smooth. Cook until thick. Add drained beans and 1/2 of the almonds. Season with Spike and dash of cayenne pepper. Top with the rest of the almonds and serve.

Can substitute onions for the almonds and sautee the same as above.

Tasty Veggie Chili

3 pounds red kidney beans
2 quarts tomatoes
2 cans tomato puree or tomato sauce
3 large chopped onions
3 stalks chopped celery
1 finely chopped garlic clove
3 chopped green peppers
2-1/2 tablespoon cummin

2 tablespoons chili powder
1/2 teaspoon onion powder
1/4 teaspoon cayenne powder
1 tablespoon sea salt
1/4 teaspoon garlic powder
2 tablespoons tamari sauce
2 tablespoons vegie or chicken bouillon
3 tablespoons Spike or 1 tablespoon sea salt

Soak red kidney beans overnight, cook until tender (Do not overcook). Add tomatoes (Chili Vegie Juice by Knudsen adds flavor in place of tomatoes or half of each) and tomato puree or tomato sauce. In a large skillet, saute in garlic oil or safflower oil; onions, celery, garlic clove and green peppers until tender, add to cooked beans. Mix cumin, chili powder, Spike/sea salt, onion powder, cayenne pepper, sea salt, garlic powder and tamari sauce into bean mixture.

You can now add more tomatoes if desired and vegie or chicken bouillon. Granulated soy protein may be added to give a meaty look and taste. Simmer on very low for 1 to 2 hours. Serve over brown rice if desired and top with grated cheese and fresh avocado. Freezes well in individual dishes to pop in oven or microwave.

Cookies

Carrot Granola Cookies

Healthy and delicious. High in beta carotene and protein.

3 cups expeller-pressed vegetable oil
3 cups firmly packed raw or brown sugar
6 eggs (see Substitute section for alternatives)
1-3/4 cups whole wheat flour
1-1/2 cups unbleached flour or 3 1/4 cups whole wheat flour
3 teaspoons aluminum-free baking powder
3 teaspoons nutmeg
1-1/2 teaspoons sea salt

6 tablespoons fruit juice
3 teaspoons vanilla
1 cup soy flour
1 cup oat flour
3 teaspoons cinnamon
3 cups raisins
6 cups grated carrots
6 cups granola
1 cup chopped nuts or sunflower seeds

Beat oil and sugar until fluffy. Beat in eggs, water and vanilla. Sift flour, baking powder, nutmeg and salt. Add to mixture along with other flours. Stir in rest of ingredients. Drop onto cookie sheet (about 1/3 cup per cookie) and bake at 350° for 12-15 minutes.

Double Peanut Butter Cookies

2-1/2 cups whole wheat flour
2 cups unbleached flour or pastry flour
1-1/2 teaspoons aluminum-free baking powder
1/2 teaspoon sea salt

1-1/2 cups expeller-pressed vegetable oil
2 cups peanut butter
1-1/2 cups honey
3 tablespoons yogurt

Mix dry ingredients. Cut in oil and peanut butter until mixture resembles coarse meal. Blend in honey and yogurt. Shape into a 2" roll and chill. Slice 1/4-1/2" thick. Place on a cookie sheet; press, spread each with 1/2 teaspoon peanut butter. Cover with remaining dough rounds, seal edges tightly with fork. Bake at 350° for 12 minutes and cool. Makes 5 dozen.
Variation: Add carob chips with the peanut butter for a filling.

Pineapple Carrot Cookies

1-1/2 cups honey or 1 can frozen apple juice concentrate plus 1 teaspoon powdered barley malt sweetener
1/2 cup molasses
1/2 cup expeller-pressed vegetable oil
1 egg or egg substitute
1 cup shredded carrots
3/4 cups finely chopped dried pineapple

1/2 cup raisins
1/2 cup chopped nuts
2 cups whole wheat flour (or half rice or oat flour)
2 teaspoons *Rumford's* baking powder (aluminum-free)
1/2 teaspoon sea salt
1 teaspoon cinnamon
1/2 teaspoon ginger

Soak raisins and pineapple for 10 minutes in hot water, then drain. Beat honey, oil, egg and molasses together and mix in carrots, pineapple, raisins and nuts. Sift together dry ingredients. Add to wet mixture and blend well. Drop from a spoon onto an oiled cookie sheet. Bake at 350° for 10-15 minutes. Makes 3 dozen cookies.

218

Fruit Oatmeal Cookies

Large recipe, good frozen and keeps well, DELICIOUS!

6 cups whole wheat flour
8 cups oats
2 teaspoons baking powder
1 tablespoon cinnamon
1-1/2 teaspoons ginger
4 eggs or egg replacer
2 cups nuts

2 cups expeller-pressed vegetable oil
3 cups honey or maple syrup
1-1/2 cups apple juice concentrate
2 teaspoons pure vanilla
2-1/2 cups date sugar or other dry sweetener or fructose

Combine dry ingredients. Mix the wet in a separate bowl, then combine together. Fold in fruit and nuts, if desired. Drop by tablespoons full on an oiled cookie sheet and press down slightly. Bake at 350° for 12-18 minutes. This is a popular cookie in health food resturants and stores.

Apple Cider Spice juice, in health food stores, is good to use in place of the applejuice concentrate or you can substitute any fruit juice.

This recipe is fun to work with. You can add nuts, nut butters, raisins, carob chips, peanut butter chips, seeds and any kind of dried chopped fruit. Try different ones. This recipe is good for the holidays, divide the mixture in half before adding the nuts and/or fruit. Take each half and make different kinds of cookies mixing in different ingredients like carob chips and nuts, chopped dried apples and raisins.

All Honey Cookies

Egg-free.

2 cups honey or liquid fructose
2 cups expeller-pressed vegetable oil
7-1/2 cups sifted whole wheat flour or 3-3/4 cup each of unbleached and whole wheat (can substitute oat or soy)

3 tablespoons aluminum-free baking powder
1 teaspoon cinnamon
1 teaspoon cloves
1 teaspoon allspice

Warm honey and oil together about 1 minute. Cool. Combine sifted flour, baking powder, spices, and sift together. Add to first mixture. Chill dough. Roll 1/8 inch thick. Slice 1/2" thick and bake on ungreased baking sheet in moderate 350°, 8-10 minutes. Dough may be formed into 2 1/2 " balls and stored in the refrigerator. Omit chilling if in a hurry. Makes about 6 dozen cookies.

Variations: Add peanut butter, finely chopped nuts, fruit or make a cookie sandwich and put a filling in the center (fruit, jelly, peanut butter) and seal the edges with a fork.

Notes

Bavarian Carob

Very rich, so not for every diet, contains eggs and cream.

1 tablespoon unflavored gelatin
1/2 cup coconut, almond milk or plain water
3 tablespoons honey
4 egg yolks

1/2 cup carob powder
2 teaspoons vanilla
2 cups heavy cream

Soften gelatin in the milk. In another bowl, separate the eggs and beat the yolks, adding the vanilla and the carob, fold into the gelatin mixture and chill for a couple hours. Beat the egg whites until stiff. Whip the cream until stiff. Fold mixtures together gently. Now gently fold into gelatin mixture and chill. Top with finely chopped nuts, slivered almonds, or fruit.

Honey Peanut Butter Cookies

4-1/2 cups honey
3 cups raw sugar (or use all honey)
3 cups expeller-pressed vegetable oil
6 eggs or egg substitute
3 teaspoons sea salt

4-1/2 cups peanut butter or any nut butter
9 cups flour (whole wheat or unbleached or your
  choice)
3 teaspoons aluminum-free baking powder
1 cup chopped peanuts *(optional)*

Whip honey and sugar and oil together until light and fluffy. Add eggs and beat well. Add peanut butter and blend. Add salt and baking powder to sifted flour and sift together. Add to sugar mixture and blend until smooth. Drop by spoonfuls onto greased cookie sheet and press with floured fork. Bake in 350° oven for 10-12 minutes. Makes about 6 dozen 3" cookies.

Honey Pecan Carob Chip Cookies

2 eggs or egg substitute
2 cups expeller-pressed vegetable oil
2 cups honey
1 cup raw sugar (or all honey)
1 teaspoons cinnamon
1 teaspoons cloves

1 teaspoons allspice
1 cup chopped pecans
2 cups of carob chips
8-9 cups flour
3 teaspoons aluminum-free baking powder

Blend eggs, oil, honey or raw sugar, and mix dry ingredients and combine. Mix in nuts and chips. Chill dough. Roll out to 1/2 inch thick and using cookie cutter or a glass, cut out cookies and place on a greased cookie sheet. May top with a pecan half centered on each cookie. Bake at 350° for 8-10 minutes.

Healthy Tip
Instead of bleached, white flour use whole wheat flour, amaranth, barley, millet, quinoa, spelt, rye, corn, oat, and rice flours. White flour has very little nutritional value and it tends to clog the body with excess mucus.

Double Rich Brownies

3 cups sweetened carob chips
8 tablespoons expeller-pressed vegetable oil
2 beaten eggs or egg substitute
1/2 cup honey or any natural sweetener

1 teaspoon vanilla
3/4 cup unbleached or whole wheat flour
3/4 teaspoon aluminum-free baking powder
1 cup chopped walnuts or any nuts

Heat oil and 2 cups of the carob chips over low heat, stirring constantly, until all the chips are melted. Blend eggs, honey, vanilla and add to carob mixture. Combine all dry ingredients, stir into carob mixture. Fold in nuts and 1 cup carob chips. Bake at 350° for 30-40 minutes until a toothpick comes out clean. Use a well-greased oblong or square cake pan. Frost with carob frosting and sprinkle a few chips and nuts on top.

Gingersnaps

2-1/4 cups expeller-pressed vegetable oil
3 cups raw sugar or brown sugar
1-1/4 cups molasses
3 eggs or egg substitute
7 cups whole wheat flour

1-1/2 teaspoons sea salt
3 teaspoons ginger
3 teaspoons cinnamon
1-1/2 teaspoons cloves
3 teaspoons baking powder

Cream together oil, sugar, molasses and eggs (or replacer) until fluffy. Mix dry ingredients before adding wet mixture, blend. Form in small balls and roll in raw sugar and place 2" apart on cookie sheet. Bake at 375° about 10 minutes.

Date Nut Granola

6 cups rolled oats
1 cup shredded coconut
1 cup toasted wheat germ
1/2 cup sesame seeds

2/3 cup powdered soy or almond milk
1 cup honey or pure maple syrup
2 cups slivered almonds or any nuts
1 cup date pieces

Combine oats, coconut, wheat germ, sesame seeds and powdered milk. Warm honey, add to dry ingredients, stirring until well mixed. Pour mixture into large well-oiled baking pan. Spread mixture evenly. Place in 350° oven and bake 45 minutes, stirring every 20 minutes. Remove from oven and add almonds and dates. Allow to cool before storing in air tight container. Makes 3 quarts.

The recipes in this book are highly nutritious. Children as well as adults love these cookies and desserts. Best of all, you won't miss the sugar, fat and chemicals found in commercially-prepared desserts because these taste wonderful. Learn to substitute different sweeteners and flours in your recipes for variety and nutrients.

Pineapple Drop Cookies

2-1/4 cups expeller-pressed vegetable oil
3 cups raw or sweetener of your choice
3 eggs or egg substitute
3/4 cup pineapple preserves

6-3/4 cups unbleached flour
3 teaspoons baking powder
1-1/2 teaspoons sea salt *(optional)*

Mix oil and sugar together. Beat in eggs and preserves. Mix dry ingredients together and add to wet ingredients mixing well. Drop from spoon, 2" apart on a cookie sheet. Bake in 375° oven for 10 minutes. Cool 10 minutes. Top with a dab of preserves in the middle and place half a walnut on each. You may make this ahead, form into a roll and store in waxed paper in the refrigerator.

High-Protein Soy Cookies

4 eggs or egg substitute
1 cup honey
1/2 cup expeller-pressed vegetable oil
2 cups cooked, pureed soy beans
1/2 cup date sugar
1/2 cup dry molasses
6 cups whole wheat flour

1 teaspoon baking soda
1 teaspoon allspice
1 teaspoon ginger
1/4 teaspoon ground cloves
1 teaspoon cinnamon
1 cup soy nuts or sunflower seeds

Mix the wet ingredients, then the dry, combine together and form into patties. Bake at 350° for about 15 minutes. You may use part oat or soy flour.

Banana Date Cookies

3 cups mashed bananas
1 teaspoon vanilla
6 cups oats
1/2 teaspoon sea salt

2 cups dates
1 cup nuts
1/4 cup apple juice or applesauce (if dates are
	hard, soak in one of these for a few minutes)

Mix all together, drop by spoonfuls on your cookie sheet, and press flat. Bake at 350° until, 15 to 18 minutes.

Healthy Tip

You can omit the salt in any recipe in this book. We do not recommend the use of added salt but have included it for those who prefer salt.

Granola Bars

2 cups honey, or maple syrup or part molasses
    or juice concentrate
2/3 cup expeller-pressed vegetable oil
2 cups oats
1 cup finely shredded coconut
1 cup chopped dates

1 cup raisins
1 cup finely toasted wheat germ
1/2 cup oat bran
1/2 cup oat flour
1 cup whole raw almonds or any nut

Melt honey and oil together, set aside. Mix rest of ingredients and pour honey-oil mixture over it and stir until well coated. Press the mixture densely into oiled cake pans, 1" high. Bake in 300° oven for 45 minutes. Cool slightly and slice into squares before completely cool.

Variation: Substitute diced dried apples, in place of dates and add a little cinnamon for a different bar.

Carob Chip Cookies

3 cups whole wheat pastry flour
3/4 teaspoon sea salt
3/4 teaspoon nutmeg
1-1/2 cups expeller-pressed vegetable oil
2 cups carob chips

3 cups sugar or fructose or raw sugar or your
    choice
1-1/2 teaspoons vanilla
3 eggs or 3 egg whites or 1 tablespoon arrowroot
    powder mixed with 2 tablespoons water

Mix dry ingredients. Cream together oil, sugar, vanilla, and eggs. Fold in dry ingredients; add nuts and chips. Drop spoonfuls of dough on greased cookie sheets. Bake at 375° for 10 minutes. Makes 3-4 dozen.

Apricot Layer Bars

Apricot filling:
1/2 cup chopped dates
2 cups dried, diced apricots
3/4 cup raw sugar or brown sugar or honey or
    maple syrup

3 whole or 1/4 teaspoon powdered cloves
1/2 cup dried coconut
Topping: same as Peach Crisp, use a double
    recipe.

Preheat oven to 400°.

Put chopped apricots in a saucepan with cloves and sweetener, add 1/2 cup water. Cook until thick and mushy. Remove cloves and puree the mixture. Set aside. Put a layer of topping in an oiled 9x13" pan. Spread apricot filling over mix. Sprinkle dates and coconut over all. Bake for 20-30 minutes or until top is lightly brown. Cut into squares.

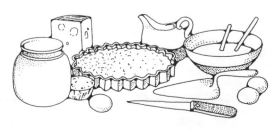

Whole Wheat Fig Bars

Filling:
1-1/2 cups chopped figs
1/2 cup chopped dates or use 2 cups of one kind
2 cups fig, orange or apple juice (from health food store)

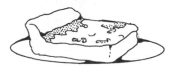

Cookie layers:
2 cups whole wheat flour
1-1/2 cups quick cooking oats
1/4 teaspoon aluminum-free baking powder
3/4 teaspoon nutmeg
1/2 teaspoon ginger
2 eggs or equivalent
3/4 cup expeller-pressed vegetable oil
1-1/2 teaspoons vanilla
1-1/2 teaspoons cinnamon
1/4 cup honey, rice syrup or barley malt
1/2 cup chopped figs combined with 1/2 cup fig juice or apple juice blended until smooth

Blend the filling ingredients in a food processor adding the juice, a little at a time until smooth. Mix in 1 cup chopped nuts by hand (*optional*) set aside for filling.

Combine dry cookie ingredients. Blend wet ingredients and add to the dry, mixing well. (Do not use the first fig mixture yet). Grease a 9x12" pan and spread half the mixture, pour in filling mixture, cover with remainder of cake mixture. Bake in preheated 350° oven until lightly browned for 30-40 minutes, cool. Frost with orange frosting, if desired.

Figs have been noted to help expel parasites, besides being high in fiber and nutrients.

Frosted Apricot Bars

1 teaspoon cinnamon
1/2 cup toasted wheat germ
1-1/2 cups graham cracker crumbs
1/2 cup expeller-pressed vegetable oil
1-1/2 cups dried apricots, chopped
1 cup crused pineapple (with juice)
1 cup quick cooking oats

1/2 cup dry powdered soy milk, or milk powder
14 ounces frozen apple juice concentrate or condensed canned cream
1 cup chopped walnuts or other nuts
1/2 cup shredded coconut
1-1/2 cups carob chips (*optional*)
1 cup date sugar (*optional*)

Mix the first six dry ingredients. Coat a 15x9" baking pan with oil. Spread the dry ingredient mixture on the bottom of the pan. Sprinkle chopped apricots over mix and poured thawed apple juice concentrate over all. Top with coconut, carob chips and nuts. Bake at 325° for 20-30 minutes.

Healthy Tip
Try adding toasted sesame seeds to pie and pastry crusts. Prepare the seeds by sprinking a thin layer in a frying pan and toasting them over a low heat, stirring until golden brown. Remove from pan and add to dry ingredients. They taste delicious.

Healthy Drinks

Mint Green Freeze
---

1 teaspoon spirulina powder or 2 teaspoons liquid
   chlorophyll or juice your own greens, i.e.
   spinach, lettuce, kale, etc.
1 cup fresh carrot juice

3 cups frozen yogurt or plain low-fat yogurt
1/2 teaspoon spearmint flavoring or 1/4 cup mint
   tea (extra strong) or 2 tablespoons unsweetened mint jelly

Mix all together. Enjoy
*This is good for high or low blood-sugar disorders and weight problems, between meals or as a meal
substitute. Good also for yeast infections, digestive or colon disorders, cancer, and vitamin deficiencies.*

Cranberry Cream

1/4 cup *Hain's* frozen undiluted Cranberry
   concentrate

3 cups frozen or plain low-fat yogurt
1/4 cup frozen undiluted apple juice concentrate

Blend and be sure to drink this three times daily for kidney and bladder problems. Bacteria cannot live in
an acid medium.
Eat live yogurt to replenish the friendly bacteria that have been destroyed by antibiotics.

Pineapple Carrot Freeze

1-1/2 cups fresh carrot juice
3 cups frozen plain low-fat yogurt

3 tablespoons unsweetened pineapple preserves or
   chopped fresh pineapple

Blend and enjoy your beta-carotene (vitamin A).
Good for those on antibiotic therapy, cancer, digestive disorders, eye and skin problems, and inflamation..

Apricot Buzz
---

8 ounces apricot juice or fresh mashed apricots
4 ounces almond or soy milk

1/4 cup almond butter, fresh and raw, if possible
1 cup low-fat plain yogurt

Blend till smooth.
Good for a bland diet and extra protein.

Also see the Healing Juices section.

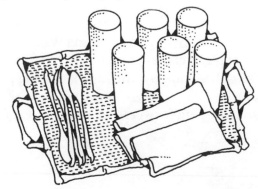

Carob Protein Delight

3 cups frozen plain low-fat yogurt
1/4 cup carob syrup or powder
1/4 cup soy or almond milk

2 tablespoons protein powder, use soy or almond
  powder or mashed tofu
2 tablespoons honey or blackstrap molasses (optional)

Blend and enjoy your protein. *Good for tissue repair, protein deficiencies, and as an energy drink.*

Banana Power

Loaded with the potassium found in bananas and yogurt. A real energy booster. Good for the very weak or ill, supplying all needed nutrients for healing.

1 frozen banana (peeled bananas and cut into chunks
  before freezing)
1-1/2 cups frozen or creamy plain yogurt
1/2 cup soy or almond milk

1 tablespoon wheat germ
1 tablespoon honey or blackstrap molasses
1 tablespoon granulated or liquid lecithin (optional)
1 tablespoon brewer's yeast (optional)

Mix in blender.

Strawberry Cream Freeze

1 cup frozen, sliced strawberries*
1-1/2 cups frozen or plain low-fat yogurt1/2 cup nut
or soy milk

2 tablespoons unsweetened strawberry preserves or
  sweetener of your choice

Blend together and enjoy.
You may substitute any fruit for strawberries, since all fresh fruits make good shakes. Bananas are a great thickener. Try blackstrap molasses for sweetness, children and women in particular need the extra iron and minerals.
Latest research indicates that strawberries are good cancer fighters. Spread cleaned, sliced strawberries on cookie sheet, freeze, bag, and use as needed.

Make Your Own Soda Pop

Kids love it!

Add one of the following to sparkling water:
Cranberry, apple or cherry concentrate, fresh lemon, lime or any fruit juice and a sweetener or soak cinnamon sticks or sassafras bark overnight in sparkling mineral water and add a sweetener and pure vanilla extract, if desired.
If you use barley-malt sweetener you will add fewer calories; it's good for diabetics and hypoglycemics.

Carrot Power

6 ounces fresh carrot juice plus 4 ice cubes
4 ounces of almond milk, can substitute any type nut
   or soy milk or low-fat plain yogurt

1 tablespoon blackstrap molasses
1 tablespoon pure garlic extract

This is excellent for smokers, anemics, arthritics, those with cancer and heart problems. It is high in beta carotene, vitamin A, iron and minerals, protein, and also L-cysteine and selenium. Kyolic liquid garlic is found in health food stores and is tasteless and odorless.

Nutritional Energy Booster

This drink is excellent for the ill or those who want a most nutritious drink. It is great for breakfast, and is a tremendous energy booster.

1 pint plain or frozen yogurt, nut or soy milk
3 ice cubes
1 banana, 1/2 fresh papaya, peach or desired fruit
1 tablespoon blackstrap molasses
1/2 cup mashed tofu or 1 tablespoon soy powder
10 drops of unsaturated fatty acids, flax seed oil is
   good
1 tablespoon lecithin granules
1 tablespoon raw wheat germ
1 tablespoon bee pollen granules

1 teaspoon buffered, powdered vitamin C
1/4 teaspoon powdered acidophilus, optional if you
   are using plain yogurt
1/4 teaspoon powdered kelp and/or
1 tablespoon powderd alfalfa or barley grass or
   wheatgrass
1 tablespoon brewer's yeast - **If you have not taken
this yeast before, start with 1/2 teaspoon
and gradually increase the amount.**
Powdered multi-vitamins can be added.

Put all the ingredients in a processor or blender.
This is a very good drink for the elderly who have problems swallowing and/or chewing. It will supply more nutrients than required daily. Do alternate the fruit used from day to day and the sweetener. Never use sugar, that would ruin this cadillac of drinks. This is a powerful drink for athletes, those who exercise, and a powerful healing drink. **Do not consume raw eggs.** You will deplete your body of the important nutrient, Biotin, a B vitamin, which can result in hair loss and many other problems. This formula will not need raw eggs for needed nutrients. It is complete!

Island Smoothie

8 ounce bottle pina colada juice or pineapple juice
4 ounces papaya juice or fresh mashed
1 banana mashed

1/4 cup almond butter. Make fresh if possible,
   using raw almonds.

Blend till smooth. *Good for all colon disorders, digestion, and cancer.*

Pineapple Flip

4 ounces coconut milk, or almond milk, fresh is
best

8 ounces pineapple juice, fresh is best
1 cup mashed papaya

Blend till smooth. *Good for needed enzymes, inflamation, heart and all colon disorders.*

227

Nut Milks

These milks are highly nutritious and have no animal fat. Use on cereals, in baking and in creamed soups, in health shakes and any time you need milk.

Almond Milk

Keep nut milks refrigerated.

If you do not have a grinder or food processor, soak the nuts overnight in the water to soften the nuts first. If you have a grinder, grind the nuts before adding the water and other ingredients. Use only raw nuts that have been in a tightly sealed container. Do not use nuts exposed to light and air, like those in bins and in heated show cases. The good oil in raw nuts becomes rancid in these environments and are toxic to the body.

1 cup almonds
3 cups water
1/2 fresh papaya optional, good for babies
1 teaspoon pure vanilla extract *(optional)*

1 tablespoon blackstrap molasses *(optional)* good mineral source
1 tablespoon brewer's yeast or wheat germ or both *(optional)*

Blend almonds into a powder and add rest of ingredients, while blending. Using the molasses and the papaya makes it a complete milk for infants, especially for those who have a milk allergy. Add 1/2 teaspoon of brewer's yeast or wheat germ to start and increase slowly to 1 tablespoon for adults, if it's used as a drink. Omit if it is used for cooking, cereals, etc.
This is an excellent addition to children's and infant's diets, substitute almond milk in place of soy, if an allergy to soy exists. It is also good for adults.

Sesame Milk

Use this recipe for cashew and sunflower milk also. It is sweet enough without additional sweetener.

1 cup sesame seeds
1-1/2 cups of water

4 pitted dates
1 tablespoon flaxseed

Grind or blend sesame seeds and flaxseed to a powder, then slowly add the rest of the ingredients. *This is excellent for bowel problems.* You can substitute soaked prunes for the dates, if constipation is a problem. Try adding different fruits and even fresh carrot juice for a refreshing and nutritious breakfast. High in protein and the needed essential fatty acids.

Easy Soy Milk

Soak 1 cup soy powder (from health food store) in 3-1/2 cups of distilled water for three hours. Place in a double broiler and simmer for fifteen minutes. You can strain this or use it as it is. The following ingredients will improve the flavor and texture.

1 teaspoon pure vanilla extract
1 cup of fresh white grape juice is also good here

1- 8 ounce bottle of *R.W. Knudsen's* papaya juice or fresh papaya. (*Optional* if milk is used for cooking.)

Keep refrigerated. This can be used in all cooking recipes in place of cow's milk, its good on cereals and any place calling for milk.

228

Hors d'Oeuvres

Garlic Butter Mushrooms

Great as a side dish, over chicken, baked potatoes,with brown rice, or you can add to casseroles.

1/2 cup virgin olive oil
3 cloves finely chopped garlic
4 cups small whole or thickly sliced mushrooms
2 tablespoons chopped fresh parsley or
2 teaspoons dried parsley

3 finely chopped green onions and tops
1 cup toasted wheat germ or whole wheat bread
  crumbs
1 tablespoon tamari
1 tablespoon wine (*optional*)

Place oil in a skillet, add the garlic and mushrooms and saute for a couple minutes. Add the parsley and green onions, stir constantly. Stir in the wine and tamari and simmer for four minutes. Put in a casserole dish and top with the bread crumbs or wheat germ and sprinkle some garlic powder, Spike, parsley and soy parmesan cheese, if desired. Bake for 10-15 minutes and serve.

Cheesy Nachos

4 cups (one large bag) tortilla chips
2 cups grated soy monterey jack or other cheese

1 cup salsa sauce or diced tomato and 2 small jalapeno chilies

Spread chips out on a cookie sheet or a large flat pan. Sprinkle with salsa sauce and the grated cheese. Place under the broiler (not too close) until the cheese melts and is bubbly. Bake at 375° for 5 minutes or until cheese is bubbly. You may place mashed beans or chili under the cheese.

Croutons

3 slices whole wheat bread
2 cloves of garlic, minced and pressed (or pinch of
  granulated or powdered, not garlic salt)

1 teaspoon dried parsley
2 teaspoons soy parmesan cheese or your choice
3 tablespoons olive oil or your choice

Cut bread into 1" cubes, add to hot skillet with oil and garlic. Sprinkle with cheese and parsley, tossing continually until golden brown. Great on salads, soups and top of Italian or tomato-zucchini casseroles.

229

Hush Puppies

1-1/2 cups ground cornmeal
3/4 cup whole wheat flour
1 teaspoon sea salt
2 teaspoons aluminum-free baking powder

1/2 chopped onion
1/2 cup water
1/4 cup corn germ *(optional)*
2 teaspoons dried parsley *(optional)*

Combine dry ingredients; add water. Drop by teaspoonful into hot oil. Fry until golden brown.

Apricot Preserves

1 pound dried apricots (or peaches, pineapple or any dried fruit), rinse in boiling water
2 cups water

1 cup honey or sweetener of your choice (2 teaspoons barley malt sweetener for no-sugar diets)
Dashes of cinnamon and ginger

Simmer in a small, covered sauce pan for 30 - 40 minutes or until soft and mushy. Mash and jar. Will keep for weeks in refrigerator.

Anytime Pancakes

1 cup whole wheat flour
1-1/2 teaspoons aluminum free baking powder
2 eggs, slightly beaten or 3 egg whites or egg replacer
2 tablespoons vegetable oil to which 1 tablespoon of maple syrup or honey has been added

1 teaspoon vanilla
1-1/2 cups buttermilk, yogurt, soy, almond, or cow's milk
1 cup finely chopped pecans
1 teaspoon cinnamon
1/2 cup unbleached flour

Mix add dry ingredients. Mix all wet ingredients. Mix together until all flour is just moistened. Put on hot griddle to which a little oil has been added. When bubbles form on top and edges are dry, turn over. Serve with heated maple syrup and chopped pecans with a dab of Hain's safflower margarine or butter in the middle.
Note: These are also good rolled up with fruit in the center and topped with the pecans and syrup.

Golden Cheese Ball

2 cups (16 ounces) natural shredded cheddar cheese or soy cheese may be substituted
1 cup chopped dates

1/2 cup softened sweet butter or margarine
1/2 cup chopped nuts or sliced almonds

Combine all ingredients except nuts, beat till smooth (use a food processor, if you have one). Shape into a large ball and roll in nuts, refrigerate.

Party Cheeseballs

2-8 ounce packages cream cheese or
    drained, plain yogurt
2 cups shredded swiss or your choice

1/4 cup date pieces
1 cup finely chopped nuts

Mix all ingredients, using only 1/2 cup nuts. Chill for about one hour. Form into balls and roll in the rest of the nuts. Serve with crackers or any way you like. Good with fruit.
You may substitute chopped green onions, a dash of Spike, a dash of cayenne pepper, 1 tablespoon tamari in place of dates and nuts, and form into balls. Chill and serve.

Avocado Dip

2 ripe avocados
1 lemon
2 teaspoons granulated or powdered garlic (not
    garlic salt)
2 teaspoons horseradish powder (or fresh, grated)
2 teaspoons Spike seasoning or dash of sea salt

2 teaspoons tamari
2 cups plain yogurt
2 tablespoons chopped fresh dill or 2 teaspoon
dried dill
Dash cayenne pepper

Mash avocados with the juice of 1 lemon. Blend all in processor or by hand. Great with fresh vegetables or on sandwiches or over stuffed avocados. Party idea: arrange a platter of carrot strips, celery, green peppers, broccoli and cauliflower and place a dish of avocado dip in the center.

Avocado Dip II

1 avocado
1 or 2 cloves minced garlic
1 finely chopped green onion

1 diced tomato
Dash of Spike seasoning or sea salt

Mash avocado and mix in garlic and green onion. Add Spike and tomato. Mix with a food processor or by hand.

Hush Puppies

1-1/2 cups ground cornmeal
3/4 cup whole wheat flour
1 teaspoon salt
2 teaspoons aluminum-free baking powder

1/2 chopped onion
2 teaspoons dried parsley (*optional*)
1/4 cup corn germ (*optional*)

Combine dry ingredients, add water. Drop by teaspoonful into hot oil and fry until golden brown

Cheesy Italian Party Snacks

Dough Mix:

2 cups dry biscuit mix

3/4 cup to 1 cup plain yogurt, soy, almond or milk
of your choice.

12 cup muffin pan, lightly greased

Preheat oven to 400°

Mix ingredients and knead dough about 20 times
or put in processor bowl with plastic blade and
mix. Roll out and cut with a 4" cutter. Press into
muffin cups.

Filling:

1 pound sliced mushrooms

1 chopped green pepper

1 chopped red pepper

1 chopped onion

1/2 cup chopped celery

15-1/2 ounces spaghetti sauce

A few sliced black olives

12 ounces mozzarella cheese

Saute mushrooms, peppers, onions, and celery. Add sauce and olives, mix and put in pans. Cover with
shredded Mozzarella cheese and bake for 15-20 minutes until golden brown.
This makes a great luncheon. Even kids love it. Serve with a crisp raw salad.

Small Pizzas

Fast, good for snacks, children's parties, and hors d'oeuvres.

Preheat oven to 375°.

Use a bread dough recipe (see Whole Grain Goodness section), or canned biscuits if you are short of
time. Roll out dough. Cut with biscuit cutter or use inverted glass. Top with a little pizza sauce and your
choice of mushrooms, onions, olives, green peppers and cheese. Bake until bubbly and light brown,
about 15 minutes.

Cheesy Party Rye

1 cup mayonnaise

1 cup soy parmesan cheese or your choice

1/2 cup plain yogurt or sour cream

Dash tabasco sauce (or use cayenne pepper)

2 teaspoons minced onion

1 teaspoon Spike seasoning

1 teaspoon horseradish powder or grated fresh

Blend ingredients together. Spread on sliced party rye bread and put under broiler for a few minutes
until bubbly and hot. Serve immediately.

In all recipes it is possible to substitute certain ingredients, such as eggless mayonnaise, for mayonnaise.
For more information on how to substitute ingredients to meet your dietary needs, see the Substitutions
section. Products you are not familiar with can be found in a health food store.

Main Dishes

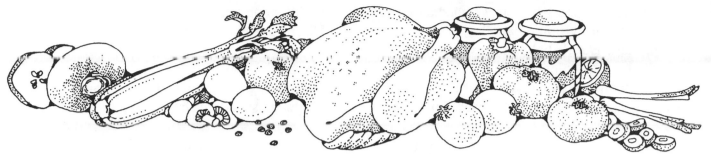

Kiddie Pocket Sandwiches

Things to stuff in pita bread:
Cream cheese or mashed tofu and nut butters
Sliced bananas and almond butter
Chopped, diced dates and a nut butter
Jelly and sliced bananas
Pineapple, rings, cream cheese and
    chopped nuts

Add sprouts and tomato to the following:
Chicken salad
Tuna salad
Egg salad
Eggless egg salad
Hummus
Nut loaf
Chicken dog and melted cheese

You may top with grated cheese and broil for a minute.

Salmon Burgers

12 ounce can of water packed salmon
1 cup fine crackers or bread crumbs
1/4 cup finely chopped celery
1/4 cup finely chopped parsley
2 teaspoons Spike seasoning or a dash of sea salt
1 tablespoon tamari sauce

1/4 cup finely chopped onion
1 tablespoon powdered or freshly
    grated horseradish *(optional)*
1/4 cup toasted wheat germ *(optional)*
2 eggs beaten lightly or only egg
    whites *(optional)*

Drain and flake tuna. Add the eggs, chopped onion, celery, 1/2 cup of the bread crumbs, parsley, Spike, horseradish powder and tamari sauce. Shape into patties and roll in the rest of the bread crumbs. Cook in hot oil till nicely browned on both sides or put under broiler and broil. Serve topped with cheese, as a sandwich or try basic sauce with fresh peas as a main dish. If you omit the eggs, do not add the crumbs to the mixture, just roll the patties in 1/4 cup of crumbs.

Vegetarians
We have included animal protein in the recipes because some people have a desire to consume it or feel they need to prepare a conventional dish for company. For vegetarians, leave the meat out. Find the recipes that fit your tastebuds and your dietary requirements and use your preferred proteins. We have included vegetarian dishes that are complete proteins.

Cream of Chicken or Turkey Bake

6 chicken or turkey breasts, skinned removed
4 tablespoons virgin olive oil
1 package *Hain's* Italian Dressing mix or
   Italian Seasoning mix
1 teaspoon Spike or a dash of sea salt
2 cans undiluted cream of mushroom soup

1 tablespoon tamari sauce
1/2 cup low-fat plain yogurt
1/2 cup kefir cheese or yogurt cheese
1/2 cup Sauterne or white cooking wine
3 chopped green onions, including stems
1/2 pound sliced mushrooms

Saute mushrooms lightly with chicken and 1/2 package of the dressing mix until lightly browned. Put into a large baking dish. Mix the rest of the ingredients and pour over the chicken or turkey and bake at 350° for one hour, basting a few times. Serve over brown rice or noodles.

Marinated Chicken Delight

Soak chicken breasts in tamari or teriyaki sauce for 15-20 minutes. Dip in seasoned mustard like Grey Poupon with White Wine. Dip in low-fat plain yogurt, then roll in bread crumbs or the breading of your choice. Put in a baking pan and bake at 350° until tender and golden brown.

Fast Frybake Chicken

3 pounds chicken or turkey pieces, skin removed
1 package *Hain's* Italian Salad Dressing or
   Italian Seasoning mix
1/2 cup *Hain's* Safflower Mayonnaise or
   expeller-pressed oil

1/2 cup whole wheat bread crumbs
Dried parsley
Dash of cayenne pepper *(optional)*

Mix one package *Hain's* Italian Salad Dressing mix with 1/2 cup mayonnaise or cold-pressed canola or safflower oil. Place chicken or turkey pieces in a shallow baking dish or a casserole and spread mixture over each piece and turn to cover both sides, sprinkle 1/2 cup bread crumbs over all. Sprinkle with dried parsley and a dash of cayenne pepper. Bake in covered casserole at 325° for about one hour. Uncover after the first 20 minutes. Try corn germ for a crunchy and nutritious coating, dipping in honey first.

Read the section on Immortal Mushrooms to find out how you can use shiitake and reishi mushrooms in all your recipes.

Turkey Marsala

1/2 cup canola or safflower oil
1 sliced red pepper
1 cup whole wheat or oat flour
1 lemon
1 tablespoon tamari sauce
1 large sliced onion
2 cups sliced mushrooms
1 green sliced pepper

4 cloves minced garlic
1 package *Hain's* dry Italian Salad Dressing mix
   or 1 tablespoon Italian seasoning mix
1 cup red wine or white wine or sherry or
   cooking wine
4 turkey breasts, skin removed
1/2 cup chopped or dried parsley
1 tablespoon bouillon in 1 cup water *(optional)*

Mix the juice of the lemon with tamari sauce and wine and sprinkle over turkey breasts; set aside. Reserve the liquid. Slice vegetables, mince and press the garlic. Place flour in plastic bag. Shake turkey breasts one at a time in flour bag, until coated. Place in hot oil in your skillet and brown lightly. Remove turkey and add 1/4 cup oil to the pan drippings and all the vegetables. Saute for a few minutes and add Italian dressing mix, stirring constantly. Add chicken, wine sauce and bouillon, cover and simmer for 25-30 minutes. Sprinkle with dried parsley. Serve over brown rice or noodles.

Creamed Chicken Breast

4 chicken breasts, skin removed
Dash cayenne pepper and Spike seasoning
Juice of one lemon
1 package *Hain's* dry Onion Soup mix

1 clove crushed garlic
2 teaspoons minced ginger root or 1/2 teaspoon
   ginger powder
1-1/2 cups plain yogurt or sour cream

Place chicken in baking pan and pour lemon juice and Spike over it. Blend remaining ingredients in a blender or processor until smooth, and pour over chicken. Bake for 25 minutes in 400° oven. Serve over brown rice with steamed broccoli. If you're in a hurry, pour canned mushroom soup mixed with a little sour cream and top with sliced mushrooms, bake as above. Good as a crock-pot dish.

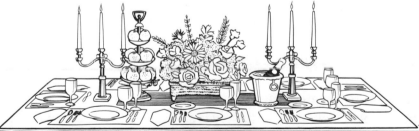

Healthy Tip
On a fat-free diet? Use tamari sauce and a little water, instead of oil, to saute mushrooms or onions. The flavor is excellent.

Apple Glazed Chicken or Rock Cornish Hens

6 Rock Cornish Hens or 2 chickens, cut up, skin removed

1/2 tablespoons fresh ground ginger or 1-1/2 teaspoons powder

8 ounces frozen undiluted pure apple juice concentrate or *Hain's* bottled apple juice

1 tablespoon arrowroot powder

1 teaspoon ground cinnamon

1 teaspoon barley malt sweetener or 2 tablespoons honey

2 sliced apples

1 tablespoon lemon juice

1 cup chopped celery

1 cup chopped mushrooms

1 peeled, chopped apple

4 cups cooked brown rice

1 tablespoon tamari sauce

3 tablespoons canola or safflower oil

1 teaspoon Spike, sea salt, dash cayenne *(optional)*

Saute mushrooms and celery in oil, add a 1/4 cup of the chopped apples (2 slices) to the cooked rice. Add the sauteed mushrooms and celery, toss everything gently. Sprinkle Spike over the chicken pieces or inside and out of cornish hens. If using cut-up chicken, place rice mix in the bottom of the oiled 13 x 9" baking dish. Place chicken pieces on top.

If using hens, stuff rice mix inside hens and place snugly in your baking dish. Pour apple concentrate in a sauce pan, add honey, cinnamon, ginger and lemon juice. Mix arrowroot powder with a little of the juice in a cup, blend until smooth, and pour into the rest of the juice. Cook over medium heat until thick, stirring constantly. Cover chicken and bake in a 350° oven until tender, about 35 minutes.

Uncover, place sliced apples over each piece or 2-3 slices over each hen. Baste with the apple concentrate mixture for the hens, or pour 1/2 over chicken or as much as needed to cover each piece, put back in the oven and bake until lightly browned, about 15 minutes, basting once again.

Serve with a steamed vegetable and garnish plate with a fresh slice of red apple.

Variation: For orange chicken, substitute one large can of frozen orange juice concentrate and prepare the same way. Use orange slices in place of the apple slices. This is great with steamed broccoli, fresh peas, or any green vegetable.

Bacteria Alert

Campylobacter bacteria can live up for up to three weeks in a refrigerator. So be careful of any juices that escape from fresh or defrosting birds. A piece of lettuce, fruit or cheese that touches these juices and is then eaten uncooked provides a perfect way to contract the bacteria. Don't assume you can smell if a chicken or turkey is contaminated. Campylobacter doesn't have an odor.

Wearing disposable or washable rubber gloves when handling raw poultry is a good practice.

Campylobacter is sensitive to freezing. Buy frozen rather than fresh chickens or freeze your fresh chicken for a few days before using. Be sure to thaw chicken completely to avoid cold spots.

Tuna Bake

2 cans white water-packed albacore tuna
3/4 cup toasted wheat germ, crushed crackers
   or bread crumbs
1/2 cup almond or soy milk
2 fresh eggs or egg replacer
1 cup riccotta or cottage cheese
1/2 cup sour cream or kefir cheese
1 box frozen peas

1/2 cup chopped, sauteed celery
1/2 cup chopped, sauteed onion
1/2 cup grated parmesan cheese (*topping*)
1 tablespoon lemon juice
2 teaspoons tamari sauce
Dash sea salt, Spike and cayenne pepper
1/2 cup diced mushrooms (*optional*)

Beat eggs and mix with cheeses, sour cream and milk. Add the tuna, sauteed vegetables, peas, bread crumbs and seasoning. Pour into casserole dish and top with parmesan cheese and bake for 30-45 minutes at 350°

Quick Tuna Vegetable Bisque

1/2 cup chopped onion
1 package frozen vegetables
2 tablespoons canola or safflower oil
7 ounce can of tuna
1 package *Hain's* Mushroom Soup
2-1/2 teaspoons lemon juice

2 cups prepaired *Hain's* Cream of Potato
   Soup
1/2 teaspoon cayenne pepper
2 cups soy or skim milk
1/4 teaspoon sea salt or Spike seasoning

In a 2-quart pan, saute onion in oil until tender. Add remaining ingredients and heat, stirring occasionally, for about 15 minutes.

Turkey or Chicken Kabobs

2 pounds cubed turkey or chicken
8 whole small white onions
8 whole cleaned mushrooms
3 quartered green peppers
8 whole cherry or 2 large quartered tomatoes
2 zucchinis

Marinade:
3/4 cup olive oil
1/2 cup apple cider vinegar
1 crushed minced garlic
1 tablespoon Spike seasoning or Italian
   seasoning

Cut zucchinis in half and in half again. Mix well and place cubed meat in a shallow baking dish, pour olive oil over the meat and let it stand for 1 hour or overnight in the refrigerator.

Place vegetables in the olive oil to coat well, remove the meat and vegetables from the oil and alternate one piece at a time on each skewer. Broil under broiler for 20 minutes, turning several times. With the left over oil, baste a couple times.

237

Quick Company Turkey Scaloppine

8 thin slices turkey or chicken breasts, skin removed
1 sliced onion
1 fresh minced garlic clove
2 packages *Hain's* dry Brown Gravy mix or 4 cups homemade gravy

Dash of Spike seasoning
1/4 cup flour of your choice
8 ounce box *De Boles* Fettuccine or noodles of your choice
1/2 cup cold-pressed vegetable oil
1 pound sliced mushrooms

Cook noodles according to directions, do not overcook. You can put a little oil in the boiling water to keep it from boiling over. Drain noodles and toss with a tablespoon oil.

Coat the turkey with flour and brown it lightly in the oil on both sides. Remove it from the pan and put the mushrooms, minced garlic and chopped onions in the pan and lightly saute. Mix the 2 packages of dry gravy mix with 4 cups water and add to fry pan with the turkey. Stir well till thickened. Turn the heat down as low as it will go and simmer for 25-30 minutes. Serve over the noodles.

Variation: You can add 1/2 cup of sour cream or yogurt and 1/4 cup of wine for a different gourmet flavor.

Easy Chicken

6 - 8 chicken or turkey breasts, skin removed
1 large sliced onion or whole small white onions
1-1/2 pounds new potatoes with skins
5 quartered carrots
5 cloves minced garlic
1 teaspoon dried thyme
1 cup rice wine vinegar

1-1/2 cups chicken stock or water
1-1/2 tablespoons bouillon
3 tablespoons vegetable oil
2 tablespoons dried parsley or fresh, chopped parsley
Dash cayenne pepper *(optional)*
1 tablespoon Spike seasoning or dash of sea salt *(optional)*

Add bouillon to water or stock. In a large 17x15" pan, place the vegetables, top with chicken. Mix seasonings, garlic, wine and stock. Pour over all and sprinkle with parsley and oil. Bake at 475° for 1 hour or until chicken or turkey is lightly browned, turn chicken or turkey once. May use canned soup in place of chicken stock. Serves 6.

Fish Marinade

Great for salmon or your favorite fish.

2 tablespoons virgin olive oil
1 teaspoon fresh lemon juice
1/4 cup grated onion
2 teaspoon minced garlic

Sprinkle with Spike, sea salt, and cayenne pepper *(optional)*
1 teaspoon freshly grated ginger *(optional)*

A good marinade for firm-fleshed fish like tuna, swordfish, or salmon. Also great for skinless chicken and turkey breasts.

Cheddar Salmon Loaf

2 cups salmon with bones for extra calcium
1 tablespoon chopped or dried parsley
2 tablespoons finely minced onion
3 tablespoons oat flour or your choice
1/2 cup finely diced celery
1-1/2 cups soft bread crumbs or cracker crumbs
1 egg
1 cup cooked sweet or short grain rice

3 tablespoons water
1/2 cup grated cheddar or cheese of your choice
2 teaspoons miso
3 tablespoons water, if needed to form a loaf
1/4 teaspoon garlic granules or powder (no garlic salt)
2 teaspoons Spike, sea salt
Dash cayenne *(optional)*

Combine tamari and miso, add rest of ingredients, then add the water, if needed. Pack into an oiled loaf pan or make into patties and place in a muffin pan for faster cooking time and if you like them crisp on the outside. Add frozen peas to a sauce and place over the loaf or patties if desired. See Cheese Sauce recipe for topping. Bake at 350° for 45-55 minutes. May cover with cheese sauce before serving.

Halibut a la Greco

4 fresh or frozen halibut steaks, 3/4 inch thick
2 tablespoons virgin olive oil
2 teaspoon arrowroot powder or 1 egg white
1/2 cup soy milk or skim milk
1 cup crumbled feta cheese
1/8 teaspoon cayenne pepper

1 large fresh, chopped tomato
1/4 cup chopped pitted ripe olives
1/4 cup toasted pine nuts or slivered almonds
1 tablespoon snipped parsley
Dash of Spike or sea salt *(optional)*

Thaw halibut in refrigerator, if frozen. In a large skillet cook halibut in olive oil over medium-high heat for 3 minutes on each side. Halibut will be only partially cooked.

Place in a baking dish. In a small bowl stir together egg and soy milk. Stir in cheese and cayenne pepper; spoon over halibut. Sprinkle with chopped tomato, olives, and nuts.

Bake uncovered, in a 400° oven for 10 minutes. Sprinkle lemon juice, parsley, and cayenne pepper on top before serving.

Go easy on the cayenne, it is very hot, but good for circulation and heart disorders. Makes 6 servings.

Perhaps the most common food-poisoning mistake is to put freshly barbecued meat back on the same platter that was used to carry it from the house to the grill. Use two platters.

239

Garlic-Honey Turkey Stir-fry

3 tablespoons expeller-pressed canola oil
1-1/2 pounds boneless, skinless turkey breast
1 cooked acorn squash
1 cup broccoli florets
1 cup brussels sprouts, separated into leaves

Sauce:
1/2 cup honey
3 cloves minced garlic
2 teaspoons fresh grated ginger
1/4 cup tamari sauce
3 tablespoons sesame oil
3 tablespoons umeboshi paste or whole
   crushed plums
1/4 teaspoon cayenne pepper to taste
Chopped green onion for garnish

Cut the turkey into 1 inch pieces or slice thinly. Heat half the oil in a large skillet or wok over moderate heat. Add the turkey and cook, stirring, for 5 to 8 minutes, until the meat is just cooked through and has a white color. *Overcooking will toughen the turkey, just be sure it is done.*

Place the turkey to a covered bowl. Add to the skillet: broccoli, brussels sprouts, and squash, cook over moderately high heat, stirring, until the broccoli is bright green and tender but still firm, about 5 minutes. Peel and cut the cooked squash into 1 inch cubes.

Combine vegetables and turkey. Combine the honey, garlic, tamari, sesame oil, umeboshi paste, and cayenne pepper. Then add to the skillet and heat, stirring. Return turkey and vegetables and toss to coat with the sauce. Garnish with chopped green onion and serve.

Flounder Florentine

2 tablespoons expeller-pressed canola oil
1/4 cup chopped onion
10 ounces fresh chopped spinach
1 tablespoon fresh dill or 1 teaspoon dried

1/4-1/2 cup almonds
1 tablespoon fresh lemon juice
Dash Spike or sea salt and garlic powder
2 pounds flounder fillets

Saute the onion in oil until transparent. Add spinach, cover and cook until spinach has barely wilted. Remove from heat. Next add lemon juice, seasoning, almonds, and let cool.

Rinse the flounder. Place each fillet with the skin side flat on a board. Divide the filling up, spoon onto each fillet, and roll it up. You can use a toothpick to hold the roll together, if it will not stay rolled. Place each roll seam side down, in a oiled baking dish and cover. Bake at 375° for 20-25 minutes, until the fish is tender and flaky.

Healthy Tip
Fresh herbs can be chopped and frozen for later use in cooked dishes. Freezing will help keep them flavorful and there's no need to defrost before using.

Salmon with Julienne Vegetables

4 salmon steaks (2 pounds)
2 tablespoons lemon juice
3 medium carrots
1 medium size zucchini
1 medium size yellow squash

4 tablespoons virgin olive oil
1 tablespoon whole wheat flour
1/4 teaspoon sea salt or Spike seasoning
1/2 cup water
1/2 cup soy milk

Cut carrots, zucchini and squash into thin strips. Wash and pat salmon dry. Cut salmon crosswise into 1 inch slices, then place them in the lemon juice, turning a few times. Set aside.

In a large skillet, heat 2 tablespoons oil. Add carrots, stir until they are coated with oil. Cover and cook for 5 minutes, until almost tender. Add the zucchini and squash and cook covered a few minutes more. Set vegetables aside in serving dish, cover and keep warm.

Heat the remaining oil in a skillet, add the salmon, and cook on medium heat. Cover to steam the salmon, when it flakes easily in about 15 minutes, add the vegetables. See the recipe for White Sauce and pour over the vegetables and salmon.

Brown Rice Chicken or Turkey Soup

Grandma's cold and flu remedy.

1/4 cup expeller-pressed safflower oil
2 thinly sliced carrots
2 cups diced celery
2 quarts (8 cups) stock or water
1 skinless turkey or chicken breast

3/4 cup uncooked brown rice
1/4 cup dried or finely chopped parsley
2 teaspoons Spike seasoning
Dash cayenne pepper
1 tablespoon tamari (*optional*)

Saute carrots and celery in oil just until barely tender. Heat chicken stock to boiling, add rice and simmer for 30 minutes, then add sauteed vegetables and seasonings. Simmer another 15-30 minutes.

You may substitute barley for the rice and add 1 cup of azuki beans. Add 1 large onion to the vegetables and you have a delicious barley-bean soup. Also use 3 cups lentils in place of the rice or the barley and beans for lentil soup.

Eggs Benedict

2 poached or steamed eggs
1 package *Hain's* Cheese Soup mix or use the
   Cheddar Sauce recipe
1/2 cup plus 4 tablespoons of plain yogurt
1/2 cup soy or cow's milk
1 cup shredded cheese

1 teaspoon horseradish powder
Dash cayenne pepper
1 teaspoon Spike seasoning or dash of sea salt
1 tablespoon tamari sauce
1 teaspoon mustard powder

Spoon over poached egg and toast. You may add cooked asparagus or broccoli under egg. When it gets hot, add the rest of the ingredients, stirring constantly.

241

Sesame Turkey Balls

1 pound cooked chicken or turkey, skin removed
2 tablespoons finely chopped onion
2 tablespoons finely chopped celery
2 teaspoons prepared mustard
1/2 cup mayonnaise or Avocado Dressing

1 teaspoon honey or dash of barley malt
   sweetener
1/2 cup toasted or plain sesame seeds
1/4 teaspoon cayenne pepper *(optional)*

Put all but the seeds through a processor or mix everything without the seeds. Form into 1" balls and chill for two hours or more, then roll in sesame seeds. Stick a toothpick in each one for serving. *Good for leftover turkey or chicken hors d'oeuvres.*

Deviled Eggs

6 hard boiled eggs
1/4 cup sweet pickle juice from your pickle jar
   or 1 tablespoon honey or 1 teaspoon barley
   malt sweetener

1/4 teaspoon dry mustard
1 teaspoon tamari sauce
1/4 cup homemade mayonnaise (or store-bought)

Cut boiled eggs in half, lengthwise. Take the yolks out, being careful not to break the whites. Mash the yolks with a fork and add all other ingredients, blending until smooth. Scoop yolk mixture back into the whites and sprinkle with paprika, if desired. Place on a bed of crisp lettuce and decorate between the eggs with sprouts or sliced tomatoes.

Fast Party Casseroles

1 cup chopped mushrooms
1 chopped sweet red pepper
10 cut up chicken breasts or 16 mixed pieces
1 chopped onion
1/2 cup butter or cold-pressed oil
1 can *Hain's* Mushroom Soup
1 can *Hain's* Cream of Chicken Soup or use
   Hain's dry soup mixes, but use only half of
   the liquid

1 can salsa sauce
2 cups chicken stock or 1-1/2 tablespoons
   chicken bouillon in 2 cups water mixed
   with 2 tablespoons arrowroot powder or 3
   tablespoons whole wheat flour
12 tortillas cut in large pieces
4 cups grated jack or Swiss cheese or your
   choice

Spread tortilla pieces on bottom of pan. Mix other ingredients, reserve some cheese to sprinkle on the top and pour over the tortillas. Place some tortilla chips on top and sprinkle with reserved cheese. Bake at 350° for 25 minutes. Serves 10
Good for leftover turkey or chicken.

Salmon Steaks

4-6 thick salmon steaks
Spike and a dash cayenne pepper
Juice of lemon
2 tablespoons vegetable or olive oil
2 tablespoons oat flour or whole wheat flour
1-1/2 cups yogurt or sour cream

2 teaspoons dried dill
2 large sliced sweet onions
1 red pepper sliced thin or canned pimentos
1 tablespoon eggless mayonnaise *(optional)*
2 teaspoons horseradish powder *(optional)*

Preheat oven to 400°. Place fish in casserole dish and season with Spike cayenne, and lemon. Put oil in a small saucepan and stir in the flour and the seasonings. Add the yogurt or sour cream and stir until just boiling and remove from heat. Arrange onion and pepper slices over steaks. Pour sauce over it all and bake covered in oven for 15 minutes. Uncover and bake another 5-10 minutes. Check by using a fork, fish should flake easily, do not overcook. Sprinkle with dried parsley, if desired.

Easy Halibut

4-5 pounds halibut steaks
1 can tomato soup or *Hain's* dry soup mix plus
    1/2 cup water
Spike seasoning or sea salt
Dash cayenne pepper
Dash of garlic powder

1 cup plain yogurt
1 large chopped onion
1-1/2 cups chopped celery
Slice of thick tomato for each serving
1 tablespoon dried or fresh, chopped parsley

Season steaks with Spike and place in a shallow baking dish. Mix all ingredients, except the fresh tomatoes, and pour over fish. Top each with a slice of tomato, a sprinkle of parsley and dash of garlic powder.
    Bake at 350° for 35 minutes, check for doneness in 25 minutes. Bake until fish flakes easily. Do not overcook or fish becomes tough.

Seasoned Baked Fish

2 pounds white fish fillets
2 cups fine bread crumbs
3 tablespoons vegetable oil
2 tablespoons apple cider vinegar or apple juice
1 teaspoon Spike seasoning or sea salt

1 tablespoon fresh or dried chopped parsley
3/4 teaspoon ground coriander
Dash of powdered garlic (1/8 teaspoon)
Dash cayenne pepper *(optional)*

Preheat oven to 375°. Mix all the dry ingredients, add the cider and oil, set aside. Oil a baking dish small enough for the fish to fit snugly. Layer the thawed fish in the dish, top with mixture and drip on additional oil (about 1-2 tablespoons). Bake from 20-30 minutes until crumbs are lightly browned. Serves 4.

Breaded Fish

Use any fish, perch, haddock, white fish fillets, etc. See recipe for croutons, put them in a processor and make fine crumbs, or use cracker crumbs and bread crumbs, or *Grainfield* Corn Flakes purchased in your health food store.

Place fish, washed and patted dry, on a platter and squeeze lemon over it, sprinkle with a dash of garlic powder or granules and *Spike* seasoning or sea salt. Let set a minute while you fix croutons. Put the crumbs in a plastic bag and shake to coat evenly. Place each fish on a well-oiled baking dish.

Sprinkle with dried parsley. Bake at 350° for 25-35 minutes. Cook just until fish flakes easily and all signs of translucency have disappeared; it should look solid white.

Great for a meal or as a sandwich. See Tartar Sauce recipe and serve with fish.

Easy Broiled Fish

Place fish on a oiled baking dish. Season with a pinch of garlic powde, not garlic salt, Spike seasoning or sea salt and cayenne pepper. Dot with a little oil. Squeeze lemon juice over the fish and sprinkle 1 tablespoon of tamari sauce on top. Broil until lightly browned and fish is cooked appearing solid white and not translucent. Baste once. Sprinkle with dried or fresh parsley. Place over brown rice with a lemon wedge. Serve with steamed broccoli or any vegetable of your choice.

Variations: During the last few minutes, top with a banana sliced lengthwise and/or slivered almonds for a more exotic dish.

Try tomato soup placed over the fish before baking with chopped onion, celery and green peppers.

Chicken or Turkey Broccoli Bake

Delicious for buffets and company dinners.

6 pounds cubed chicken or turkey	4 tablespoons flour of your choice
10 cups cooked brown rice	1 teaspoon horseradish powder
5 eggs or egg substitutes	1-1/2 teaspoons sea salt
1 tablespoon tamari sauce	2 cups shredded cheese
1/2 teaspoon garlic	3 bunches broccoli
1/2 cup dry parsley	1 tablespoon Spike seasoning or 1 teaspoon sea salt *(optional)*

Combine above ingredients reserving one cup of the cheese. Top with reserved cheese and almonds. Bake at 350° for 30-40 minutes. For your own convenience, place in individual bowls and freeze. Serves 16.

Note: The eggs can be omitted if using short grain brown rice (brown rice sticks together).

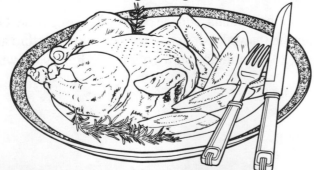

Easy Turkey Pot Roast

1 large turkey breast, skin removed
1/2 head cabbage
6-8 carrots
2 stalks celery
2 onions

3 turnips
6 potatoes
1 package *Hain's* dry Onion Soup mix
2 packages *Hain's* Brown Gravy mix
2-1/4 cups water

Place turkey breast in a roasting pan and brown lightly in oil on all sides and sprinkle with Spike. Place quartered cabbage, whole carrots, celery stalk cut into 4 pieces, onions cut in half, whole turnips, potatoes with skins, use whole potatoes about the size of large lemons and place them around the roast. Mix the onion soup and the two packages of the gravy mix together with the water, pour the mixture over all.

Cover and bake at 350° in a preheated oven for 2-3 hours, depending on size of roast. Baste after 1-1/2 hours. You will have a delicious thick gravy. Try this recipe using other kinds of meat you prefer.

Cabbage-Baked Chicken

Cabbage is good for colon , ulcers and all types of cancer, add more to you diet!

1 chicken or turkey breast, skin removed
Garlic powder to taste
Spike seasoning
2 teaspoons caraway seed
Lemon juice
1 head green cabbage cut in 1 inch slices
3 red cooking apples

2 sliced onions
2 halved turnips
3 sliced carrots
1/2 cup vegetable oil
1 package *Hain's* dry Onion Soup Mix
1-1/2 cups water

Heat oil in a large fry pan, sprinkle spices over chicken and lemon juice, brown on both sides. Heat oven to 375°. Oil a 9x13" baking pan and place cabbage and the rest of the ingredients on the bottom. Place the chicken on top. Mix the dry soup mix with the water and pour over top and cover. Place in oven for 30 to 45 minutes. When chicken is tender, sprinkle 1-1/2 cups Swiss cheese on top and bake in oven till melted, about 5 minutes.

U.S. cattle ranchers received a surprise when news from the European Common Market arrived, telling them that Europe would not buy any more meat that had been treated with hormones.

245

My Favorite Low-Fat Quick Meals

This will take a whole turkey. I buy them ahead and freeze them at Thanksgiving, farm fresh. I take one out of the freezer (always defrost meat in the refrigerator, never at room temperature) and prepare as follows: I use my large canning pan. Use the largest one you have. Wash and clean the turkey and place breast side down in the pan and cover with water. Bring to a boil and turn down heat and cook 6 hours or till tender. Add water to keep the turkey covered. When tender, take the turkey out of the broth and put the broth in the refrigerator till cooled. Put the turkey there also.

When cooled, slice the breast, wrap separately and freeze for later use. Freeze the rest in individual servings to make the **Broccoli Bake**, turkey salad **sandwiches**, **Turkey a la King**, and other favorite recipes.

Turkey melts are most popular. Open up a pocket bread and place egg salad, or tofu eggless salad on the bottom half, top with pieces of turkey and then cheese, place under broiler for a few minutes, remove and top with sliced tomatoes and alfalfa sprouts and place the top half of pita bread on top.

Hot Manhattans and **casseroles** use the sliced white meat.

Make **Turkey Brown Rice** or **Turkey Noodle Soup**. Place broth in a large pan and add the following: 1 pound brown rice or whole wheat noodles. Add 3 cups water to broth also. Saute in hot safflower oil, 2 sliced carrots, 1 onion chopped, 3 stalks celery chopped just till tender, add to soup, season with Spike seasoning or sea salt and cayenne pepper to taste. Turkey prepared in this manner has very little fat. This can be in any fat-free diet. Be sure to skim the fat from the broth after it cools so you can easily remove it.

Turkey has more nutrients than chicken and less calories and fat. Experiments have shown turkey to be an anti-depressant and high in tryptophane.

Greek Moussaka

Meat-free or with meat.

2 large eggplants
2 tablespoons olive oil
Dash sea salt
1 cup chopped onions
1 clove minced garlic
8 ounce can tomato sauce or chopped tomatoes
1 tablespoon snipped parsley
1/4 teaspoon oregano or Italian seasonings

1/4 teaspoon cinnamon
4 beaten eggs or egg substitute
1/4 cup vegetable oil
1/4 cup flour
1 teaspoon sea salt or Spike seasoning
2 cups soy milk or your choice
1/2 cup soy Parmesan cheese

Peel and cut eggplant into 1/2" slices. Saute oil, salt, onions, and garlic. Brush both sides of eggplant slices with oil, sprinkle with sea salt or Spike. Brown eggplant in skillet about 1-1/2 minutes on both sides, drain and set aside. In the same skillet cook onion and garlic until brown and tender. Drain off the fat. Stir in tomato sauce, parsley, 1 teaspoon sea salt or Spike, oregano and cinnamon. Simmer, uncovered for 10 minutes.

In a saucepan add oil, stir in flour, 1 teaspoon salt, add milk all at once, cook and stir until thickened and bubbly. Gradually stir the hot sauce into eggs.

In 3x9x2" baking dish arrange half the eggplant. Pour the tomato sauce over all, add remaining eggplant, pour on milk mixture. Top with parmesan cheese and additional cinnamon. Bake at 325° for 40-45 minutes. Top with additional parsley when serving. Makes 10 servings.

Variations: You can add ground turkey, chicken, or beef and saute it with the garlic and onions.
This is the way the true Greek Moussaka is prepared.

Macaroni and Cheese

This can be made with non-dairy products using tofu cheese and blended tofu.

12 ounce elbow, spiral, or wide noodles
2 cups shredded cheese
4 thick slices of tomatoes
1/2 stick *Hain's* Safflower Margarine or
   vegetable oil
1/2 cup oat or whole wheat flour

1 cup plain yogurt
1-1/2 cup soy or cow's milk
2 teaspoons Spike seasoning
Dash cayenne pepper
1 tablespoon chopped parsley
1 package *Hain's* dry Cheese Soup mix *(optional)*

Boil macaroni about 7 minutes until tender (do not over cook, test for tenderness), drain. Melt the margarine in a skillet and add the flour, stirring constantly while adding the milk and the yogurt. Add the cheese soup and seasonings. Stir until thickened and add one cup of the shredded cheese. Place the macaroni into the cheese sauce, put in a casserole dish and top with the tomato slices and the rest of the cheese. Bake for 25 minutes in 350° oven or until brown on top. May add a can of tuna, peas, and garlic for a one-dish meal.

Veggie Roast

This is delicious, so packed with protein and nutrients that it is well worth visiting a health food store for the ingredients. Give your family a meal they will love.

2 cups cooked, mashed soybeans
2 cups cooked, mashed lentils
1 cup cooked sweet or short grain rice
1/2 teaspoon poultry seasoning
1/4 teaspoon thyme
1/4 teaspoon savory
1/2 teaspoon basil
2 cups chopped onion
1 to 1-1/2 cups chopped celery
1/4 cup ground sesame seeds or tahini
1/4 cup ground raw almonds or almond butter

1/2 cup oat bran
2 vegetable bouillon cubes
3 cups cooked and mashed carrots
1 cup whole grain bread crumbs or cracker
   crumbs
1 cup *R.W. Knudsen's* Very Veggie juice or
   catsup
3 tablespoons tamari
Spike seasoning or sea salt, to taste
1/2 cup ground raw walnuts *(optional)*

Mix all together and add more juice, if necessary to create a moist loaf. In a large baking dish, form into the shape of a roast. Top with catsup, sliced onions, and prepared *Hain's* Brown Gravy mix. This can also be made into patties for sandwiches. Bake 1-1/4 hours at 325°.

Use a different spoon for stirring raw and cooked foods, and don't taste meat, poultry, eggs, fish, or shellfish if they're raw or while they are cooking. That includes raw cake or cookie batter that contains eggs to avoid bacterial illnesses.

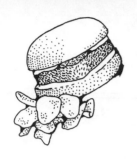

Meatless Burgers

Tofu Burgers
---

3 tablespoons cold-pressed oil
1 pound tofu
1 finely chopped onion
2 chopped garlic cloves
1/2 cup shredded carrots
2 tablespoons tamari

1/2 cup wheat germ or cracker crumbs
2 beaten eggs
1/2 cup soaked bulgur wheat
1/2 cup shredded cheddar cheese or your choice
2 teaspoons Spike
Dash cayenne pepper

Soak bulgur for 20 minutes in 1/2 cup water. Saute onions and garlic in hot oil, adding the carrots. Drain the bulgur of any excess water after soaking and add to onion mixing well. Add the tamari sauce and Spike. Remove from stove.

Mash the tofu and mix with the beaten eggs, add the cheese. Combine tofu mixture with the bulgur wheat mixture. Form into patties (they will be sticky) and roll in the wheat germ and fry in hot oil until browned on both sides. Broil or bake at 375° for 20 minutes until nicely browned.

Easy Pizza Muffins
---

4 English muffins, split half or use French bread
1 cup pizza sauce, tomato paste, or tomato
    sauce
1 cup shredded mozzarella, parmesan or Swiss
    cheese
1/2 green pepper or sliced zucchini
1/2 cup sliced black olives

1/2 cup sliced mushrooms
1/2 cup chopped onion
Sprinkle of granulated garlic or powder
Sprinkle of oregano
1 can anchovies *(optional)*

Place muffins or French bread on shallow baking pan, top with sauce, spices, vegetables and top with cheese. Bake at 400° for 15-20 minutes. Make ahead and freeze.

Soy Burgers
---

1 cup cooked mashed soy beans
1 chopped onion
1 cup uncooked oats
1 chopped green pepper
1 cup shredded carrots

1 teaspoon garlic powder
1 teaspoon Spike or a dash of sea salt
2 teaspoons dried or fresh oregano
1 cup grated cheese
1 teaspoon dried or fresh basil

Mix well. The batter should be quite stiff. To make patties, roll mix into a ball slightly larger than a golf ball. Flatten ball to 1/2" thick. Saute in hot oil so they will be crisp.

For cheeseburgers, put cheese on top and broil until cheese melts.

Quick Chili Tortillas

This takes 5 minutes to make.

2 whole-wheat tortillas
1 can *Health Valley* Chili or homemade chili
2 slices monterey jack or cheese of your choice

Shredded lettuce
1/2 tomato, chopped
1/2 avocado, sliced

Put tortilla on large plate, spread each with 1/2 can chili and put a slice of cheese on top. Put under broiler for about 2-3 minutes until hot and bubbly. Remove from oven and top with shredded lettuce, chopped tomatoes and sliced avocados. Dab salsa sauce over all.

You may add shredded cabbage, carrots, black olives, guacamole in place of avocados, any tomato hot sauce or chili peppers. Serves 2.

Cheese Nutburgers

1 cup whole wheat crackers or bread crumbs
3/4 cup ground nuts
1 cup shredded soy cheddar cheese or your choice
1/4 cup vegetable broth or soy milk

2 beaten eggs or egg substitute or 1/2 cup cooked short grain brown rice
1 tablespoon tamari
1 teaspoon Spike and dash cayenne pepper

Mix all ingredients. Shape into patties. Bake on an oiled cookie sheet. Bake at 350° for 20-35 minutes. You may put it in an oiled loaf pan and top with catsup and sliced onions and bake like meatloaf.

Cornmeal Bulgur Patties

2 cups cornmeal mush
1 cup cooked bulgur wheat
1/2 cup chopped nuts

1/4 cup sesame seeds
Vegetable salt or kelp to taste

Combine in the order given and form patties. Put on lightly greased cookie sheet and bake at 350° for 30 minutes. Make smaller patties for a great cocktail hors d'oeuvres.

Nature's Burger is a wholesome, economical, and easy to make alternative to hamburgers and other fast foods. It is a protein food with whole grains, vegetables, legumes and seeds, yet it contains no products of animal origin, preservatives, or colorings. Nature's Burger can be found in most health food stores.

Open-Faced Zucchini Burger

The best sandwich ever!

2 slices toasted whole-wheat bread
1 cup spaghetti sauce
1/2 cup sliced mushrooms
1/4 cup soy parmesan cheese

1/4 cup shredded soy Mozzarella cheese
2 large slices zucchini
1 tablespoon cold-pressed oil
1 teaspoon honey *(optional)*

Dip zucchini slices in the beaten egg and then in the flour and saute in hot oil for a couple of minutes on each side, until lightly browned. Place zucchini on top of the toast and place on a baking dish. Mix the sliced mushrooms and honey in the spaghetti sauce. Pour over the zucchini and top with cheeses and broil for a few minutes until lightly browned and bubbly hot.

Good Things spaghetti sauce is great. Omit mushrooms and honey and top with the sauce. Egg plant is great in place of the zucchini.

Bulger Soy "Sausage" Patties

Try these patties crumbled over pizza or in a spaghetti sauce as meat balls. This recipe can fool almost anyone, it tastes so much like sausage, can also be used on pizzas.

3 cups cooked bulger soy grits
1/4 cup whole-wheat flour
1-1/2 tablespoons crushed basil leaves
1/2 teaspoon sage
Dash cayenne pepper

1 tablespoon tamari
1-1/2 tablespoon poultry powder
1 tablespoon Spike seasoning or dash of sea salt
1/2 cup cold-pressed oil
3/4 cup grated cheese *(optional)*

Mix the cooked bulgar soy grits, egg *(optional)*, flour, basil, sage, poultry seasoning, cayenne, Spike, tamari, and garlic powder together. Form nto patties and fry in small amounts of oil until lightly browned.

Ground turkey can be substituted for the soy grits. Saute the ground turkey with the seasonings. You can also use any type of vegetarian meat substitute and/or soy granules.

Variation: Make cocktail-ball size and serve with sweet and sour sauce.

Notes

Muffins

Banana Raisin Muffins

1-1/2 cups whole wheat flour
1 cup honey or desired sweetener
2 tablespoons *Rumford's* aluminum-free baking powder
3 cups whole bran or bran cereal-oat, wheat, or rice
1/2 cup expeller-pressed vegetable oil

3 beaten eggs or egg replacer
3 cups mashed bananas
3/4 cup soy or skim milk
1 cup chopped nuts
1 cup raisins
1-1/2 teaspoons sea salt *(optional)*

Sift together dry ingredients. Stir in bran. Combine other ingredients, then add all at once to flour mixture, stirring just until flour mixture is moistened; fold in nuts. Bake at 400° for 20-25 minutes.

Apricot Nut Muffins

1 cup whole wheat flour
3/4 cup unbleached flour
2 teaspoon aluminum-free baking powder
1/2 cup expeller-pressed vegetable oil
1/2 cup honey or maple syrup

1/2 cup soy or skim milk
1 cup diced dried apricots
1 beaten egg *(optional)*
1/2 teaspoons sea salt *(optional)*

Mix dry ingredients together, mix wet ingredients, then combine the two. Do not beat, stir until smooth. (Add 1 cup chopped nuts or seeds, if desired. Soak apricots in warm water before dicing.) Bake in 350° oven for 20 minutes. Fill muffin cups 2/3 full.

Apple Corn Honey Muffins

Large recipe, freeze the extra.

3-1/3 cups corn meal
1/2 cup corn germ or wheat germ
6 cups sifted flour
2 tablespoons *Rumford's* aluminum-free baking powder
1-1/2 teaspoons sea salt

5 eggs or egg substitute
3 cups soy, almond or cow's milk
2 cups honey or pure maple syrup
3/4 cup expeller-pressed vegetable oil
1 cup apples

Slice apples thin, then chop. Mix dry ingredients in one bowl and wet ingredients in another bowl, then combine. Fold in expeller-pressed vegetable oil and apples. Fill well-oiled muffin pans 2/3 full. Bake at 400° for 15-20 minutes.

**Soya-lecithin spread can be used as a butter substitute.
It is made from lecithin, unhydrogenated soybean oil, and beta carotene.**

251

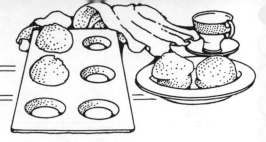

Apricot-Bran Muffins

High in vitamin A and fiber.

2 lightly beaten eggs or egg substitute
2 cups apricot or peach juice
4 tablespoons expeller-pressed vegetable oil
2-1/2 cups whole bran, cereal or flakes
2 cups whole wheat flour
1 cup mashed apricots or peaches

1/2 cup honey or liquid fructose
2 tablespoons *Rumford's* aluminum-free baking
  powder
1-1/2 cups dried apricots chopped
1/2 cup chopped nuts
1/2 teaspoon sea salt *(optional)*

Mix all wet ingredients first, then dry ingredients. Combine and bake at 400 ° for 25-30 minutes.

Carrot Muffins

High in protein, beta carotene, iron and fiber.

2 cups whole wheat flour
2 teaspoons *Rumford's* aluminum-free baking
  powder
1 teaspoon cinnamon
1/2 cup chopped raisins
1/2 cup chopped nuts
1 to 1-1/2 cups grated carrots or sweet potatoes

1/2 cup yogurt
1 egg or egg substitute
2 tablespoons expeller-pressed vegetable oil
1 cup soy milk or fruit juice
1/2 cup maple syrup
1 teaspoon vanilla

Preheat oven to 375°. Sift together flour, baking powder and cinnamon. Add raisins and sweet potatoes.
Combine egg, oil, milk, yogurt, maple syrup and vanilla. Add to flour mixture and stir gently and quickly.
  Coat muffin tins with non-stick spray or liquid lecithin and divide batter among them. Bake 25-30
minutes. Makes one dozen muffins.

Apple-Bran Muffins

2 lightly beaten eggs or egg substitute
2 cups skim, soy or *Rice Dream* milk
4 tablespoons expeller-pressed vegetable oil
2-1/2 cups whole bran cereal or flakes
2 cups unbleached or a whole wheat flour
1 cup chunky applesauce or a chopped fresh apple
1/2 cup frozen apple juice concentrate
  (undiluted) or honey

2 tablespoons *Rumford's* aluminum-free baking
  powder
1-1/2 cups dried apples, soaked in hot water and
  chopped or chopped fresh apple
1/2 cup chopped nuts
1/2 teaspoon sea salt *(optional)*

Mix all wet ingredients first, then the dry together. Combine and bake at 400 ° for 25-30 minutes.

Cooking Tip
**Making extra quantities of these muffin mixes and freezing what you don't use immediately will
save you time and effort. To thaw frozen dough, simply remove from freezer, allow to stand at
room temperature for about 1 hour, or you can freeze muffins after baking.**

Bran Apple Muffins

High in fiber, low in fat.

1 cup wheat bran
1 cup frozen apple juice concentrate or plain
    juice
1-1/2 cups whole-wheat flour
2 teaspoons *Rumford's* aluminum-free baking
    powder
1/2 teaspoon cinnamon
1 egg or egg substitute

1 grated medium unpeeled apple or 1 cup
    applesauce
1/2 cup raisins
1/2 cup chopped nuts
2 tablespoons expeller-pressed vegetable oil
1/2 cup molasses or honey
1-1/2 teaspoons vanilla

Preheat oven to 375°. Soak bran in apple juice for 10 minutes. Meanwhile, sift together flour and baking powder. Mix in apple and raisins. In a separate bowl, combine egg, oil, molasses, and vanilla.

Add bran mixture to flour mixture. Then add egg mixture, combining all gently and quickly.

Coat muffin pans with oil or use paper baking cups. Divide mixture and fill muffin cups 2/3 full. Bake 20-25 minutes. You may substitute 2/3 cup of chopped dried fruit for the grated apple.

Banana Oat Muffins

3 cups whole wheat flour
3/4 cup fructose or honey
3 tablespoons baking powder
1 cup oat bran or whole wheat bran
3 beaten eggs or egg substitute
3 cups mashed bananas

3/4 cup soy or skim milk
3/4 cup expeller-pressed vegetable oil
1/2 teaspoon nutmeg
1 tablespoon cinnamon
1/2 teaspoon sea salt *(optional)*

Sift together the flour, baking powder, and salt. Stir in the bran. Combine the egg, banana, milk, oil, and honey. Add liquids all at once, stirring just until flour mixture is moistened. Add 1 cup chopped nuts, if desired. Bake at 400° for 20-25 minutes. Makes 3 1/2 dozen muffins.

Instead of bleached, white flour, use whole wheat flour, Vita-Spelt, or rye, corn, oat, rice flours. White flour has very little nutritional value and it tends to clog the body with mucus.

Pies and Pie Crusts

Quick Fruit Pies

Sugar-free.

Line a pie pan with the crust of your choice and fill it with sliced fruit. Take one 11-ounce can of frozen apple juice concentrate or bottled concentrate undiluted and pour into a saucepan and thicken with two tablespoons tapioca or arrowroot powder. Cook until thick like pudding, add a pinch of cinnamon. Pour over fruit in your pie crust.

If a sweeter pie is desired add one to two teaspoons powdered barley malt sweetener. Place the top crust over fruit or sprinkle with your favorite crumb mixture. Bake for 45-55 minutes in 350° oven.

Lemon Meringue Pie

Eggs needed.

1 pre-baked pastry for a single-crust pie
1-1/2 cups honey
2 tablespoons arrowroot powder or corn starch

3 tablespoons unbleached white flour
2 cups soy milk or cow milk
2 eggs-separated

4 tablespoons lemon juice

Pre-bake crust. Combine arrowroot, honey, flour, and egg yolks in sauce pan. Heat milk to boiling and slowly add to mixture, stirring constantly. Return to pan and cook over medium heat. It will take about four minutes after it starts to boil for it to become smooth. Remove from heat and add lemon juice. Pour into baked shell and top with meringue recipe below.

Beat egg whites until soft peaks form, gradually adding fructose and vanilla. Put filling in pie shell and top with the egg white mixture and bake 5 minutes or until meringue is golden brown in a 375° oven.

Yogurt Fruit Pie

No cooking required.

1/2 pound small curd cottage cheese or mashed
    and drained tofu
1 teaspoon vanilla
1 cup fruit flavored yogurt

1/2 cup low-fat dry milk powder or soy powder
Fresh blueberries, strawberries
1 sliced banana
1/4 cup strawberry jelly *(optional)*

Line a pan with your favorite crust recipe. Place the fruit in the crust. Blend the other ingredients together and pour over the fruit. Chill at least 2 hours before serving.

Substitution Tip

You may substitute your favorite healthy sweetener in these recipes. If a recipe calls for dry ingredients and you substitute honey, ADD 1/2 cup more flour to the dry ingredients. If you have a dry sweetener, and the recipe calls for honey, SUBTRACT 1/2 cup of the flour or largest dry ingredient.

Strawberry-Banana Ice Cream Pie

No cooking required.

3 large cookies
8 ounces yogurt cheese (see Yogurt section) or
   1-1/2 cups plain or strawberry yogurt
1/2 cup tofu
3/4 cup honey or sweetener or your choice
   (fructose makes firmer pie)

1/2 cup instant non-fat powdered milk or soy
   powder
1 teaspoon vanilla
2 bananas
2 cups fresh strawberries (sliced)

Crumble the cookies and press in an oiled pie dish. Blend all but the cookies the following in a processor or blender reserving 1/2 cup of the strawberries for the top of the pie. Pour into pie crust, top with 1/2 cup of the strawberries and freeze. If strawberries are out of season, substitute strawberry preserves and omit the honey.

You may use a granola crust. See Pie Crusts in this section to choose a crust.

Peanut Cream Pie

Kids and grownups love this pie, no cooking.

8 ounces cream cheese
8 ounces tofu or yogurt
2 large ripe bananas

1/2 cup honey
1/3 cup carob powder
1 cup peanut butter or almond or cashew

Blend all ingredients together in the order listed, with a blender or by hand. Crumble any kind of cookies, press on bottom of a well-oiled pie plate, pour mixture on top and chill for a few hours. Top with peanuts and carob chips, if desired. Put in the freezer and take out 15-30 minutes before serving.

Cranberry-Pecan Pie

This should be served as a side dish, not as dessert.

Crust Mix:
1/2 cup wheat germ
1/2 teaspoon cinnamon
1/2 cup fine or flaked coconut

Filling:
12 ounce can apple juice concentrate
1 tablespoon arrowroot powder or cornstarch
1 bag fresh cranberries
2/3 cup pecans
1 cup maple syrup or honey
3 eggs *(optional)*

Press crust mix into well-oiled pie pans, use enough oil to moisten. Put one 12-ounce can of frozen or bottled apple juice concentrate in a pan on stove, add 1 tablespoon arrowroot powder or cornstarch and mix. Put whole, cleaned cranberries (about 1 bag) into juice and cook for a couple minutes until thick and hot, but don't overcook. Now pour into your crust and arrange pecans on top. Mix together 3 eggs and 1 cup maple syrup or honey and pour over pie. Bake at 325° for 25-30 minutes. Let cool for 10 minutes or so before serving.

255

Coconut Cream Pie

This is my favorite pie, without wheat, eggs or dairy products.

1 quart soy or almond milk
3/4 cup honey or maple syrup
1 1/2 cups fine flaked coconut
2 teaspoons vanilla
6 tablespoons arrowroot powder or cornstarch

1-1/2 tablespoon agar agar flakes or unflavored
   gelatin
1/4 cup water
1 teaspoon barley malt sweetener *(optional)*

Mix milk, honey, coconut, vanilla, thickener, and sweetener in blender until smooth. Pour into a saucepan and cook, stirring constantly until thickened.

In a pan, put 1-1/2 tablespoon of agar agar flakes or 1 tablespoon of unflavored gelatin into 1/4 cup of water, stir and boil for one minute until dissolved. Add to first mixture. Pour all into a crumbled cookie crust or any crust of your choice and chill.

Variation: Add mashed bananas to first mixture and line a pie shell with sliced bananas and coconut. Also top with fresh or dried coconut and/or whipped cream or tofu whipped cream.

Sugarless Blueberry Pie

2 pints fresh or frozen blueberries
11 ounce can of undiluted apple juice concentrate

3 tablespoons arrowroot powder or cornstarch
Juice of one lemon or 1 tablespoon *(optional)*

Heat apple juice concentrate until boiling. Add arrowroot to a small amount of juice to make a paste and add to juice concentrate, stirring constantly until thick (should be real thick to absorb the juice from the blueberries while baking.) Add lemon juice, fold in blueberries and pour into unbaked pie shell. Top with pie crust and slit the top. Bake at 375° for 30-40 minutes.

Easy Pumpkin Pie

1 cup plain yogurt
1/2 cup date sugar or brown sugar
2 eggs or egg substitute
1 teaspoon cinnamon
2 cups cooked or canned pumpkin

3/4 teaspoon nutmeg
1/8 teaspoon ground cloves
1/2 cup honey
1/2 cup molasses

Preheat oven to 350°. Mix ingredients and pour into a pie shell. Bake 50-60 minutes or until a knife comes out clean.

Variations: You may substitute two cups of cooked, mashed soybeans in place of the pumpkin. The pie will still taste like pumpkin and be high in protein.

Healthy Tip
Try adding toasted sesame seeds to pie and pastry crusts. Prepare the seeds by sprinkling a thin layer in a frying pan and toasting them over a low heat, stirring until golden brown. Remove from pan and add to dry ingredients. They taste delicious.

Pineapple Chiffon Pie

Requires whole eggs.

5 egg yolks
3/4 cups honey or desired sweetener
1 tablespoon unflavored gelatin
1 cup canned pineapple juice (not fresh)
1-1/2 cup crushed, drained pineapple

1/2 cup yogurt or sweet cream
4 egg whites
1/4 teaspoon sea salt
1/4 cup fructose or honey

In sauce pan, mix yolks, honey, gelatin, and pineapple juice. Cook over medium heat, stirring until mixture starts to boil. Remove and add drained pineapple. Chill, stirring once in a while until thick. Beat egg whites till stiff. Fold yogurt and 1/2 cup of the whites into pineapple mixture, using an under/over motion. Fold in the rest of the egg whites. Put in a baked pie shell and chill. Sprinkle with toasted coconut, if desired.

Coconut Custard Pie

Requires whole eggs.

9'' unbaked pie shell
1/2 cup milk or soy powder
1-1/4 cups water or use soy milk
3 lightly beaten eggs

1/4 cup honey
1/4 teaspoon sea salt
1/2 teaspoon vanilla
3/4 cup unsweetened coconut

Combine milk powder and water. Add eggs, honey salt and vanilla. Then add coconut and pour into the pie shell. Bake at 375° about 10 minutes, then reduce heat to 325° and bake until firm, about 20 minutes.

Lemon Meringue Pie

Requires whole eggs.

9'' baked pie shell
5 tablespoons arrowroot or cornstarch
1/2 teaspoon sea salt
3/4 cup boiling water
2 teaspoons grated lemon rind

3/4 cup lemon juice
4 beaten egg yolks
4 egg whites
6 tablespoons fructose
1/2 teaspoon vanilla

Mix arrowroot, salt and honey in the top of a double boiler. Add boiling water and cook over direct heat until the mixture boils, stirring constantly. Place over hot water in a double boiler, cover and cook for 20 minutes or until thick. Beat egg whites while gradually adding fructose and vanilla until soft peaks form. Put filling in pie shell and top with egg white mixture, bake five minutes in 375° oven.

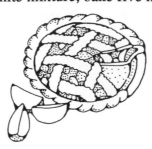

Quick Apple Pie

Sugar-free.

6 apples or other fruit
12 ounce can undiluted frozen apple juice
   concentrate

2 tablespoons arrowroot powder or corn starch
1/2 teaspoon cinnamon
1 teaspoon barley malt sweetener *(optional)*

Core and quarter fruit. Simmer until thick, all but the apples. Pour over apples, arrange in the pie crust. Cover with top crust. Bake at 375° for 40 minutes.
Apple juice concentrate is delicious as a sweetener for any fruit pie.

EZ-Pie Crust

2 cups whole wheat flour
1/2 cup warm water

1/2 cup Safflower oil

Mix together, roll out between waxed paper. Just remember twice the amount of flour to liquid

No Cholesterol Pumpkin Pie

21 oz. drained tofu
1 cup honey or rice/barley malt syrup
1 3/4 cups canned or fresh baked pumpkin
2 teaspoons ground cinnamon
1/2 teaspoon ground allspice

1/2 teaspoon nutmeg
1/2 teaspoon ginger
1 tablespoon arrowroot powder
1/4 teaspoon salt *(optional)*

Preheat oven to 400°. Blend tofu until creamy smooth in a food processor or blender. Add the honey(taste for sweetness), spices and pumpkin and blend together. Pour into a prepared pie shell. Bake for 1 hour. To test, insert a knife in center and withdraw. Knife should come out clean when pie is done.

Note: Can substitute any brand of dry soup mix for Hain's dry soup mix

Zucchini Crust

4 cups grated zucchini
3 beaten eggs or egg replacer
1/2 cup brown rice flour or your choice of flour

1 teaspoon Spike seasoning and dash cayenne
or kelp
1 cup grated cheese of your choice

Drain and pat zucchini dry. Mix all ingredients together and pat into a pie pan. Bake at 350° for 25 minutes. Brush with expeller-pressed vegetable oil and bake 8 minutes more.

Rice Crust

Wheat-free.

2-1/2 cups cooked sweet or short grain brown
rice
3 tablespoons expeller-pressed vegetable oil
2 tablespoons sesame seeds
3 tablespoons chopped onions
1/2 cup parmesan cheese or grated cheese of

your choice
1 teaspoon Spike seasoning or dash of sea salt
Dash cayenne pepper *(optional)*
1/4 cup carrots *(optional)*
1 teaspoon tamari sauce *(optional)*
1 beaten egg *(optional)*

Mix all ingredients and press into an oiled pie pan. Bake for 15 minutes in a 350° oven until brown.

Graham Cracker Crust

No bake.

1 cup graham cracker crumbs
1/2 cup finely shredded coconut

1/2 cup wheat germ
3/4 cup expeller-pressed vegetable oil

Combine dry ingredients, add oil. Place in oiled pie pan. Mix all and press evenly over bottom and sides.

Coconut Crust

1 cup finely ground dried coconut
4 cups quick cooking oats
1 cup whole wheat or 1/2 cup soy flour

3/4 cup honey or maple syrup
3/4 cup expeller-pressed vegetable oil

Mix all together and press in bottom of pie pan.
Good as a topping over fruit also.

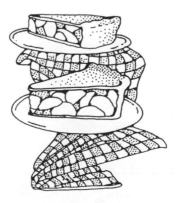

Wheat-free Crust

4 tablespoons canola or safflower oil
4 tablespoons water
Dash salt

1-1/2 cups soy, millet or barley flour
1 teaspoon baking powder

Mix all ingredients together and roll out on oiled or floured board.

Vegetable Crust

1 cup grated carrots
1 cup grated zucchini
1 cup grated potatoes
3 beaten eggs or egg replacer

1 cup grated cheese
1/2 cup brown rice flour or another flour
Dash cayenne pepper and dash sea salt *(optional)*

Drain the carrots, zucchini and potatoes and pat out all excess water. Mix all together and press into oiled pie pan. Bake at 350° for 30 minutes. Makes 2 crusts.

Nutty Crust

A moist crust.

1/3 cup expeller-pressed vegetable oil or *Hain's*
    Safflower Margarine
1 cup finely chopped nuts
1/2 cup honey or maple syrup

1-3/4 cup whole wheat flour or
    1 cup whole wheat and 3/4 cup quick cooking
    oats

Mix all together and with floured hands, press into a pie pan. Flute edges and poke holes in bottom with fork to prevent bubbles. Bake for 15 minutes at 350°.

Notes

Puddings

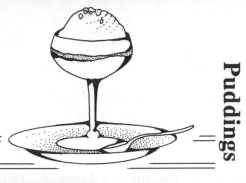

Peach-Rice Custard

1-1/2 cups soy or cow's milk
2 eggs or egg replacer
1/2 cup honey
1/2 teaspoon nutmeg

1/2 teaspoon cinnamon
2 cups cooked brown rice
4 cups fresh or frozen peaches

Preheat oven to 350° and oil a 2-quart casserole. Heat milk until lukewarm. Beat eggs lightly, add honey and spices then pour slowly into warm milk and cook, stirring constantly with a wooden spoon for 15 minutes or until it starts to thicken.

Remove from heat and add rice. Pour half of the rice mixture into the casserole, top with peaches, rice and more peaches. Bake for 10-15 minutes until the custard is set. Serve warm or cold with milk.

Millet-Vanilla Pudding

Wheat free, sugar free, dairy free.

2 cups hot moist millet
2 cups crushed pineapple with juice
2 teaspoons vanilla

1 banana
1 tablespoons barley malt sweetener *(optional)*

Blend all ingredients until smooth. Chill. Top with crushed nuts.
Variations: Cover bottom of dish with granola and pour pudding on top.
Use crumbled cookies on the bottom.
May add 3/4 cup raisins and 1 teaspoon cinnamon.
Delicious served for breakfast or served in half a papaya or cantaloupe.

Maple Rice Pudding

3/4 cup uncooked rice
1-1/2 cups water
1 tablespoon expeller-pressed oil
1/2 cup raisins or diced, dried fruit
2-1/2 cups almond, soy or cow's milk or 1/2 cup
   dry milk and 2 1/2 cups water
1/2 cup pure maple syrup or honey

3 tablespoons whole wheat flour or 1 tablespoon
   arrowroot
1 teaspoon vanilla
3/4 teaspoon cinnamon
1/4 teaspoon nutmeg *(optional)*
1/4 teaspoon sea salt *(optional)*

Cook rice in water and oil for 25 minutes. Bring to a boil, cover and simmer on lowest heat. Add raisins, milk, maple syrup and salt. Simmer 15 minutes more.

Add thickener to a little of the mixture and return to pan, stirring constantly until desired thickness is reached. Stir in cinnamon, nutmeg and vanilla. Serve warm or chill. If using almond milk, top with slivered almonds.

Coconut Rice Pudding

This recipe is great for allergies--no milk, wheat, eggs or sugar.

1 quart coconut milk, soy, or almond milk
1/4 cup plus 2 tablespoons raw brown rice
1/2 teaspoons sea salt
1 tablespoons arrowroot powder or cornstarch

Grated peel of half a lemon
1/3 cup honey *(omit if using coconut milk)*
1 cup grated fresh coconut
1 tablespoons expeller-pressed vegetable oil

In 1-1/2 quart baking pan combine milk, mix the arrowroot with a small amount of the milk before adding, rice, lemon peel and honey. Bake uncovered at 300° for 3 hours total. At the end of two hours, add coconut and oil. If you use the coconut milk, it contains no sugar.

Bread Pudding

Eggs required.

3 fresh eggs
3 tablespoon expeller-pressed vegetable oil
1 teaspoon pure vanilla extract
3 cups soy or skim milk

8 slices of your favorite bread
1 teaspoon cinnamon
3/4 cup fructose or raw sugar (if using honey use
    1/2 cup less of milk)

In mixer or by hand beat eggs and sweetener, add vanilla. Barely warm milk, then add to the egg mixture, stirring constantly.

Spread oil on the bread, cut it into cubes and place a layer on the bottom of a 2- to 3-quart casserole dish. Sprinkle a little cinnamon over the bread and add some raisins, if you desire. Pour egg mixture over the bread and sprinkle with cinnamon. Bake in a 350° oven for 20 to 25 minutes. Serve warm or chill.

Notes

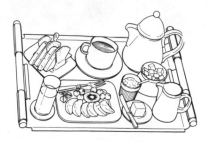

Quick Lunches

Green Pepper Omelets

Requires whole eggs or egg whites.

4 eggs
1/8 cup chopped green peppers
1/8 cup sliced mushrooms
1/2 cup shredded cheese

1 teaspoon Spike seasoning
Dash cayenne pepper
3 tablespoons yogurt, sour cream, or milk

Beat eggs, add Spike and yogurt and put into an oiled skillet or omelet pan. Cook until firm, but still moist in the center. Add chopped vegetables and cheese, flip over and cook a couple of minutes on low heat. Top with a pinch of parsley and sprinkle with shredded cheese. Serves 2 or 3 people.

Avocado Dreaming Sandwich

Alfalfa sprouts
1 slice cream cheese or yogurt cheese (*see section on Yogurt*)

1 sliced tomato
1 sliced onion
1/2 avocado

Mash the cream cheese and the avocado together. Spread in pocket bread or on sliced whole grain bread. Top with the onion, tomato and sprouts. Great tasting and fast.

Italian Omelet

Great as a lunch or light dinner. Requires whole eggs or egg whites.

1/2 cup cottage cheese, low-fat plain yogurt or
   milk
4 eggs or egg whites
1/2 cup parmesan cheese
1/2 cup spaghetti sauce
1/2 cup chopped onion
6-8 slices zucchini
1 tablespoon parsley

1 teaspoon Spike seasoning
1 chopped tomato
Dash garlic powder
3 tablespoons butter or oil
1 teaspoon Italian seasoning or 1/2 teaspoon
   oregano and 1/2 teaspoon basil
1/2 cup mushrooms (*optional*)

Saute onions, zucchini and mushrooms in oil and seasonings. Beat the eggs, dairy and Spike. Cook in skillet or omelet pan until firm, but moist in center. Add sauteed vegetables a dash of garlic and spaghetti sauce. Top with thickly sliced tomatoes sprinkled with parmesan cheese and put under broiler for just long enough to have cheese melted and bubbly hot. Top with a sprinkle of parsley. Serves 2-4.

Salads

Indonesian Salad

Salad base:

3 cups cooked brown rice
2 chopped scallions
1/4 cup toasted sesame seeds
1/2 cup raw cashews or nuts of your choice
1/2 cup raisins or chopped dried apricots
1/2 cup sliced water chestnuts
1 cup fresh mung beans

1 cup pineapple chunks or 1 cup snow peas and
    bamboo shoots or both
1/2 cup coconut
1 chopped green pepper
2 stalks chopped celery
Fresh parsley

Toss lightly and serve with the Indonesian dressing on page 277.

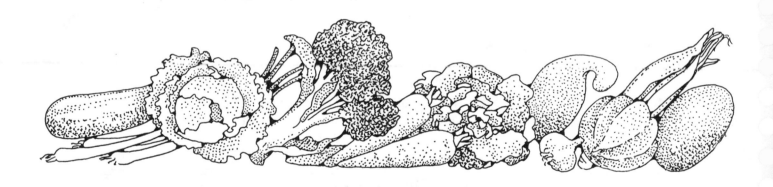

Tabuleh

A great salad or sandwich stuffer.

1 cup bulgur
1 cup boiling water
1/2 cup cucumber, peeled, seeded, and chopped
4 minced fresh tomatoes
1-1/2 cups chopped fresh parsley
1/2 cup chopped celery

1/2 cup chopped onions
1/2 cup olive oil
1/3 cup lemon juice
2 teaspoons tamari
1 teaspoon Spike seasoning or sea salt
1/2 teaspoon taco mix seasoning *(optional)*

Pour boiling water over bulgur in a large bowl. Let stand for 15 minutes, drain off excess water. Mix all ingredients together and toss. Serve chilled over a bed of lettuce, in a taco shell, or in a pocket bread with shredded lettuce. Olive oil and lemon juice may be replaced with Good Things Dressing recipe.

Rice Salad

What a refreshing way to serve rice that gives you all the needed nutrients for a meal.

2 cups cooked brown rice
1 cup shredded carrots
1/2 cup shredded red cabbage
Sprinkle garlic powder
1/2 cup fresh chopped parsley
1 package frozen green peas or fresh peas slightly steamed
1/2 cup chopped onion
Cut up cherry tomatoes
1/2 cup chopped celery
1 cup Good Things Salad Dressing (see recipe in Salad Dressings section)
Cook rice, add remaining ingredients, toss, and chill before serving.

> When a recipe calls for <u>brown rice</u> remember you have a choice of short or long grain. The short is best in recipes that need to hold together, it is stickier while long grain stays separate better. The long grain is best served as a side dish or as in fried rice or vegetables. In salad either short or long grain is good.

Spinach Salad Supreme

Makes 4 large salads

1 package fresh spinach or 1 pound spinach
1 large sweet red onion
4 - 6 sliced large mushrooms

1 can sliced water chestnuts
Artichoke hearts
Alfalfa or mung bean sprouts

Clean and wash spinach. Drain and place in 4 salad bowls. Arrange vegetables attractively. Any vegetable is appropriate, use those you like. Can top with sliced almonds or sunflower seeds.
The Good Things Dressing is great for this salad, it's sweet and sour, just right, find it in the Salad Dressings section.

Summer Rice Salad

Another nutrient packed salad, good for all, particularly good for healing.

1/2 cup sliced mushrooms (try reishi or shiitake)
1/2 cup chopped celery
1 green pepper diced
1 cup chopped fresh pea pods or slightly steamed
4 cups cooked brown rice
3 tablespoons chopped fresh parsley or dried
1 tablespoon dill weed
Dash of cayenne pepper

3/4 cup cold pressed safflower or eggless mayonnaise and 2 tablespoons apple cider vinegar with 1 teaspoon barley malt concentrate sweetener
2 cups cherry tomatoes cut in half or large tomatoes diced *(optional)*
2 teaspoons Spike seasoning or sea salt *(optional)*
I also like half "Good Things Dressing and half eggless mayonnaise."

In a skillet, saute mushrooms, celery and green pepper in garlic oil. Add peas, cooked rice and seasonings, cook 2-4 minutes and allow to cool. Add rest of ingredients and the dressing. Serve on a bed of lettuce or stuffed in an avocado or tomato and chill before serving or serve warm. You can add broccoli or cauliflower, slightly steamed. *If you have arthritic problems omit the tomatoes and use another vegetable of your choice.*

Corn Relish Salad

3 cups cooked fresh cut off the cob or canned corn
1 cup finely chopped red peppers
1/2 cup finely chopped green peppers
1/2 cup chopped celery
1/2 cup chopped onion
1 teaspoon Italian seasoning

1 cup Good Things Salad Dressing or 3/4 cup
   expeller pressed canola or olive oil
1/4 cup honey or any sweetener of your choice (I
   use barley malt)
1 teaspoon celery seed (optional)
1/2 teaspoon turmeric (optional)

Mix together all the ingredients and chill. Good served in half an avocado or stuffed tomato.

Cool Salad

3 avocados, halved, pitted and peeled
1/4 cup raisins
1-1/2 cups cooked brown rice
1/2 cup sesame seeds

1 cup shredded carrots
2 sliced green onions
1/2 cup diced celery
1 teaspoon Spike or sea salt (optional)

Toss chilled, cooked rice with carrots, celery, onions, and Good Things Salad Dressing or yogurt or Avocado Dressing (see recipe in Salad Dressing section) or a dressing of your choice. Place avocado halves on a bed of lettuce, fill with rice mixture and top with seeds and raisins. For a change try adding chopped tofu. Makes 6 servings.
Spike is a terrific seasoning, use in place of salt. You will love it in all your foods It can be purchased in a health food store.

Tempeh Salad

1 package frozen tempeh or homemade
2 teaspoons mustard
1/4 teaspoon turmeric
1/4 teaspoon garlic powder
   1/3 cup chopped celery
1/4 cup chopped parsley

3 green onions chopped
1/3 cup tofu mashed with 1/3 cup of eggless
   mayonnaise or all mayonnaise
1 teaspoon tamari sauce
Dash Spike seasoning and cayenne (optional)

Cut tempeh into small cubes, brown in a little oil with part of the green onions. Cool, add rest of the ingredients, chill.
Tempeh, derived from soybeans, is a good source of protein.

See the recipes on how to prepare tofu and yogurt mayonnaise. You can purchase eggless or tofu mayonnaise in a health food store. Raw eggs, as found in most supermarket mayonnaises should not be consumed. See the section on Meat and Dairy. Raw eggs not only can cause salmonella poisoning but also deplete the body of needed B vitamins and biotin, which can cause hair loss.

Tabuleh Taco Salad

2 cups of bulgur (cracked) wheat
1 package *Hain's* dry Taco Seasoning
2 cups chopped cucumber
1/2 cup chopped fresh parsley
1-1/2 cups cherry tomatoes, cut in half or chopped large tomato
4 green onions, diced, including stems
2 teaspoons Spike seasoning (optional)

Dash cayenne pepper (optional)
1-2 cups Good Things Dressing or
Dressing: Mix together
3/4 cup expeller-pressed canola or safflower oil
3 tablespoons lemon juice
Dash garlic powder
1 teaspoon basil
1 teaspoon Italian seasoning

Cover bulgur with cold water and soak 30-40 minutes. Mix seasoning with the parsley, green onion, cucumbers, toss with the bulgur wheat (remove any excess water) add the dressing and the tomatoes, toss all lightly. Serve on a bed of lettuce or stuffed in a pocket bread, tomato or avocado. Also good on top of a large garden salad or in tacos.

24-Hour Marinated Honey Cukes

1 large red sweet pepper, cut into strips
6 cups sliced cucumbers
2 sliced white sweet onions
1 tablespoon Spike seasoning or 2 teaspoons sea salt
1 tablespoon tumeric powder

1/2 cup honey or 1 teaspoon barley malt sweetener
2 tablespoons finely chopped parsley
1/2 cup apple cider vinegar
1 cup water

Mix the cucumbers, onion and red peppers with rest of the ingredients and refrigerate for at least 4 hours. It's best when left to stand overnight. Add broccoli, cauliflower or any vegetable of your choice. Do not throw out the liquid, just keep adding vegetables. Make a little extra liquid to keep a jar ready. Marinated vegetables are good snacks and side dishes. The vegetables keep much longer because of the acid content in the vinegar.

Greek Salad

1 sliced green pepper
1 cubed cucumber
1 cup cauliflower florets and/or broccoli
2 cups chopped celery
2 cups cherry tomatoes
1 cup sliced ripe black or Greek olives
8 ounces (2 cups) feta cheese, cubed or tofu

1 teaspoon Spike and dash cayenne pepper
2 tablespoons lemon juice
2 teaspoons dried oregano leaves
3 cloves garlic, finely minced
1 cup pure unrefined olive oil
1/2 teaspoon kelp (optional)

Mix all vegetables and toss in the cheese. Put all spices, oil, garlic, lemon juice, parsley etc., in a jar and shake well. Pour over the vegetables and marinate at least one hour. Sprinkle with soy parmesan cheese, if desired.

Waldorf Nut Salad

5 large ripe red apples with skins
1-1/2 cups chopped celery
2 cups coarsely chopped raw walnuts
1-1/2 cups whole green seedless grapes

Dressing:
1 cup eggless mayonnaise
1/2 cup low-fat plain yogurt
2 tablespoons honey or sweetener of your choice
1 juiced lemon

Core and quarter apples. Toss with lemon juice. Mix in celery, walnuts, and grapes.

Mix dressing ingredients together and fold into apple mixture. Serve on a crisp bed of lettuce, if desired. Can add raisins, sunflower seeds and/or grated coconut, if desired.

Pasta Salad

1 pound spiral pasta *spinach, tomato, varieties are nice and colorful*
2 tablespoons olive oil
1 stalk chopped celery
1/2 chopped cucumber
1 large chopped tomato
1/2 cup sliced black olives

2 cups red kidney beans
1 chopped sweet red or green pepper
1 cup tofu or crumbled feta cheese (*optional*)
1/2 cup Good Things Salad Dressing (see Salad Dressing recipes)
2 tablespoons eggless mayonnaise,

Mix together mayonnaise and Good Things Salad Dressing. Toss pasta lightly with all above ingredients, fold in the dressing. Can sprinkle with dried parsley.

Garden Macaroni

1 pound whole wheat or vegetable shell macaroni
1 large chopped zucchini
1 large chopped green pepper
1 quart home canned or fresh tomatoes
1 cup diced celery

1 cup shredded carrots
1 cup Italian dressing or Good Things Dressings
1 large chopped onion
1 cup eggless mayonnaise (*optional*)

Peel and chop tomatoes. Cook macaroni till tender, test often, whole wheat or vegetable cooks quicker. Do not overcook. Blend together mayonnaise and Italian dressing. Toss with all of the above . Chill and serve. May add cubed tofu or cheese, if desired.

In all recipes calling for dried fruit, remember to soak the fruit in boiling water for a few minutes before using. This will not only soften the fruit, but will also kill bacteria and mold that forms on fruits during the drying process

Potato Salad Vinaigrette

2 pounds boiled potatoes with skins
1/8 cup fresh parsley, chopped fine
1 tablespoon celery seed
1 teaspoon Spike seasoning or sea salt
1/4 cup apple cider vinegar
1 tablespoon lemon juice

2 teaspoons Dijon mustard or your choice
2 cloves garlic, minced and mashed
2 tablespoons olive oil
1/2 cup thinly sliced onions and celery
1/4 cup diced red pepper

Clean the potatoes (peel if desired), place in a sauce pan and cover with cold water. Boil and cook for about 30 minutes, until they can be easily pierced with a fork, but are not mushy. Drain, rinse with cold water, and dice. Place in a bowl and gently toss with parsley and seasonings. In a separate bowl, mix vinegar, lemon juice, mustard, and garlic. Slowly stir in the oil. Pour the dressing over the warm potatoes. Toss lightly to coat all the potatoes with dressing and cool. Add celery, carrots, onions, and red pepper. Mix well

Sprout Salad

1 pound mixed bean sprouts and alfalfa sprouts
1 chopped apple or onion
1 stalk chopped celery
1/2 chopped cucumber
1 cup shredded carrots

1 cup shredded turnips
1 cup shredded red cabbage
1/2 cup raisins
1/2 cup sesame or sunflower seeds

Toss ingredients lightly with Good Things dressing *(see Salad Dressing recipes)* or one of your choice. High in all nutrients and especially good for the healing of cancer, arthritis, and colon disorders.

Cranapple Mold

2 cups undiluted frozen apple juice concentrate
2 cups undiluted frozen cranberry juice concentrate
8 ounces unflavored gelatin
1 cup blueberries

1 cup seedless grapes
3/4 cup slivered almonds
1 cup sliced bananas or fruit of your choice

Bring cranberry concentrate to a boil, add the gelatin, remove from stove. Stir in the apple concentrate and chill about one hour. Stir in the rest of the ingredients. Pour into an oiled mold, if desired. Chill until firm, about four hours. Unmold onto a crisp bed of lettuce, garnish with grapes and/or fruit.

This Jello® made with all cranberry concentrate is great for kidney and bladder disorders. Try using all apple juice for the gallbladder. Omit the fruit for the very ill or when fasting.

See the recipes on how to prepare tofu and yogurt mayonnaise. You can purchase eggless or tofu mayonnaise in a health food store. Raw eggs, as found in most supermarket mayonnaises should not be consumed. See the section on Meat and Dairy. Raw eggs can not only cause salmonella poisoning but also deplete the body of needed B vitamins and biotin, which can cause hair loss.

Honey Fruit Boat

2 red sweet grapefruits
2 bananas, sliced (prepare last)
2 cantaloupes or honeydew
1 pint fresh strawberries
1 small bunch seedless grapes

1 cup finely grated coconut
1 cup honey
3 tablespoons lemon juice
1 cup chopped nuts, optional
1 pint fresh blueberries (optional)

Cut melon in half and remove the seeds. Peel grapefruit, pull apart by the sections and coat with honey, roll in finely grated coconut and set aside. Mix lemon juice, honey and coconut together, stir in the fruit (except the grapefruit sections) and fill the melon halves. Top with creamy yogurt and place grapefruit sections on top, sprinkle with nuts. This is great for that special luncheon and fast to prepare. Serve in a bowl with lettuce leaves arranged around it. Omit the honey for a sugar-free diet, substitute with rice or barley malt syrup.

Lentil Salad

3 cups cooked lentils
1 teaspoon curry powder
1 stalk chopped celery
1/2 chopped green pepper
1 clove crushed garlic

1/2 cup chopped onion
1 cup cherry tomatoes
1/4 cup chopped fresh parsley
1 tablespoon tamari
1/2 cup of Good Things Dressing (see recipe)

Cut cherry tomatoes in half. Mix all together and serve on a bed of lettuce, in a pocket bread, stuffed in a tomato, or in half an avocado. This salad is a good source of protein, fiber and nutrients.

24-Hour Cabbage Slaw

1/2 medium cabbage
1 small halved sweet or red onion
1/2 medium green pepper
2 carrots
1/2 teaspoon Italian seasoning

2/3 cup apple cider vinegar
1/3 cup vegetable oil
Dash barley malt sweetener
1/2 teaspoon Spike seasoning or sea salt (optional)

Slice cabbage wedges, onion, and pepper. Shred carrots and add to cabbage mix. Add remaining ingredients together and stir into cabbage mix. Refrigerate at least 8 hours before serving. At serving time, stir thoroughly and drain any excess liquid. Makes 6 one-cup servings. You may make this a day or two in advance. Raw cabbage is good for colon disorders, ulcers, and cancer.

Avoid foods containing the following additives: sodium nitrite, sodium nitrate, BHA, BHT, propyl gallate, saccharin, acesulfame K (artificial sweetener), MSG, artifical colorings and flavorings, and all preservatives. These additives are all potentially harmful to the body.

Hawaiian Fruit Jello

1-1/2 tablespoons unflavored gelatin or agar agar
3 cups pineapple juice
1/2 cup finely grated coconut

2 bananas
1 cup pineapple, crushed or cut in rings *(optional)*

Mix 1/2 cup juice with gelatin, set aside. Bring to a boil one cup juice and add to the gelatin, stir until dissolved. Add rest of juice, refrigerate until it starts to gel, then add bananas, coconut, pineapple and fold in lightly. Return to refrigerate until firm. Check occasionally to be sure fruit is well mixed before it sets.
Do not use fresh or frozen pineapple-the acid prevents jelling. Can sprinkle top with grated coconut and chopped nuts.

Yogurt Cukes

2 large sliced white sweet onions
4 sliced cucumbers
2 teaspoons Spike seasoning or sea salt
1/2 cup apple cider vinegar
1/2 cup low-fat plain yogurt

1-1/2 teaspoons dried or fresh dill weed
2 teaspoons horseradish powder or fresh grated
1/4 teaspoon barley malt sweetener or 2 teaspoons honey
1 tablespoon chopped parsley, fresh or dried

Place onions and cucumbers in a bowl and sprinkle with the Spike or sea salt, and the dill. Combine the yogurt and the vinegar, barley or honey. Fold in cucumbers. Top with the parsley and chill.

Potato Salad

10-15 medium new red potatoes with skins
1 cup chopped celery
1 cup chopped green pepper
1 cup chopped onion
2 tablespoons chopped parsley
1 cup tofu or eggless mayonnaise
1/4 cup low-fat plain yogurt

1 tablespoon honey or 1/2 teaspoon barley malt sweetener or sweetener of your choice
2 teaspoons whole celery seed *(optional)*
2 tablespoons sesame seeds *(optional)*
2 teaspoons Spike seasoning or sea salt *(optional)*
1/4 cup chopped sweet red pepper *(optional)*
5 hard boiled eggs *(optional)* or diced tofu

Scrub potatoes well and cut out eyes as they can upset the stomach. Boil potatoes until tender, but not mushy. Drain and set aside to cool. May make a day ahead and cool in the refrigerator. Cut potatoes into bite-size chunks, add chopped vegetables and spices. Mix mayonnaise, Spike, yogurt, and sweetener together. Stir all together and chill.

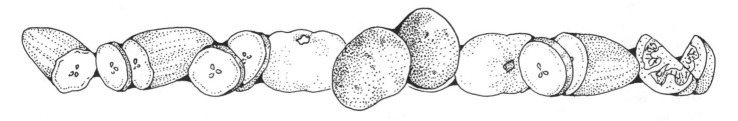

Eggless Egg Salad

1 pound tofu cubed
1/2 onion, minced
1 stalk celery, chopped
1/2 teaspoon dill
1/4 teaspoon mustard
1 teaspoon Spike seasoning or a dash of sea salt

1/4 teaspoon turmeric
1/4 teaspoon celery seed
1 teaspoon horseradish powder
1 tablespoon chopped parsley
1/4 cup chopped sweet honey pickles or pickle relish

Use tofu mayonnaise or *Hain's* eggless mayonnaise, can mix half plain yogurt with the mayonnaise and a little sweetener if desired. Toss all together lightly. Chill and serve on a bed of greens, stuffed in a pocket bread or on whole grain bread. High in protein.

Avocado Delight

2 avocados
1/2 cup halved cherry tomatoes
1/2 chopped onion

1 cup alfalfa sprouts
1 stalk chopped celery
1 cup cubed soy or raw-milk monterey jack cheese

Peel and slice avocado, mix remaining ingredients with Avocado Dressing (see Salad Dressing recipes) and top with sliced avocados. Place on a bed of lettuce, stuff in a large tomato or pocket bread.
May use mayonnaise as dressing. **Those with high cholesterol or diabetes should not consume avocados often** because of the fat content; although they have good fatty acids and are beneficial for hypoglycemic individuals.

Quick Jello

3 cups unsweetened fruit juice
1 tablespoon agar agar *(seaweed gelatin)*

3/4 cup nuts (optional)

Mix agar agar in 1 cup of fruit juice and simmer while stirring for 5-10 minutes. Add remaining juice and cook a couple minutes longer, fold in fruit, if desired. Pour into a mold or bowl and refrigerate until set. Serves 6. If you like it sweeter, add 1/4 cup fructose or a sweetener of your choice.
Agar agar is high in minerals.

Sweet Red Bean Salad

4 cups cooked red kidney beans
1/2 cup chopped celery
1/2 cup chopped onions
1/2 cup honey pickle relish
1 cup diced tofu

1/4 cup low-fat plain yogurt
1 tablespoon honey or touch of your choice of
   sweetener
1/4 cup tofu or eggless mayonnaise

Combine the mayonnaise, yogurt, sweetener, and Spike with cayenne. Mix rest of ingredients and combine both together.
Variation: Use three different kinds of beans and add the Good Things Dressing.

Anti-Cancer Root Salad

1 cup shredded cabbage	2 small diced beets
3 diced radishes	2 diced turnips
1 diced parsnip	1 minced onion or garlic
2 tablespoons apple cider vinegar	2 tablespoons olive oil
1/4 cup minced fresh parsley	2 tablespoons fresh thyme
1/2-1 tablespoon grated fresh horseradish	

Place washed beets in a pan with enough water to cover, boil 30 minutes. Drain, cool, peel, and dice. Steam or boil the remaining root vegetables and cabbage in another pan until tender, drain. Mix the onions, vinegar, oil, thyme, horseradish, and cayenne pepper (optional). Whisk into a creamy dressing. Toss together, top with parsley and serve.

Choice Salads

Choose one from the left list and combine with ingredients in the list on the right:

Tuna	1 can sliced or chopped water chestnuts
Salmon	1 cup chopped celery
Chicken	1/2 cup diced onions
Turkey	1/2 cup pickle relish or chopped sweet pickle
Tofu	1/2 cup red or green pepper
Fresh peas	1 cup eggless mayonnaise or Good Things Dressing
Boiled red potatoes or white, with skins on	
Cooked beans	
Cooked brown rice	1 cup shredded or cubed cheese
Cooked pasta	1/2 cup chopped nuts
Spaghetti	3 chopped hard-boiled eggs(*optional*)

Different ways to serve it:
- stuffed in a tomato or avocado
- in celery
- stuffed in pocket bread
- on a bed of lettuce
- rolled in crepes
- alone as a side dish
- as a sandwich
- topped with cheese sauce
- on crackers

When having a buffet, chop enough ingredients from the right list to make several salads, using one ingredient from the left list for each salad. It's fast and easy!

> **Forget about fish being brain food. The latest research shows that fruits and vegetables will keep you mentally sharp. A *U.S. Agriculture Department* study indicates that boron, a mineral found in leafy vegetables and most fruits, but not meat or dairy products, can dramatically improve a person's mental agility. Fifteen people, aged 44 to 69, were put on a boron-rich diet for seven weeks and then tested. The result was little short of astounding, up to a 30 percent improvement in mental alertness, STAR, March 31, 1992.**

Salad Dressings

Garlic Oil

Take one quart cold-pressed or expeller-pressed safflower oil, canola, or pure virgin olive oil, add as many cleaned garlic cloves as you like. **Drop them briefly into boiling water to kill and mold or bacteria that may have developed on the surface. Keep the jar in the refrigerator** and use the oil and cloves as needed. You now have a valuable garlic oil that is good for the heart, colon, circulation, arthritis, candida, and many other ailments. Use this oil in salad dressings and for sauteing.

Shallot Oil
---

2 cups chopped shallots
1 quart cold- or expeller-pressed safflower or canola oil

Peel shallots and chop. Place in 2-quart jar with a tight lid. Pour safflower oil over shallots and place the lid on tightly. **Store in refrigerator** until ready to use in a recipe that calls for shallots or seasoned oil. As you use the oil, refill the jar. Do not add shallots until all shallots are used. The shallots will keep for a month. Use the same way as the garlic oil.

Good Things House Dressing
---

3 cups apple cider vinegar
3 tablespoons minced dry onions
3 packages dry *Hain's* Italian dressing mix or
   6 tablespoons dry Italian seasonings
1/2 teaspoon powdered garlic or granules

1 cup water
2 tablespoons dried parsley
1 cup honey or 2 teaspoons barley malt
   sweetener
1 tablespoon liquid lecithin *(optional)*

Place all ingredients, except the oil, in a gallon jar. Shake well, fill up the rest of the jar with expeller-pressed canola, olive, or oil of your choice. The olive oil is the best for lowering cholesterol. Always store oils after opening in the refrigerator, shake before each use. This oil is called for in many recipes and will supply your daily needs for unsaturated fatty acids. Make sure the olive oil is pure virgin olive oil.

Lecithin is a wonderful brain food, high in choline, inositol, and the B vitamins. It is an emulsifier that holds water and oil in suspension so they will not separate. This is why it is found in so many processed foods.

Sesame Miso Dressing

1-1/2 tablespoons sweet white miso
2 teaspoons white rice vinegar or white wine
2 teaspoons honey or 1/4 teaspoon barley
   malt sweetener or rice syrup

3 tablespoons tahini butter or fresh ground
   sesame seeds
1 teaspoon tamari
1 cup tofu

Mix all together in blender or processor. Substitute any nut butter you wish for the tahini.

Avocado Dressing

1 avocado
1/2 cup yogurt or sour cream
1 teaspoon lemon juice
1/2 teaspoon Spike

Dash of cayenne pepper
1/8 teaspoon garlic powder or granulated
1/3 teaspoon barley sweetener or 1 tablespoon
   honey

Pour lemon juice over mashed avocado and mix well, add the rest of the ingredients (a processor or blender works well).

Use on sandwiches, in salads, over baked potatoes and great as a dip for fresh vegetables.

Natural Russian Dressing

1-1/2 cups eggless mayonnaise or yogurt or
   mix half and half
1/2 cup homemade ketchup
2 teaspoons mustard
1 tablespoon honey or 1/4 teaspoon barley
   malt sweetener

1/2 cup finely chopped green onion
3 hard-cooked eggs, chopped fine
1 tablespoon apple cider vinegar
2 teaspoons tamari
1/2 cup sweet pickle relish
1/4 cup chili sauce

Chop the eggs fine. Combine all ingredients in a jar, and refrigerate. Keeps a month

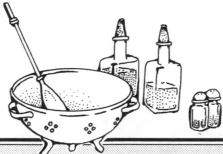

"Mayonnaise can be a breeding ground for salmonella poisoning, a nasty intestinal infection," reported *American Health Magazine*, October 1991. **Mayonnaise (store-bought or home-made) made with fresh eggs carries a risk. Restaurant salad bars that have salad dressings made with mayonnaise should be avoided.**

Tofu Eggless Mayonnaise

The first 6 items listed are the main ingredients:

1/2 pound tofu

1 teaspoon Spike

Dash of cayenne

3/4 cup cold-pressed oil

2 teaspoons lemon juice or apple cider
vinegar

2 teaspoons prepared mustard

3 tablespoons yogurt

1 teaspoon tamari

1 teaspoon horseradish powder *(optional)*

Dash of granulated or powdered garlic
(optional)

1 teaspoon liquid lecithin *(optional)*

3 tablespoons honey or 1/2 teaspoon barley
malt sweetener *(optional)*

2 tablespoons sesame tahini *(optional)*

Mix all ingredients until smooth and store in the refrigerator. If oil seperates, just stir again. (Use within two weeks.)

If making by hand, use egg whip and follow these instructions:

Let all ingredients sit at room temperature for about one hour. Drain and pat tofu dry. Beat egg yolks in large bowl until lemon colored and thick. Beating all the time, add mustard and vinegar, add a little at a time 1/2 cup oil, do not stop beating. Mix the rest of the vinegar and lemon juice. Adding a drop at a time each of the oil and lemon mixture until thick and smooth.

If it does not thicken, add another beaten egg yolk, a drop at a time, beating constantly. Stir in 1 tablespoon of honey, if desired.

Mayonnaise

We added this recipe for those who consume raw eggs. We do not recommend consuming raw eggs.

2 whole eggs

2 teaspoons sea salt

3 cups oil

2 tablespoons lemon juice or vinegar

In processor or blender, add egg, juice, and salt. Blend, about 2-3 seconds. While blending add oil very gradually. When mayonnaise thickens, taste for additional needed ingredients. Pour into covered jar and refrigerate. **Use within 10 days.**

If mayonnaise should happen to separate, blend in 2 egg yolks and slowly add the separated mayonnaise to the eggs, blending constantly. Makes about 3 1/2 cups.

It is easier to make in a processor, but it can be made by hand:

Let all the ingredients sit at room temperature for about one hour. Beat egg yolks in large bowl until lemon colored and thick. Beating all the time, add vinegar, 1/2 cup of the oil stir in a little at a time. Mix in the rest of the vinegar and lemon juice.

If it did not thicken, add another beaten egg yolk, a drop at a time, beating constantly. Stir in 1 tablespoon of honey, if desired.

Bleu Cheese Dressing

Bleu cheese is the most nutritious of all cheeses.

1 cup eggless mayonnaise or your choice
1/2 cup sour cream or yogurt, kefir
    or cottage cheese
3/4 cup crumbled bleu cheese or roquefort

Dash of Spike or cayenne pepper
Dash of garlic powder
2 teaspoons dried parsley

Mix and serve.

Vinaigrette with Dijon Mustard

3/4 cup light olive oil
1/4 cup Japanese vinegar or sherry wine
    vinegar

4 tablespoons Dijon mustard
Italian parsley, chopped
Dash of Spike and cayenne pepper to taste

Mix vinaigrette, whisking or shaking until creamy.

Poppy Seed Dressing

6 ounces tofu
2 tablespoons poppy seeds
1/4 to 1/2 cup honey or 1 teaspoon barley
    malt sweetener

1/2 cup Good Things Dressing or 1/4 cup oil
    and 1/4 cup apple cider vinegar
1 cup yogurt

Mix all ingredients in your processor or blender and blend until smooth.
Good on fruit salads also. If you omit the tofu, substitute extra yogurt or sour cream.

Indonesian Dressing

1/2 cup pineapple juice
1/2 cup expeller-pressed canola or safflower oil
2 tablespoons sesame oil
1/4 cup tamari
Juice of one lemon

2 cloves minced garlic or 1/4 teaspoon
    powdered garlic
1 teaspoon freshly grated ginger or 1/4 teaspoon
    powered ginger
Dash of Spike seasoning or sea salt *(optional)*

Combine all ingredients, chill. Place a serving of the Indonesian Salad on a bed of lettuce, top with dressing before serving. Good on many salads.
If using fresh pineapple juice, it will aid in digestion and be good for inflamation,

277

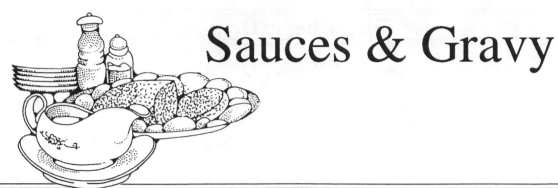

Sauces & Gravy

Basic Sauce

2 tablespoons arrowroot powder
2 cups almond or soy milk or low-fat plain yogurt
2 tablespoons oil

1/8 teaspoon cayenne pepper
1/2 teaspoon Spike or sea salt
1/2 tablespoon dried parsley

Mix a little milk with arrowroot to blend into a paste. Slowly add the rest of the milk. Warm oil in a skillet and add the milk. Bring to a boil, stirring constantly until thickened, add seasonings.

Tomato Sauce

6 cups fresh or canned tomatoes
1 finely chopped onion
1/2 teaspoon basil
1/2 cup chopped green pepper
2 teaspoons Italian seasoning
2 cans tomato paste
1/4 cup fresh chopped parsley or
    2 tablespoons dried parsley
1/4 cup honey or barley malt sweetener
2 teaspoons Spike

Dash cayenne pepper
2 bay leaves
1 teaspoon oregano
2 cloves minced garlic or
    1 teaspoon garlic powder or granules
4 tablespoons cold-pressed safflower, canola, or
    olive oil
1/2 teaspoon sea salt *(optional)*
1 can tomato sauce *(optional)*

Put tomatoes through a processor with skins. Saute onions and garlic in oil for 2-3 minutes. Do not burn or overcook the garlic, it will make the sauce have a bitter taste. Add green pepper and seasonings, tomatoes and sauces. Simmer for an hour or so on very low heat.
Variation: Add sliced mushrooms with garlic and onions for a mushroom sauce.

Quick Salmon Sauce

2 packages dry Onion Soup mix
Dash Spike
1/2 pound mushrooms

3 cups water
2 cups yogurt or sour cream
1 cup shredded cheese

Saute 1/2 pound mushrooms in 2 tablespoons of oil. Mix water and onion soup and add to mushrooms, add cheese and yogurt or sour cream. Mix well and place over the salmon.
Pour over any fish, meat or vegetables.

Cashew Sauce

Great over steamed vegetables, brown rice, tofu dishes, and any time you need a sauce.

1 cup raw cashew butter or ground raw cashews
3 tablespoons oil
3 finely chopped green onions
2 teaspoons dried parsley or
  2 tablespoons chopped fresh parsley
3-1/2 tablespoons any flour or
  1 tablespoon arrowroot powder
2 teaspoons Spike
Dash cayenne pepper
3 cups water or stock

> **Keep whole grain flour, crackers, and breads in the refrigerator to protect the oils from becoming rancid and mold occurring.**

Variation: 1 tablespoon vegetable bouillon or soy milk
Saute the onions lightly in oil, about 2 minutes. Add the cashew butter and the flour, stirring constantly. Stir in the liquid and seasonings. Simmer until thick.
For an almond sauce, use almonds and almond milk for stock.

Teriyaki Sauce

2-1/2 tablespoons white wine or rice vinegar
1-1/2 tablespoons sesame oil or cold-pressed
  safflower or canola oil
2 teaspoons grated fresh ginger root or powdered
  ginger
3 cloves minced garlic or 1 teaspoon granulated

2 tablespoons honey or barley malt sweetener
1/2 teaspoon dry mustard
1 teaspoon horseradish powder
2 tablespoons tamari sauce
4 tablespoons miso (any kind)
2 teaspoons Spike *(optional)*

Mix all ingredients together. *Variations:*Use as a baste on shish kabobs, sauteed tofu, vegetables, or any meat substitute, fish, or poultry. As a dip for fried tofu, fish sticks, any meat or meat substitute.

Salsa Sauce

1 quart home canned Italian tomatoes or
  6 freshly diced.
1 sweet finely diced red or green pepper
1 large or 2 finely chopped medium onions
3 minced garlic cloves

2 teaspoons Spike seasoning or
  Dash of sea salt and cayenne pepper
1/2 cup chopped fresh parsley or
  2 tablespoons dried parsley or cilantro
1 tablespoon lime juice

Mix all ingredients and chill.

> **Don't store acidic foods like tomatoes or citrus juices in open cans. Any lead in the solder can leach into the food.**

Homemade Double Tahini

3 cups sesame seeds.
1/4 to 1/2 cup expeller-pressed sesame oil

Grind seeds while slowly adding oil until desired consistency is reached (like peanut butter).Use *Protein-Aide* sesame seeds, they have a secret method for processing and packaging that protects the freshness. *Variations:* Add wheat germ, peanuts, chopped nuts, make a sauce, dressing, add to veggie meat loaves, and casseroles. Use on toast or as you would butter, its healthier. You may use any nuts, like almond, cashew or peanuts, by adding oil and processing.Try adding chopped dates to your butters, it tastes great.
Cashew is one of my favorite butters a real dessert on crackers.
Sesame seeds are great for quick energy and contain a high amount of protein, and the amino acid tryptophan.

Sweet and Sour Sauce

1-1/2 cups crushed or chunked pineapple chunks
  or crushed
3 tablespoons apple cider vinegar
1 cup frozen apple juice concentrate
1/2 cup water

1 tablespoon miso
2 teaspoons grated ginger root
3 tablespoons ketchup
1 teaspoon Spike or sea salt
2 tablespoons arrowroot powder or corn starch

Mix arrowroot in small amount of liquid before adding to the recipe.
Combine all ingredients in a heavy saucepan and bring to a boil, stirring constantly for a few of minutes until thick.
It's great over vegetables and brown rice, vegetables and noodles, egg rolls, tofu chunks, tofu patties, finger food dips, baked turkey, chicken breasts, or whole chickens.

Dill Yogurt Cream Sauce

3 cups low-fat plain yogurt
2 teaspoons Spike or sea salt
Dash cayenne pepper
6 finely chopped green onions
1/4 cup apple cider vinegar

1 bunch finely chopped fresh dill or
  2 tablespoons dried dill
1/2 teaspoon horseradish powder or 1 tablespoon
  grated fresh horseradish

Mix together, and store in the refrigerator in a jar with a tight lid. This will keep a couple of weeks. Use over tofu patties, fish, sliced cucumbers or tomatoes, green vegetable salads and boiled whole new potatoes.
Great in potato skins.

Cheese-Mushroom Sauce

1-1/2 cups water
2 packages *Hain's* Cheese Soup mix
1 cup sauteed mushrooms
Sprinkle of parsley
Dash of cayenne pepper

1 tablespoon horseradish powder
2 teaspoons Spike seasoning
1 cup low-fat plain yogurt or sour cream
1-1/2 cups grated soy cheese or cheese of your choice
1 tablespoon tamari *(optional)*

Blend all ingredients and cook over low heat, stirring constantly until thickened. *Great over vegetables, Eggs Benedict, baked potoes, steamed broccoli, fish, tofu, turkey or chicken breast.*

Cheddar Sauce

Add the following to the basic sauce recipe while still hot, stirring constantly until cheese melts:

1 cup shredded cheese
1 cup yogurt or sour cream

1 tablespoon powered or freshly grated horseradish
Dash of Spike and cayenne pepper

You can use kefir or goat's milk cheese, cottage cheese, swiss cheese, or monterey jack.
Variations:

    1) Great over meatloaf, sandwiches, baked potatoes, vegetables, and fish.

    2) Poach eggs, place on a slice of toast, pour sauce on top and broil for a few minutes.

    3) For chicken ala king, add chicken ot turkey or meat substitute, one cup sauce, and one box frozen peas. Serve over biscuits or brown rice.

    4) add sauteed mushrooms and onions to basic sauce. Pour sauce over layers (alternately) of sliced potatoes and onions and bake at 375° for about an hour. You may add tuna, salmon, cooked chicken, turkey, or tofu hot dogs (in health food stores).

Easy Tartar Sauce

1/2 cup mayonnaise
1/2 cup pickle relish
1/2 cup chopped onion

2 tablespoons lemon juice
Dash Spike seasoning
1/4 cup chopped green pepper *(optional)*

Mix all ingredients. Great with fish, in any sandwich, or potato, bean, and other salads.

Herb-Lemon Sauce

Juice of a lemon
4 teaspoons fresh dill
2 tablespoons chopped parsley or 1 tablespoon dried

1/2 cup low-fat plain yogurt
2 teaspoons horseradish powder *(optional)*

Add the above to make herb-lemon sauce for fish, chicken or vegetables.
Variation: Add 1 cup shredded cheese for cheese sauce
Great with sauteed or steamed vegetables.

Natural Ketchup

5 pounds fully ripe tomatoes
1/3 red pepper, chopped
1/3 green pepper. chopped
1 stalk celery, cut up
1 large onion, chopped
1 teaspoon mustard seed
1 teaspoon ground dry basil
3/4 teaspoon ground all spice
1/3 teaspoon granulated garlic or powder (not garlic salt)

1 large whole bay leaf
1 teaspoon cinnamon
2/3 cups raw, brown sugar, honey, or sweetener of your choice
1 teaspoon paprika
1/3 cup apple cider vinegar
Dash cayenne pepper *(optional)*
1 teaspoon Spike seasoning or 1 teaspoon sea salt *(optional)*

Put tomatoes through a food processor. Add peppers, onions, celery, and process a portion at a time until smooth. Add spices except whole bay laef and cinnamon while processing and apple cider vinegar. Put all in a heavy pan. Add bay leaf and cinnamon.

Simmer on low heat for a couple of hours until thick. Remove bay leaf. Jar and keep refrigerated or can for later use. Makes 2 quarts.

Miso Gravy

1 cup minced onions or use *Hain's* dry Onion Soup mix and increase water to 2 cups, omitting soy milk
3 tablespoons oat, whole wheat flour or arrowroot
3 tablespoons garlic or vegetable oil
Dash garlic powder (omit if using garlic oil)
1/2 cup water

2 tablespoons miso
1 cup soy milk
1/2 tablespoon tamari
Dash cayenne pepper *(optional)*
1 teaspoon Spike seasoning *(optional)*

Place oil in a frying pan, add onion, saute until transparent, add flour, stirring constantly. Add the rest of the ingredients, stirring until thickened (about 3 minutes)

This is also good to pour over a roast before baking.

A quick wat to prepare a basting sauce like this, is to combine one package of dry Onion Soup mix and one package *Hain's* Gravy mix and 2-3 cups water to use with type roast or with vegetables or pasta dishes

---

Notes

Soups

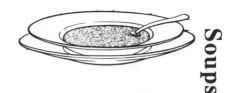

Hearty Lima Bean Soup

3 tablespoons expeller-pressed oil or garlic oil
1 pound lima beans
1 chopped large onion
2 stalks chopped celery, hearts, and leaves
1 chopped large carrot
3 tablespoons chopped fresh parsley or 1 tablespoon dried

2 tablespoons vegetable bouillon or miso
1 whole bay leaf (remove when soup is done)
2 tablespoons tamari
2 teaspoons Spike seasoning or a little sea salt
Dash cayenne pepper
1 cup potato flakes (*optional*)

Put 1-1/2 quarts water over the soaked beans and soak overnight; bring to a boil and turn down to a simmer. Simmer about 1-1/2 hours, test for tenderness to see if they are done. Add vegetable bouillon. Saute onions, celery and carrots in hot oil. May use garlic oil or add a crushed garlic clove. Add seasonings and stir in potato flakes, they add to the flavor and thickness or boiled potatoes mashed or place raw cubed potatoes in soup while cooking. Test beans to be sure they have completed cooking.

Black Bean Soup

2 cups black beans
6 cups water
2 tablespoons expeller-pressed oil

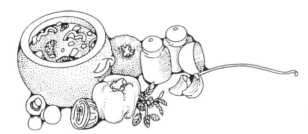

Saute:
1 large chopped carrot
2 chopped onions
2 stalks chopped celery
1/2 teaspoon sea salt or 2 teaspoons Spike and dash of cayenne
1 whole bay leaf, remove before serving
1 teaspoon celery seed
1/4 teaspoon basil
Juice of one-half lemon
1 tablespoon tamari sauce

Soak beans overnight in pressure cooker. Pressure cook beans 1-1/2 hours in soaking water or cook slowly for 2-3 hours with the bay leaf, remove the leaf before blending the beans. When done puree beans in a blender; add the salt, herbs and sauteed vegetables. Simmer 15 minutes more and add the juice of one half lemon and the soy sauce. Garnish with a dash of plain yogurt or sour cream and chopped chives.

> **Sauted onions, celery and carrots are flavorful seasonings, no need for meat. Add to all your soups.**

Barley Bean Soup

Azuki/anasazi beans are highest in nutrients of all beans.

1/2 pound azuki or anasazi beans
1/2 pound barley (or 1 pound barley, if no beans are desired)
2-1/2 quarts water
2 tablespoons garlic oil or safflower oil
2 diced carrots
1 diced large onion
2 chopped stalks of celery

6 tablespoons vegetable broth, or 2 tablespoons miso mixed with 4 tablespoons water
1-1/2 tablespoons Spike seasoning or dash of sea salt
Dash of cayenne pepper (*optional*)
1/2 cup dried veggies or 1 box *Hain's* dry Vegetable Soup mix (*optional*)
1/4 cup parsley, chopped or dried (*optional*)

Bring beans to a boil and simmer covered for 1-1/2 hours.

Saute carrots, onion, and celery in oil and add to barley along with bouillon or miso. Barley swells a lot, so it may need additional water. Stir in Spike, cayenne, dried veggies, and parsley.

One quart *R.W. Knudsen* Very Veggie juice is good for extra flavor or a *Very Veggie Chili* juice which is good if you like a more spicy flavor. Vegetarians will especially like the added flavor from these juices.

Onion Miso Soup

1/2 cup garlic oil or expeller-pressed safflower oil
4 large onions, quartered and cut in half
2 quarts water or stock
1 tablespoon Spike seasoning
Cayenne pepper to taste
3 tablespoons miso

1/4 cup soy parmesan cheese or your choice
2 slices whole grain bread
1-1/2 tablespoons vegetable oil
1/4 teaspoon garlic powder
1 tablespoon vegetable bouillon (*optional*)

Cut bread into 2" squares. Saute onions in oil for 3 minutes or until transparent, not brown, set aside. Heat water or stock in four-quart pan. Add cup of stock to the miso and mix well, working out lumps, add to the stock. Add bouillon, cayenne, and Spike. Taste for flavor, may need more Spike or bouillon. Add sauteed onions.

In frying pan, mix oil, garlic powder, 2 tablespoons soy parmesan cheese, toss squares of bread into pan for a minute until lightly browned. Top soup with croutons and sprinkle with Parmesan cheese.

Top with a slice of toast and one or two slices of soy or plain Swiss cheese, put under broiler for a few minutes until cheese melts, for French Onion Soup.

Alkalizing and Healing Broth

3 stalks celery or bok choy
3 carrots
1 cup spinach leaves

Parsley
1 large onion or 2 cloves garlic
6 new unpeeled potatoes

Cover with water in a soup pot. Let cook until broth has a rich flavor. Strain and drink hot or cold. *This is a powerful healing broth, rich in beta carotene, potassium, sodium, calcium, iron, manganese, magnesium and sulfur.*

Cream of Tomato Soup

6 ripe tomatoes
4 tablespoons whole wheat flour
3 tablespoons soft Hain's Margarine or vegetable
   oil
2 teaspoons Spike seasoning
1 tablespoon vegetable broth

1 cup soy milk or powered milk
1 cup yogurt or sour cream
1 teaspoon dried parsley or fresh
Dash cayenne pepper (optional)
1 teaspoon horseradish powder (optional)
1 tablespoon honey (optional)

Simmer tomatoes, that have been peeled and put through a processor or chopped fine, over low heat until tender (about 15 minutes). Blend in the flour with the margarine and mix into tomatoes, stirring until thickened. Add seasonings, yogurt and soy milk. Keep on the stove just until heated through. Top with chopped parsley and serve. This is also good added to cooked brown rice. Try adding *R.W. Knudsen* Very Veggie juice for a different flavor. Almond milk can be used if you have a reaction to cow or soy milk. It is best to rotate the types of milk used in cooking.

Creamed Tomato Soup

2 tablespoons vegetable oil
2 chopped onions
1 tablespoon arrowroot paste
3 tablespoons whole wheat flour in 1/8 cup cold
      water or1/2 cup dried potato flakes to thicken

5 quarts tomatoes
1 quart heated soy milk or your choice
1/2 teaspoon parsley
1/2 teaspoon basil
1/2 cup tamari

Saute onion in oil, add tomato and heat until softened. Press through sieve or put through a food mill to remove the seeds. Add arrowroot paste to tomato mixture and cook until thickened, stir often. Add remaining ingredients and simmer gently for 20 minutes. For a creamier soup, add more soy milk to taste.
This soup is best when made a day ahead.

Mushroom Soup

Rich in all minerals, protein, and vitamins. Use reishi or shiitake mushrooms to make a soup for those suffering from cancer or any disease.

2 tablespoons expeller-pressed oil
2 pounds sliced mushrooms
1 diced onion
1-2 tablespoons dulse or any sea vegetable

3 packages mushroom soup mix or
   3 tablespoons miso
6 cups water
Dash of cayenne pepper (optional)

Saute mushrooms and onion in expeller-pressed oil. Combine soup mix with water and heat. Add sauteed vegetables and spices.
Variation: 2 cups of plain yogurt and 2 cups of soy milk may be added, in place of the 4 cups water added last.

For quick, delicious soups try *Taste Adventure* pre-cooked, instant soup mixes. *Take my word for it, they are like home-made and all you do is add water.* The mixes are available in health food stores. PB

Minestrone (Italian Soup)

1 cup dried red kidney beans or other beans
5 quarts water
1 tablespoon Spike seasoning
2 tablespoons tamari
Dash cayenne pepper
2 tablespoons miso
2-1/2 cups chopped onion
1 clove minced garlic
1-1/2 cups diced celery

2 cups finely shredded cabbage
1-1/2 cups diced carrots
2 medium potatoes, unpeeled, cubed
1 tablespoon parsley (fresh or dried)
1-1/2 cups thinly sliced zucchini or yellow squash
1-1/2 cups green beans
1 quart tomatoes
1-1/2 cups uncooked spaghetti, broken up

One quart *R.W. Knudsen* Very Veggie or Chili Veggie Juice, can substitute for tomatoes or tomato juice. Mix together: grated soy parmesan or romano cheese with a pinch of crushed basil (set aside one tablespoon). Place beans, water and seasonings in a large kettle and add miso paste. Simmer, covered, for 3 hours. Add onion, garlic, celery, cabbage, carrots, potato, parsley and Miso paste. Simmer covered, on low heat, until vegetables are tender, about 1/2 hour.

Add squash, green beans, tomatoes and spaghetti. Simmer on low heat until spaghetti is cooked, about 10-15 minutes. Add more Spike and tamari, if needed. Serve in bowls and sprinkle with cheese and basil mixture. Good with lasagna, spaghetti, or pizza and with salad. Makes about 7 quarts.

Carrot Onion Miso Soup

Good for the heart and healing. Rich in all minerals, protein, and vitamins.

1 onion, in large chunks
3 cups sliced carrots
3 tablespoons expeller-pressed safflower oil
2 tablespoons dried parsley (or fresh)
2 tablespoons dulse or sea vegetables of your
   choice

1 quart water (more if you want more liquid)
2 tablespoons any kind of miso mixed with 4
   tablespoon of water
2 teaspoons Spike seasoning or a dash of sea salt
Dash cayenne
1 clove minced garlic

Saute garlic, onions and carrots until only slightly soft, but keep the carrots crisp. Heat water to boiling, add carrots, garlic, and onions and simmer for 5 minutes. Add creamed miso, Spike seasoning, cayenne and parsley.

Serve topped with soy parmesan cheese and whole wheat garlic croutons. If you like more or less flavor, increase or decrease the miso.

Notes

Tofu Soup

A wonderful soup when you are not feeling well, rich in all minerals and proteins needed for healing.

1 quart vegetable stock or bouillon
1/4 cup finely chopped spinach
8 ounces cubed tofu
1/2 cup chopped celery heart (very center of stalk)
   and leaves

1 tablespoon dulse or any dried seaweed
2 chopped green onions
1 teaspoon Spike seasoning
Dash cayenne pepper
2 teaspoons tamari

Add all the ingredients together, except the tofu, to the stock and simmer for 10 minutes. Add tofu and simmer 3 more minutes. Serve with rice crackers.

Split Pea Soup

1 pound split peas
2 quarts water
2 sliced carrots
1 large sliced onion

3 stalks chopped celery
2 diced potatoes
Spike seasoning or sea salt
Cayenne pepper to taste

Bring split peas and water to a boil and simmer until tender (about 1 hour). Saute carrots in garlic oil until tender, but still crisp: May add dried mixed veggies or sea vegetables and dried parsley (has diuretic effects and helps digestion.) Add vegetables to split peas. Add 3 tablespoons of vegetable broth or miso, if desired. For thicker soup add 1/2 cup potato flakes. Never overcook the sauteed vegetables, keep them crisp, not soft.

Potato Cuke Soup

12 medium diced potatoes with skins
5 medium diced cucumbers
3 diced onions
1-1/2 cups soy milk or your choice
1/4 cup chopped chives

1/4 cup chopped green pepper
1/4 teaspoon each tarragon, rosemary, and basil
1/2 teaspoon parsley
1 cup sour cream or yogurt

Place potatoes and onions in a large pot and add just enough water to cover, simmer until half done. Add cucumbers and simmer 15 minutes more. Add milk and herbs and simmer 10 more minutes, do not boil. For added flavor, saute onions in garlic oil *(see recipe for garlic oil)* for a couple minutes and add 2 tablespoons vegetable or chicken bouillon.

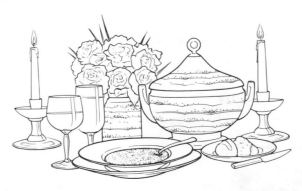

Cheesy Potato Soup

6-8 peeled and cubed large potatoes
2 chopped large onions
3 chopped stalks celery and leaves
2 chopped carrots
1/4 cup expeller-pressed safflower oil
2 quarts soy milk or your choice

2 packages *Hain's* dry Cheese Soup mix or
  2 cups shredded cheese
3 teaspoons Spike seasoning
2 tablespoons tamari
1/2 cup fresh chopped parsley or dried (*optional*)
Dash cayenne pepper (*optional*)

Saute chopped celery, carrots, and onions in oil (*I always use these sauteed vegetables in most of my soups, for the seasoning and the nutrients*). Boil potatoes in twice as much water as potatoes until tender and add sauteed vegetables. Add dry soup mix to a little water before adding to soup. Mix in the rest of the ingredients, except milk, and simmer for 15-20 minutes on lowest heat, covered. Add milk and heat, but do not boil. Watch carefully so as not to scorch. Add 2 tablespoons vegetable bouillon or miso, if desired.
I always thicken this soup with dry potato flakes; try 1 cup of flakes, it adds more flavor and body.

Instant Cream of Vegetable Soup

This is a good way to use left over vegetables.

Place 2 cups of one or any combination of the following in a processor or blender:

Asparagus	Broccoli	Carrots	Cauliflower	Corn
Cooked onions	Peas	Squash	Sweet potatoes	Tomatoes

Add 1-1/2 cups of any one or a combination of the following:

Yogurt	Milk	Soy milk	Goat's milk	Sour cream	Rice milk	Almond milk

Blend till smooth, season and serve cold or hot. A quick nourishment !

Cindy's Cream of Broccoli and Yellow Squash Soup

4 tablespoons olive oil, butter, or ghee
1 medium diced yellow onion
1 large bay leaf
2 medium crushed garlic cloves
3 cups chopped broccoli
2 cups sliced yellow crookneck squash
1 teaspoon sea salt

2-1/2 cups water or vegetable stock or miso
2 cups Original Rice Dream
1/2 teaspoon basil, thyme and marjoram
  (each)
1 cup broccoli florets
fresh chives, finely chopped (*optional*)

In a 3 quart saucepan, over medium heat, saute onions and garlic in butter/oil until onions are translucent. Add chopped broccoli, squash, bay leaf, salt and water or stock. Cover and cook for 15 minutes (or until the broccoli is tender). Using a food processor or blender, puree mixture until smooth and creamy. Return puree to pot, whisk in Rice Dream and all the seasonings and simmer over a low flame for 10 minutes. Steam broccoli florets 3-5 minutes; add to soup. Gently stir and serve immediately topped with chives. Serves 6-8

Sweet Treats

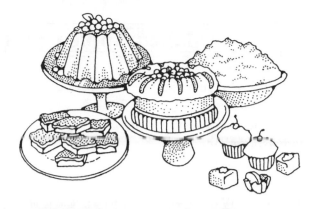

Carob-Peanut Creamsicles

1/2 cup malt or rice syrup or honey or
   maple syrup
1 cup peanut, almond or sesame butter
1 mashed banana

1-1/2 cups vanilla or plain yogurt
4 tablespoons carob powder
1 cup soy, nut or cow's milk

Combine syrup, peanut butter and banana. Mix carob and yogurt and add to the peanut butter mixture; stir in the milk. Pour into small-sized muffin tins, which are lined with muffin cups or waxed paper that will peel off. Insert sticks. Do not let them sit out of the refrigerator too long before eating or you will have to refreeze.

Cracker Jacks

4 quarts popped popcorn
1 cup expeller-pressed vegetable oil

1/2-3/4 cup molasses or honey
1-1/2 cups peanuts or pecans

Mix oil and maple syrup. Toss popcorn in mixture with peanuts. Spread on large cookie sheet or cake pans and bake for 15 minutes at 350°. Stir a time or two while baking. Cool and serve.

Hot Bananas

4 tablespoons expeller-pressed vegetable oil
   or safflower margarine
3 tablespoons pineapple juice

5 bananas
3 tablespoons pure maple syrup
Pinch of ground ginger

Halve bananas length-wise. Heat and mix all ingredients except the bananas in frying pan. Gently lay bananas on top and turn only once, brown lightly. Serve topped with honey ice cream, yogurt or spoon on top of banana cake or banana bread, or on top of baked fish.

Baked Apple Cranberry Dumplings

Pastry for a 2-crust pie
Apple coating:
2 tablespoons raw, brown sugar or Sucanat
1/4 teaspoon cinnamon
4 medium baking apples
2 tablespoons expeller-pressed oil
1 egg yolk (or egg substitute) to use later
   (optional)

Apple cranberry sauce:
1 cup cranberries, washed and stemmed
3/4 cup raw or brown sugar or sucanat
2 tablespoons pure maple syrup
1-1/2 cups chopped apples
2 tablespoons expeller-pressed vegetable oil

Form pastry into a ball, wrap in waxed paper and refrigerate. Combine 2 tablespoons of sugar and the cinnamon and put on the waxed paper. Pare and core apples, roll in cinnamon and sugar mixture and reserve the leftover mixture.

Preheat oven to 450° and oil a 13x9x2" pan. Roll pastry out to 1/4 to 1/2" thickness, place apple on dough and cut a rectangle around that will wrap around the apple, leaving a 1/2" opening around the upper edge of the apple. To seal the seams of dough around the apple, moisten overlapping edges of dough with water and press to seal. Press pastry to whole apple. Place in pan, so it does not touch the sides.

Lightly dab oil into the center of the apple. Mix egg yolk with 2 teaspoons water and brush on pastry. Sprinkle reserved cinnamon-sugar on top and bake 15 minutes, reducing the oven temperature to 350°. Brush pastry again with yolk and water. Bake 20-30 minutes longer or until apples are tender and pastry is crisp and golden brown.

Meanwhile, make the sauce. In a medium saucepan combine cranberries and sugar, mashing cranberries slightly. Add maple syrup and 1/4 cup of water, mix well and bring to boiling, stirring, about 3 minutes. Add a chopped apple and the oil, bring to a boil, reduce heat, simmer covered for 5 minutes. Remove apples to serving dish, spoon sauce over top and around base of apples. Serve warm with vanilla ice cream, fruit or flavored yogurt or tofu whipped cream (see recipe).   Makes 4 servings.

Apple Raisin Crisp

5 cups cored, sliced apples
1 teaspoon cinammon
1 cup pure maple syrup or honey
1/2 cup expeller-pressed vegetable oil

1 cup quick cooking oats
1/2 cup raisins
1 cup chopped nuts

Lightly oil in shallow baking pan. Place sliced apples over bottom and sprinkle cinnamon on top. Mix the rest of the ingredients together, except the nuts. Spread the mixture over apples and top with nuts. Bake at 350° for 30-35 minutes.

If you are in a hurry, crumbled oatmeal cookies on top are great, also!

Quick Peach Crisp

Easy and nutritious!

1 can drained sliced peaches or favorite fruit
Dash nutmeg and ginger
2 tablespoons flour or 3 tablespoons tapioca
　or arrowroot powder
1 tablespoon expeller-pressed vegetable oil or
　margarine

3 tablespoons fructose or raw sugar or 1
　teaspoon barley malt sweetener
2 tablespoons quick cooking oats
1/2 teaspoon cinnamon

Pour peaches into a small baking dish, top with rest of ingredients and mix well except oil. Brush top with oil. If in a big hurry for a quick dessert, top with apple-cinnamon granola or granola of your choice, brush with oil and bake at 350° for 25-39 minutes.

Crumble cookies on top of peaches also and top with butter and nuts. Serve after baking, topped with honey ice cream or yogurt.

Frozen Banana Supreme

3 bananas
Melt together in double boiler:
1 cup carob pieces

2 tablespoons expeller-pressed vegetable oil
1 cup finely chopped nuts
Cut bananas in half crosswise and freeze.

Put melted carob in a tall glass. Dip each banana half in carob coating and roll in the nuts and return to freezer until ready to serve.

Sugarless Date-Applesauce Dessert

2 cups quick cooking oats
3 tablespoons expeller-pressed vegetable oil
1/2 teaspoon cinnamon
1/4 teaspoon ginger
1/2 cup chopped nuts

1/2 cup date sugar, maple syrup or pre
　soaked, mashed dates
1 cup finely chopped dates
2 cups unsweetened applesauce

Mix oats, cinnamon, ginger, date sugar or maple (syrup or dates, mix in 1/2 cup finely chopped dates at this time). Add expeller-pressed vegetable oil until mixture is crumbly. Place half of the mixture in well-buttered baking dish. Press down. Spread a layer of applesauce or sliced apples, nuts, dates, and top with the rest of mixture. Bake in 350° oven for 30 minutes. Serve hot or cold.

Banana Dream

Buy the marked down bananas that are ripe, these are the best for freezing. Peel and freeze whole or in chunks. Place the frozen bananas in a blender, processor, or a *Champion* juicer and enjoy just like ice cream.

Fruit Preserves

1 pound dried apricot or peaches, pineapple
   or any dried fruit
2 cups water
 Dash of cinnamon and ginger

1 cup honey sweetener of your choice or 2
   teaspoons barley malt sweetener for low-
   sugar diets

Simmer in a small, covered sauce pan for 30-40 minutes or until soft and mushy and put in a jar. *Keeps for weeks in the refrigerator.*

Frozen Yogurt Pops

Great summer diet treat and for children!

3 cups yogurt with fruit or add your own
   fresh fruit to plain yogurt

1 cup frozen fruit juice concentrate

Stir ingredients together. Pour into ice cube trays and put a wooden popscicle stick in each. Freeze.

Easy Peanut Butter Nuggets

No wheat or eggs
1/4 cup millet or oat flour
3/4 cup peanut butter
1/2 cup fructose or honey (any liquid sweet
   ener)

1-1/2 cups crisp rice cereal
1/2 cup finely chopped cashews or other nuts
   (optional)

Mix ingredients. Roll into balls and bake for 10-15 minutes at 350°. Cool, then remove. May substitute puffed millet, puffed rice, puffed, or granola for the rice crispies.
Do not over-bake.
Variation: Dip balls in melted carob chips just from the oven, and place on waxed paper.

Not all soy non dairy products are created equal, but grated parmesan soy cheese by *Soyco* **has the taste you expect with the benefits of no cholesterol, no dairy, and no preservatives.**

Carob Nut Candy

No cooking required.

1-1/2 cups pure maple syrup or honey
1 cup peanut butter or any type of nut butter
1 cup carob powder
1 cup lightly toasted sesame seeds

1 cup peanuts or any type of nuts
1 cup shredded unsweetened coconut
1/2 cup chopped dates or raisins
1/2 cup milk powder *(optional)*

Oil an 8" square pan. Heat syrup and peanut butter together in saucepan and quickly stir in carb powder. Add remaining ingredients. Pour into shallow pan and refrigerate until firm. Cut into squares, store in refrigerator.

Fruit Nut Balls

1 cup coarse ground cashews
1 cup coarse ground almonds
1 cup date pieces
1 cup soft raisins
1 cup dried, chopped pineapple
1 cup dried, chopped apricots

1 cup fine, ground coconut
1/4 cup honey or any liquid sweetener
(barley malt syrup, maple syrup or rice syrup)
3 teaspoons lemon or orange juice.

Put all nuts through a food processor or chop. Cut dried fruit into small pieces, add honey and juice and mix well. You may put all in your food processor and blend them with just a few small bits here and there. Form into balls and coat with melted carob chips, roll in grated coconut, or chopped nuts. Wrap in wax paper and store in the refrigerator.

Foolproof Carob Fudge

Fast, easy and delicious.

16-18 ounces sweetened carob chips
14 ounces condensed milk (not evaporated)
1/2 cups nuts

1-1/2 teaspoons vanilla *(optional)*
1/2 cup any nut butter and raisins *(optional)*

In a saucepan, melt chips with milk over low heat. Stir in the rest of the ingredients. Spread into a waxed paper lined 8-inch square pan. Chill and eat.

We recommend *Hain's* soft margarine because it contains only 1/2 the amount of saturated fat as other stick margarine and is made from a quality safflower vegetable oil. You can substitute the butter, oil or any margarine of your choice in any recipe. PB

Carob Drops

Kids love 'em!

1/4 cup expeller-pressed vegetable oil
3/4 cup honey
1/2 cup your choice milk
1/2 cup carob powder

1 teaspoon vanilla
3/4 cup peanut butter
3 cups rolled oats
3/4 cup shredded coconut

Boil oil, milk, honey, and carob together for 5-6 minutes. Remove from heat and add the vanilla. Drop by teaspoons onto waxed paper.

Fig Macaroon Candy

No cooking required.

1 pound pureed figs
1-1/2 pound fine, dried coconut
1/4 cup molasses

1/4-1/2 cup honey or 1/2 cup molasses
2 teaspoons vanilla
Juice of one lemon

Puree figs in a processor or blender, slowly adding coconut. Remove half from blender or processor. While blender or processor is still running, add lemon juice and vanilla until well blended. Add molasses and honey. Stop blender or processor and push down fig mixture. If mixture is too hard for machine, remove mixture and finish by hand. Add remaining fig mixture and blend with fork. Press firmly into oblong baking dish. Cut into squares.

Kids Graham Treats

Adults love these too!

Peanut, almond, or cashew butter
Graham crackers or cookies
Carob chips

Bananas *(optional)*
Crushed nuts *(optional)*

Spread crackers or cookies on cookie sheet, top with nut butter, sliced bananas, carob chips and crushed nuts. Bake in 300° oven just until chips melt.

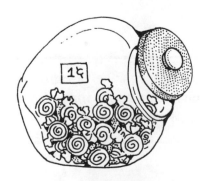

Vegetable Dishes

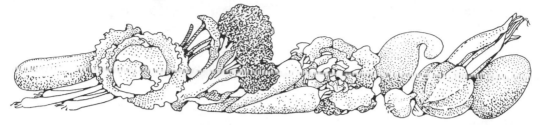

Tofu Honey Carrots

5 cups carrots,
1 cup green onions
1 pound drained and cubed tofu
1/2 cup canola or safflower oil

1/2 cup honey, maple syrup, or half of each
2 tablespoons dried parsley or fresh, chopped
1/2 teaspoon sea salt *(optional)*

Cut onions in one inch strips. Cut carrots lengthwise in one inch strips. In saucepan, steam carrots in just enough water to cover, until tender crisp (not soft) for about 5-10 minutes. In skillet, saute onions and tofu in oil for 3 minutes, stir in drained carrots, maple syrup or honey, sea salt and parsley. Add sesame seeds, if desired, for additional protein. Makes 6-8 servings.

Baked Potato Pops

1-1/2 cups mashed potatoes (can use leftovers)
1/2 cup finely chopped green pepper
1 finely chopped onion
1 cup cooked short grain or sweet brown rice
2 tablespoons expeller-pressed vegetable oil

1/2 cup shredded soy cheese or grated parmesan,
1 teaspoon Spike seasoning or sea salt
3/4 cup whole grain cracker crumbs
Dash of cayenne pepper *(optional)*
1-1/2 tablespoons ketchup *(optional)*

Preheat oven to 375°. Saute onion and green pepper in oil. Add rest of ingredients and form into 2" balls. Place on oiled cookie sheet and press with fork or bottom of glass. Bake until light brown. May add 2 beaten eggs, if desired.

Parsley Buttered Potatoes

12 small whole new potatoes with skins
1/2 cup expeller-pressed vegetable oil
4 tablespoons lemon juice
2 teaspoons Spike seasoning or sea salt

Dash cayenne
3 tablespoons chopped parsley
6 finely chopped green onions
2 teaspoons dulse seaweed *(optional)*

Scrub potatoes well, boil or steam till tender but not mushy. In skillet, saute green onions in oil, add rest of ingredients, tossing potatoes in last, serve hot. These are also good put under the broiler for a few minutes before serving.
Never eat potato eyes, they can make you sick, so cut them out. Also avoid green-tinted potatoes.

Zucchini Bake

2 sliced yellow squash
5 zucchinis sliced
1 chopped onion
1 minced clove of garlic
3 chopped stalks of celery
3 tablespoons vegetable oil
1/2 cup fresh chopped parsley or dried
2 teaspoons Spike seasoning, Vegit or 1 teaspoon sea salt

Dash of cayenne pepper
2 teaspoons Italian seasoning or oregano
1/2 cup plain yogurt or sour cream
3 tablespoons arrowroot powder mixed with a little water
3 eggs beaten slightly or egg substitute
1/2 cup mashed tofu, kefir, or cottage cheese
1 cup each, Swiss and parmesan or cheese of your choice

Saute onions, minced garlic and celery in oil for a couple minutes. Add yogurt, tofu, eggs, and 1/2 cup grated cheese, stirring constantly. Add arrowroot mixture, parsley and seasonings. Cut zucchini in half lengthwise. Place in baking dish and top with slices of yellow squash and prepared mixture. Top with grated Swiss and parmesan or your choice of cheese. Bake at 350° for 45 minutes.

Variation: May add canned salmon or tuna before the sauce.

Creamed Peas

See Basic Sauce recipe. While sauce is cooking, add one box frozen peas or 10 ounces fresh peas. Remove from heat and add cubed soy cheddar cheese or cheese of your choice.

Variation: May add slightly steamed carrot slices.

Crispy Potato Melt

Great as a side with supper, lunch or breakfast

4-6 large potatoes with skins
1/2 finely minced onion
1/2 cup shredded cheese of your choice

2 teaspoons Spike seasoning or a dash of sea salt
Dash cayenne pepper
2 tablespoons chopped parsley

Scrub potatoes and slice thin. Put potatoes in medium size pan with just enough water to cover. Boil for about 10 minutes (don't overcook). Strain and drink the liquid, great for the heart due to the potassium and for balancing the body's acidity. In an oiled heavy skillet shred half the potatoes, pushing into a circle to form a large patty. Sprinkle the cheese, Spike, dash of cayenne, finely minced onion and the parsley, press firmly.

Press last half of shredded potatoes on top and sprinkle with a little more Spike, pressing firmly forming a large patty, checking the bottom for doneness. When golden brown, flip over, being very careful to keep in a patty form. It should be nicely browned and crisp on the outside. Serve on a platter with a bunch of parsley.

Honey-Sweet Potatoes

6 large or 8 medium sweet potatoes
3/4 cup honey or 1/2 honey and 1/2 raw sugar
3 slices chopped dried pineapple rings

3/4 cup chopped walnuts or pecans
1 can unsweetened pineapple preserves or orange marmalade *(optional)*

Boil potatoes with skins until slightly tender. Slip off peelings, chunk or slice potatoes, and place in an oiled casserole.

In a small saucepan heat the honey, chopped pineapple, and orange marmalade, stirring until well mixed. Pour over sweet potatoes and bake for 35-45 minutes in 350° oven.

May top with crushed pineapple or fresh pineapple rings and a sprinkle of cinnamon and ginger.

Spanish Brown Rice

1 cup uncooked brown rice
2 cups vegetable stock or
    2 cups water and mix in one box *Hain's* dry Tomato Soup mix
2 stalks chopped celery
1 large chopped green pepper
1-1/2 cups fresh or home canned diced tomatoes

2 teaspoons Spike seasoning or a dash of sea salt
Dash of powdered or granulated garlic
1 tablespoon honey or any natural sweetener
1 large chopped onion
Dash cayenne pepper *(optional)*
2 tablespoons chopped fresh or dried parsley *(optional)*

Saute the onion and celery in 1/4 cup Good Things Garlic Oil or expeller-pressed vegetable oil until barely tender. Put 2 cups water or as suggested above in saucepan; add rice and bring to a boil, cover and simmer for 35 minutes. Add sauteed vegetables and rest of ingredients and mix well. Simmer for 15 minutes longer, until rice is tender.

If you're in a hurry you can use only Hain's dry Vegetable Soup Mix, place with the rice and water before cooking; works quickly, if you're in a hurry.

Honey Harvard Beets

10 beets with tops
1/2 cup *Hain's* soft Safflower Margarine
1/2 cup honey or barley malt or maple syrup

1 lemon
1 tablespoon arrowroot or cornstarch and 1 teaspoon Spike seasoning or dash of sea salt

Scrub beets very well, leaving tops on. Bring to boil, with just enough water to cover, and simmer until tender, but not mushy. Drain, cool and slip off peelings and cut off tops. Quarter and slice. In a pan, melt margarine, add honey, lemon juice and grated peel. While stirring, add arrowroot and seasonings, until thickened. Mix with beets.

Variation: Try using orange marmalade in place of sweetener and lemon.

The beet water is very nutritious; it can be saved for stock or drunk as a beverage when cooled.

Broiled Tomatoes

3 large tomatoes,
2 tablespoons plain yogurt or sour cream or
    eggless mayonnaise
1/4 cup soy Parmesan cheese or your choice
3 tablespoons chopped parsley

1 teaspoon Spike seasoning or a dash of sea salt
    and dash cayenne pepper
Dash garlic powder (not garlic salt)
1/4 cup toasted wheat germ *(optional)*

Slice tomatoes in 1" thick slices. Place in a layer on a lightly oiled cookie sheet or large baking pan. Mix rest of ingredients and sprinkle over each slice of tomato. Broil for a couple minutes until lightly browned. These are good placed on top of casserole dishes before baking. 6-8 servings.

Crisp Potato Skins

4 baked potatoes
3 tablespoons sesame oil
1/3 cup plain yogurt or sour cream (or 1/2 cup
    mashed tofu, or see recipe for Tofu Sour
    Cream)

2 teaspoons dried chopped parsley
3 teaspoons Spike seasoning
1/2 cup shredded soy cheese or cheese of your
    choice
Dash of cayenne pepper *(optional)*

Mix yogurt and cheese; add the Spike and oil. Put the mixture in the potato skins, covering the inside. Place on oiled cookie sheet or shallow baking dish and bake at 375 ° for 20-30 minutes, until browned and crisp.

Sesame Frybakes

5 potatoes with skins
3 tablespoons tahini

1 teaspoon tamari
1 tablespoon sesame oil

Scrub and cut potatoes into quarters. Mix sesame tahini, tamari and sesame oil. Roll each potato quarter in this mixture and spread them on lightly oiled cookie sheet. Bake at 425° for 25-35 minutes, turning a couple times. If you want real crispy fries, put under the broiler for a couple of minutes, turn and watch very closely so as not to burn.

Notes

Whole Grain Goodness

Good Things Whole Wheat Bread

Makes 11 loaves - for a smaller recipe, see Whole Wheat Bread on the following page.

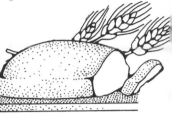

Mix and let stand:
3 quarts water, warm
3 cups expeller-pressed vegetable oil
1-1/2 cups honey
6 ounces yeast

Add:
13-1/2 ounces gluten flour
2 tablespoons sea salt
4 pounds fresh ground flour
4 pounds pre-ground flour

Mix together 10 minutes. Let rise 10 minutes, punch down and knead on oiled or floured board, adding enough flour slowly to make the dough not too sticky to handle. Turn onto floured board, let rise. Punch down, divide and place in loaf pans. Bake at 450° for 10 minutes, lower heat to 300° until done.

Spelt Flour Bread

Wheatless - makes 3 loaves

2-1/2 cups warm water
1/2 cup apple juice concentrate, warmed to the
   temperature of the water
2 packages quick-rise yeast

2 teaspoons sea salt
1/4 cup expeller-pressed vegetable oil
8 - 9 cups spelt flour

Combine the warm water, apple juice concentrate and yeast in a large bowl. Let stand for about 10 minutes or until foamy. Add 4 cups of flour and beat with electric beater on medium speed for 7 - 10 minutes. During the beating the gluten joins forming long strands in the dough and the dough becomes a cohesive ball that begins to climb the beaters. Discard the beaters and continue using a spoon.

Beat in the oil and salt. Stir in another 1 - 2 cups of flour, until dough reaches a consistency you can handle. Put the dough on a floured board using a cup of the remaining flour. Knead about 10 minutes, replenishing the flour on the board as needed. Let the dough absorb enough flour to make it firm and elastic.

Put the dough in a large oiled bowl and turn it over once so the top becomes oiled, too. Cover the bowl and let the dough rise in a warm place (free of drafts) until it doubles in size, about 30-60 minutes. Punch down the dough and shape it into three loaves. Put each loaf into an 8 x 4'' loaf pan. Set aside to rise again until nearly double, about 45 minutes. Put in the oven at 375° for 40-45 minutes. Immediately run a knife around the edges of the pans and remove loaves from pans.

Pizza Crust

1 ounce dry yeast
2/3 cup warm water

1/2 cup expeller-pressed vegetable oil
1-1/4 to 1-1/2 cups whole wheat flour

Mix 1 tablespoon dry yeast (1 ounce) into 2/3 cup warm water, let stand 5 minutes. Then mix in 1-1/4 to 1-1/2 cups whole wheat flour, oil and knead for 5 minutes. Roll out on floured or oiled surface, place in pizza pan, add your favorite filling and bake in preheated oven at 400° for about 15 minutes, or until done.

When making bread dough, save some for a pizza crust. Bread dough makes a great deep-dish style pizza crust.

Whole Wheat Bread

Makes 4 loaves

2 tablespoons dry yeast
1/2 cup warm water
5 cups hot water
9 cups whole wheat flour
3 cups unbleached or oat flour (can use soy, rye etc.)
2 teaspoons sea salt

3/4 cup expeller-pressed safflower oil
2/3 cup barley malt syrup or honey
Place 1/2 cup of warm water into a bowl, add yeast.
If you add 1 tablespoon sweetener (honey), it will work faster.
Let mixture sit for 15 minutes.

In a large mixing bowl combine the 5 cups of hot water with 4 cups of the flour (mix the different flours together or you can use all whole wheat.) Add another 3 cups of flour mixing by hand or on slow speed in a mixer. Add the yeast mixture, oil and sweetener until well blended. Add 3-4 cups of the remaining flour, kneading until the mixture leaves the sides of the bowl. Flour amount may vary. A stickier dough will create a moister bread, while a dryer dough will create a dryer loaf. Oil a board or counter top and your hands.

Remove the dough from the mixing bowl 1/4 at a time. Knead a few times and form into a loaf and place in oiled bread pans.

Place a small amount of oil on top of the loaves and cover with a damp cloth, place in a warm spot and let rise to 1/3 - 1/2 it's size (about 1/2 hour). Bake in a preheated 350° oven for 40 to 50 minutes. Watch the tops, if they are browning too quickly, place a piece of tin foil loosely over the tops. Do not touch the loaves or slam the oven door. When done remove the loaves from the pan and put on a rack to cool. ENJOY!

Be creative, try adding sprouts before kneading on the board for sprout bread or more honey, cinnamon, and raisins and you have raisin bread. Sunflower seeds or any nuts, sauerkraut in the rye bread, your options are endless.

High Protein Bread

Makes 2 loaves

1 tablespoon yeast (1 ounce)
2 cups lukewarm water
1/4 cup honey or raw sugar
1/4 cup unsulfered blackstrap molasses
2 eggs - *optional, if omitting add extra 1/4 cup molasses*
1/2 cup soy flour and 1/2 cup millet - or all soy

or millet
3-1/2 to 4 cups whole wheat flour
1 cup powdered non-instant milk or powdered soy milk
1/2 cup toasted wheat germ
2 tablespoons brewer's yeast
2 teaspoons sea salt

Mix yeast in lukewarm water (not too cold nor too hot) with molasses and honey, let stand for five minutes. Mix in eggs and three cups flour, beat with electric mixer or processor or by hand. Mix in the rest of the flour, reserving 1 cup whole wheat flour, wheat germ, brewer's yeast and sea salt.

Mix last cup of flour in slowly until a ball forms that is not sticky. Knead in processor or turn onto floured or oiled board and knead for about 8-10 minutes. Place dough in well-oiled bowl and put in a warm place to rise, cover with a damp towel. When it is twice its size, punch down and let rise again for 15 minutes. Divide the dough and place in two well-oiled bread pans. Let it rise until double, covered with a damp towel, Bake in a 350° oven for 45-50 minutes.

If desired, brush the top with oil when bread is done.

Sour Dough Starter

1/2 teaspoon dry yeast   1-1/2 cups lukewarm water   2 cups flour

Mix yeast with water. Add flour and stir. Put in a large glass, china, or ceramic container with a loose lid. (Never use metal.) Let it sit at room temperature for 3 days, stirring once or twice a day. The starter will "work" and will have a definite sour odor. After the starter has soured, it can be stored in the refrigerator and used periodically.

Caraway Rye Bread

Makes 1 large loaf
1 tablespoon dry yeast or 1 ounce fresh yeast
4 tablespoons molasses
1-3/4 cups warm water
1 teaspoon sea salt *(optional)*

4 tablespoons expeller-pressed safflower oil or your choice
2 cups rye flour
2-1/2 cups whole wheat or unbleached flour
2 tablespoons caraway seeds

Place the yeast in a large mixing bowl, pour the warm water over and mix lightly, never use hot or cold water because it will stop the yeast from becoming active. Stir in the molasses and let sit a few minutes. Combine the flours and the salt. Add the oil to the yeast mixture, mix lightly. Stir in the flours a cup at a time until the dough pulls away from the sides of the bowl. Add just enough flour to be able to handle, it should be slightly sticky, too much flour will give a dryer loaf. Oil your hands lightly and knead on a oiled board or you may want to flour your hands and the board. Knead in the caraway seeds. Shape into a loaf and place in a oiled loaf pan. Let it rise in a warm place until double in size. Bake in a 350° oven for 50-60 minutes.

Add 1/2 cup sauerkraut, if desired.

Zucchini Bread

This freezes well and is very moist.
3 cups honey
2-1/2 cups expeller-pressed vegetable oil
6 eggs or egg replacer
5 teaspoons vanilla
6 cups grated zucchini
4 cups whole wheat flour
1 cup oat flour

1/2 cup oat bran
2 teaspoons baking powder
2-1/2 sea salt *(optional)*
7-1/2 teaspoons cinnamon
3 cups chopped nuts
1 Tablespoon yeast in 1/4 cup warm water and a drop or two of honey

Combine ingredients in order they are given, add yeast mixture last.
Let rise for one hour in loaf pans. Bake at 300° for one hour.

Rice Bread

Eggs Required - wheat-free and yeast-free
Good for those suffering from candidiasis.
1 cup soy flour (or oat flour)
3 cups brown rice flour
4 tablespoons aluminum-free baking powder
   (*Rumford's* Aluminum-Free Baking Powder can be found in health food stores)

1/2 teaspoon sea salt
2 eggs, separated
1/2 cup rice syrup
1 cup soy milk or milk of your choice
1/2 cup yogurt
4 tablespoons expeller-pressed safflower oil

Combine all dry ingredients. Whip egg whites until stiff but not dry. Beat the yolks until creamy. Add the syrup, milk and oil to dry ingredients, mix well. Add yolks and mix well. Fold in egg whites. Bake at 350° for about one hour in well-oiled bread pan.

Flavor Treats

To add a new flavor to your cooking try substituting dried fruit, vegetables, nuts, grains, cheese, seeds, or herbs and spices for some of the flour called for in the recipe. Simply put the ingredient in the measuring cup and add the right amount of flour on top.

Sweet Potato Biscuits

A healthy way to get your beta carotene.

1 cup mashed yams *(sweet potatoes)*
2 tablespoons honey
1/2 cup vegetable oil
2 cups whole wheat flour
1/2 teaspoon ground cinnamon

2 teaspoons *Rumford's* Aluminum-Free
    Baking Powder
Dash ground nutmeg
3/4 cup low-fat plain yogurt or buttermilk

Preheat oven to 400°. In a large bowl, mix together sweet potatoes, honey, and oil until well blended. In a separate bowl, sift together dry ingredients. Add dry ingredients and yogurt to potato mixture. Mix by hand until a soft dough is formed. Do not over mix.

Place dough on floured surface and roll out to a 1/2 inch thickness. Use a 2-inch biscuit cutter and place biscuits on ungreased cookie sheet.

Bake for about 20 minutes, until lightly browned.

Anytime Pancakes

1-1/2 teaspoons aluminum-free baking
    powder
2 slightly beaten eggs or 3 egg whites or egg
    replacer
2 tablespoons vegetable oil to which 1
    tablespoon of maple syrup or honey
    has been added

1 teaspoon vanilla
1-1/2 cups buttermilk, yogurt, soy, almond,
    or cow's milk
1 cup finely chopped pecans
1 teaspoon cinnamon
1 cup whole wheat flour
1/2 cup unbleached flour

Mix dry ingredients together. Mix all wet ingredients. Combine the two until all flour is just moistened. Put on hot oil griddle. When bubbles form on top and edges dry, turn over. Serve with heated maple syrup and chopped pecans and a dab of *Hain's* Safflower Margarine or butter in the middle. *These are also good rolled up with fruit in the center and topped with pecans and syrup.*

Almond Fried Rice

1/2 cup fresh mushrooms, sliced
1-1/2 cups cooked brown rice
1 clove garlic, minced
4 tablespoons almond oil or oil of your choice
3/4 cup slivered almonds
1/2 cup mung sprouts, chopped lightly
3 green onions, chopped fine
2 teaspoons tamari sauce

1 tablespoon miso (any kind) mixed with 1
    tablespoon water
2 tablespoons chopped fresh parsley or 2
    teaspoons dried
2 tablespoons arrowroot powder or cornstarch
    mixed with just enough water to make
    into a paste
Dash cayenne pepper (*optional*)

Heat 2 tablespoons oil in a wok or heavy skillet. Add mushrooms, garlic, and onions, saute for 2 minutes (do not brown). Remove from wok and set aside. Put the rest of the oil in a wok, add the arrowroot mixture and stir a couple seconds, add rice, almonds, cook until slightly browned (about four minutes). Add garlic mixture and mix. Add miso, tamari and a dash of cayenne pepper, mix well and serve.

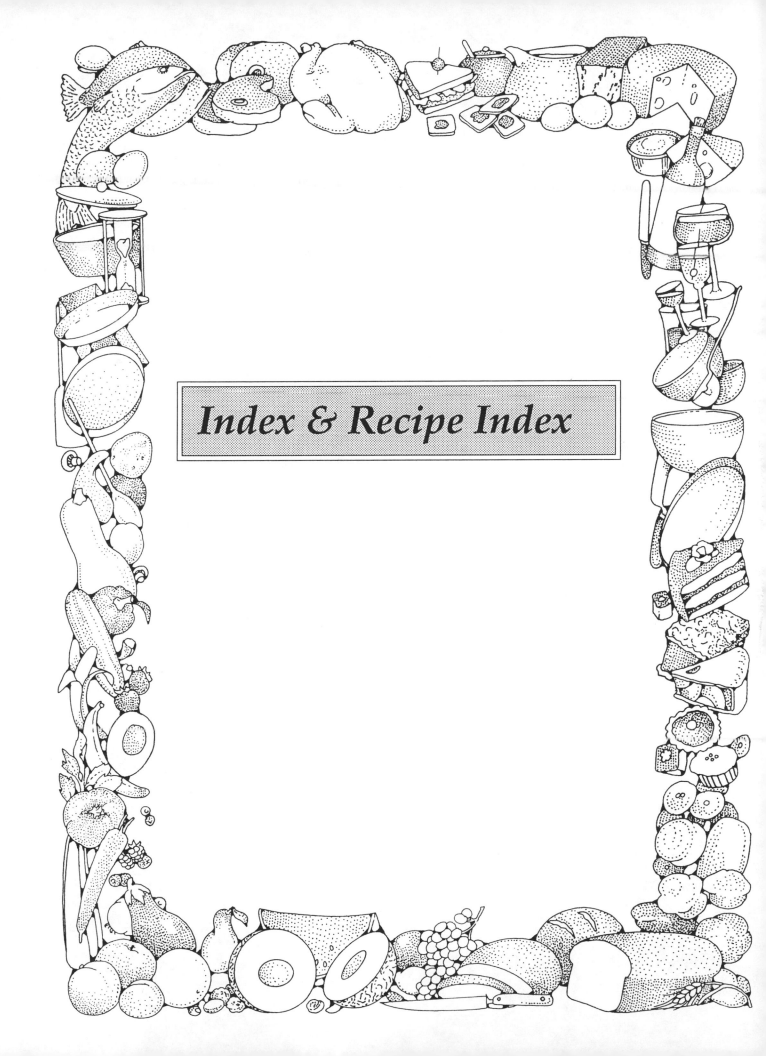

Index & Recipe Index

A

Abdominal
    Pain 21, 102, 104
    Swelling 104
Accutane 47
Acesulfame K 175, 176
Acidic 16
Acidity 64, 67, 152
Acidophilus 113
Acidosis 109, 118
Acids 98, 99, 117, 183
    Alginic 163
    Arachidonic 75
    Benzoic 109
    Bile 52, 95
    Chlorogenic 67
    Citric 77
    Ellagic 108
    Essential fatty 59, 62, 73-79, 83,
        84, 94, 124, 151, 163, 168,
        191
    Folic 97, 187
    Free-fatty 77
    Gamma-linolenic 97, 159
    Ganoderic 142
    Glutamic 164, 198
    Lactic 183, 187
    Linolenic 74, 95
    Linolic 74
    Malic 128
    Nuclecic 149
    Oleic 95, 143
    Oxalic 126
    Pantothenic 62
    Phosphoric 66
    Phytic 52, 119
    Polyunsaturate 74, 115
    Tanic 137
    Trans-fatty 84
    Urea 146, 183
    Uric 66, 67, 109, 125, 130, 146,
        183, 188
Acne 28, 109, 129, 136, 141, 146,
    177
Acopoletin 65
Acrid 66
Activated carbon 186
Acute appendicitis 66, 67
Adaptogen 136, 139
Adrenals 10, 66, 128, 129, 136, 139,
    162
Adzuki 168
Aflatoxins 41, 59, 75, 103, 113

Agar Agar 48, 94, 148, 164
Aging 84, 142, 144, 162
AIDS 6, 30, 50, 136-138, 142, 159
Air pollutants 7
Alaphagactrosidase 52, 64
Alaria 164
Alcohol 84
Alcoholism 61, 68, 106, 139
Aldicarb 106
Alfalfa 62, 73, 97, 136, 138, 167,
    168
Algin 164
Alkaline test 99
Alkalizing 61, 67, 150, 152
Alkaloids 155
Allergies 9, 11, 18, 21, 79, 96, 118,
    138, 139, 140, 141, 143, 146,
    147, 188, 189
    Children's 18, 22
Allspice 101
Almonds 8, 74-76, 81
Aluminum 148, 153, 193, 195
Alzheimer's Disease 28, 139, 142,
    153, 193
Amantadine hydrochloride 65
American ginseng 139
American Heart Association 44
Amino acids 51, 63, 96, 97, 119,
    146, 148, 159, 168, 198
Anemia 18, 60, 62, 63, 107, 128,
    130, 138, 161
Anger 178
Angina 139
Animal fat 75, 78
Antibacterial 9, 136, 138
Antibiotics 9, 20, 107, 139, 140, 144,
    150, 153, 188
Antibodies 6, 187
Antifungals 20, 137, 138
Antigens 6
Anti-histamines 20
Anti-inflammatories 9, 20, 136, 137,
    140, 143
Anti-oxidants 8, 20, 62, 63, 66, 105,
    109, 113, 115, 126, 128, 130,
    137, 142, 169
Antiseptic 107, 141
Anti-virals 9, 20, 138, 140, 142
Anus, burning 21, 152
Anxiety 9, 136, 137, 143, 178, 183
Apiol 66
Appendicitis 66, 67, 107
Appetite 61-63, 95, 102, 138

Apples 71, 93, 94, 95, 106, 110, 111,
    128
Apricots 8, 76, 94, 106, 111
Arame 164
Aromatherapy 136
Aromatic oils 77
Arrowhead Mills 58
Arrowroot powder 83, 120, 148
Arteries 19, 107, 155
Arteriosclerosis 30, 84, 85, 113, 117,
    138, 177, 183
Arthritis 6, 9, 11, 29, 61, 62, 64, 67,
    84, 94, 102, 106, 107, 109,
    113, 128, 130, 136-140, 149,
    154-156, 162, 163, 177, 183,
    194
Artichoke 157
    Jerusalem 158
Arugula 124
Asparagine 62
Asparagus 62, 69
Aspartame 175
Aspirin 73, 84
Asthma 40, 46, 60-62, 64, 66, 101,
    103, 107, 108, 113, 140, 142,
    143, 160, 162, 198
Astragalus 9, 11, 136
Astringent 141
Athlete 97, 148
Atherosclerosis 65, 84, 99, 183
Autolyzed yeast 198
Avocado 63, 74-76, 106, 111, 173

B

Backache 21, 102, 129
Bacon 79
Bacteria 6, 9, 52, 60, 85, 96, 102,
    107, 132, 142, 144, 146, 153,
    157, 177, 187, 188, 192, 193,
    196, 197, 236
    Infections 138
Bad breath 132, 136
Baking powder 148, 172, 195
Baking soda 51, 148, 153, 172, 195
Bananas 93, 106, 110, 111
Barium 168
Barley 8
    Grass 159
    Malt 140, 148, 176
Basil 101
    Sweet 101
Bass, striped 85

Recipe Index